NUTRITION AND DIET RESEARCH PROGRESS

APPETITE: REGULATION, ROLE IN DISEASE AND CONTROL

NUTRITION AND DIET RESEARCH PROGRESS

Additional books in this series can be found on Nova's website under the Series tab.

Additional E-books in this series can be found on Nova's website under the E-books tab.

NUTRITION AND DIET RESEARCH PROGRESS

APPETITE: REGULATION, ROLE IN DISEASE AND CONTROL

STEVEN R. MITCHELL
EDITOR

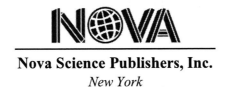

Nova Science Publishers, Inc.
New York

Copyright © 2011 by Nova Science Publishers, Inc.

All rights reserved. No part of this book may be reproduced, stored in a retrieval system or transmitted in any form or by any means: electronic, electrostatic, magnetic, tape, mechanical photocopying, recording or otherwise without the written permission of the Publisher.

For permission to use material from this book please contact us:
Telephone 631-231-7269; Fax 631-231-8175
Web Site: http://www.novapublishers.com

NOTICE TO THE READER

The Publisher has taken reasonable care in the preparation of this book, but makes no expressed or implied warranty of any kind and assumes no responsibility for any errors or omissions. No liability is assumed for incidental or consequential damages in connection with or arising out of information contained in this book. The Publisher shall not be liable for any special, consequential, or exemplary damages resulting, in whole or in part, from the readers' use of, or reliance upon, this material. Any parts of this book based on government reports are so indicated and copyright is claimed for those parts to the extent applicable to compilations of such works.

Independent verification should be sought for any data, advice or recommendations contained in this book. In addition, no responsibility is assumed by the publisher for any injury and/or damage to persons or property arising from any methods, products, instructions, ideas or otherwise contained in this publication.

This publication is designed to provide accurate and authoritative information with regard to the subject matter covered herein. It is sold with the clear understanding that the Publisher is not engaged in rendering legal or any other professional services. If legal or any other expert assistance is required, the services of a competent person should be sought. FROM A DECLARATION OF PARTICIPANTS JOINTLY ADOPTED BY A COMMITTEE OF THE AMERICAN BAR ASSOCIATION AND A COMMITTEE OF PUBLISHERS.

Additional color graphics may be available in the e-book version of this book.

Library of Congress Cataloging-in-Publication Data

Appetite : regulation, role in disease, and control / editor, Steven R. Mitchell.
    p. ; cm.
 Includes bibliographical references and index.
 ISBN 978-1-61209-842-5 (hardcover : alk. paper)
 1. Appetite. 2. AppetitexEffect of drugs on 3. Appetite disorders. 4. Eating disorders. I. Mitchell, Steven R.
 [DNLM: 1. Appetite Regulation--physiology. 2. Appetite Regulation--drug effects. 3. Eating--psychology. 4. Eating Disorders--etiology. WI 102]
 QP136.A679 2011
 615'.78--dc22
2011004574

Published by Nova Science Publishers, Inc. †New York

CONTENTS

Preface		vii
Chapter 1	Appetite Regulation in Early Childhood: The Impact of Parenting Behaviours and Child Temperament *Faye Powell, Claire Farrow, Emma Haycraft and Caroline Meyer*	1
Chapter 2	Role of Appetite Control in Metabolic Disease Conditions *Stephen D. Anton, Pamela J. Dubyak and Kelly M. Naugle*	29
Chapter 3	Appetite Regulation and Role of Appetizers *K. S. Premavalli and D. D. Wadikar*	55
Chapter 4	Association between Soup Intake and Obesity-Related Parameters *Motonaka Kuroda, Masanori Ohta, Hitomi Hayabuchi and Masaharu Ikeda*	75
Chapter 5	Serotonin Neurotransmission in Anorexia Nervosa *Darakhshan Jabeen Haleem*	97
Chapter 6	Older and Aging Consumers Diet and its Influence on Health: The Spanish Case *Teresa García and Ildefonso Grande*	113
Chapter 7	Appetite Preferences: Investigating the Roles of Relationship Satisfaction and Idealistic Thinking in Food Decision-Making Strategies of Romantic Couples *Jennifer M. Bonds-Raacke*	125
Chapter 8	Disease-Associated Anorexia as Part of the Anorexia-Cachexia Syndrome: Potential Etiologies and Interventions *Mark D. DeBoer*	135
Chapter 9	Regulation of Children's Food Intake *Gie Liem*	153

Chapter 10	Phytochemicals for the Controlof Human Appetite and Body Weight *S. A. Tucci, E. J. Boyland and J. C. Halford*	**171**
Chapter 11	Ghrelin: A Peptide Involvedin the Control of Appetite *Carine De Vriese, Jason Perret and Christine Delporte*	**217**
Index		**265**

PREFACE

Appetite is regulated by a close interplay between the digestive tract, adipose tissue and the brain. In this new book, the authors present current research in the study of the regulation, role in disease and control of appetite. Topics discussed include parenting behaviors and early childhood appetite regulation; serotonin neurotransmission in anorexia nervosa, aging consumers diet and its influence on health; appetite preferences; phytochemicals for the control of human appetite and body weight and ghrelin peptide in appetite control.

Chapter 1 - The ability to appropriately regulate appetite appears to be intrinsic from birth. However as children develop and become socialised, problems with the control and regulation of appetite are commonplace, as evidenced by the high prevalence of overweight and obesity in later childhood and adulthood. This chapter explores different theories of appetite regulation and discusses the various eating behaviour traits which have been identified during early childhood. Although there are several aspects of parenting behaviour that may contribute to a child's appetite regulation, or lack of regulation, this chapter focuses on the impact of the feeding practices that parents employ, and the feeding environment that parents provide when parenting their children, in influencing children's eating behaviours, appetite and weight. This chapter also explores the literature on child temperament and its contribution to eating behaviour and appetite regulation. Although the literatures on parenting influence and child temperament have been poorly integrated in relation to early child eating, some speculative suggestions are made about how these two aspects of behaviour may interact together to influence the regulation and control of appetite in young children.

Chapter 2 – Excessive caloric intake is a significant health concern in the United States and in industrialized countries around the world. Today, individuals are consuming significantly more food than in previous years. Epidemiological studies indicate that per capita energy intake increased by approximately 300 kcal per day from 1985 to 2000, after having remained fairly constant for the previous 75 years. If an individual's energy expenditure remained constant, a daily increase in energy intake of 300 calories would result in a weight gain of two to three pounds per month. Many studies suggest, however, that individuals are much more sedentary today than in previous years. Thus, rates of weight gain may be even greater than this estimate. In line with this, there has been a substantial increase in body weight across all segments of the U.S. population over the past few decades. Current estimates indicate that approximately 66% of the U.S. adult population is overweight or obese; an estimate that is 20% greater than 30 years ago.

Chapter 3 - Appetite is a pleasant sensation of having urge for consuming food and appetite regulation, a multifaceted phenomenon is influenced by many factors such as food intake, energy expenditure, nutrition and active ingredients such as spices and passive components as polycarbohydrates. Apart from these harmones leptin and ghrelin have an impact on appetite regulation and altitude increase shows a profound effect on increased harmonal levels thereby reduced appetite. The natural appetisers with spices as an active component and their role on leptin levels thereby appetite regulation has been dealt in this chapter.

Appetite is a psycho-physiological phenomenon in living beings which can be referred to the urge for consuming food. In general, the food pattern, quantum of food, feeling of satiety and hunger, physiological body constitution, weather conditions have the influence on appetite. In fact, appetite phenomenonly possess three distinct phases i.e., appetite control, appetite suppression and appetite regulation which have an impact on physiological actions, body weight, as well as food intake, energy expenditure and the fitness of the digestive system. Appetite reflects the synchronous operation of events and processes at three levels, neural events trigger involving a behavioral response in the peripheral physiology, in turn the same is translated into brain neuro-chemical activity which represents the strength of motivation and willingness, to eat or refrain from eating. Besides these, the psychological events of craving for food, choice of sensations as well as behavioral operations of taking meals, snacks, energy products (Blundell and Halford, 1998) have a greater impact at the holistic level of food consumption and utilization by the body. Attitude and awareness towards healthy eating is also very important besides the motivation. Hearty et al., (2007) in their study on 1, 256 Irish adults by random sampling concluded that attitude and motivation towards eating healthily was related to measured dietary behavior and lifestyle.

Appetite is a pleasant sensation that causes a person to desire or anticipate food. Appetite reflects on physiological components through hormonal control, but also possesses psychological state for arriving at a decision. Appetite is often felt in mouth or palate depending more on odour or flavor and the pleasant memory of food. In fact, appetite is product specific, whereas appetite expression is human specific, however, the appetizing effect encompasses the product, appetite expression and its mode of measurement. The whole mechanism of operations in appetite expression covers various phases for giving the judgement. Firstly, the reaction of sensory attributes which is responsible to the food characteristics reflects the judgement on the quality of food. Secondly, the physiological responses from the gastro-intestinal tract generate signals reflecting the quantity of food consumed. Thirdly, the food utilization and absorption along with energy expenditure is obtained by metabolic information. Fourthly, the adipose tissue reserves influences the appetite through lipostatic signal. Fifthly, these signals reaches the brain network, processes, organizes the functional response. Thus, the food type and feeding behavior have a greater impact on appetite; physiological responses influences the appetite control while the brain network process play a greater role in appetite regulation, while, the appetite suppression is related to the satiety signals when the physiological events are triggered as responses for not eating the food or which suppresses urge to eat for a particular period of time. However, all these states of appetite are inter-related in the physiological events as well as psychological behavior. The potential use of olibra, an appetite suppressant in dairy products, fruit drinks, soups and chocolate mixes has been discussed by Heasman and Mellentin (1998). More than these aspects, these states of appetite are influenced by various nature related factors such as altitudes, oxygen availability, living temperatures, basic tastes perception of sensory organs as well as type of food for consumption.

Chapter 4 - In this review, the authors discuss epidemiological studies examining the correlation between soup intake and obesity-related parameters. Several epidemiological studies conducted in Western countries have shown a negative correlation between soup intake and obesity-related parameters, such as body mass index (BMI), serum cholesterol, and serum triacylglycerol, suggesting that soup intake reduces the risk of obesity in Western countries. After adjusting for confounding factors, multiple linear regression in a cross-sectional study of 103 Japanese men aged 24–75 years showed that the frequency of soup intake was significantly and inversely associated with BMI, waist circumference, and waist-to-hip ratio. On the other hand, no significant associations were found with other metabolic risk factors. These findings suggest a negative correlation between soup intake and obesity-related physical parameters in Japanese men. In addition, after adjusting for confounding factors in a cross-sectional study of 504 Japanese adults aged 20–76 years (103 men and 401 women), multiple regression analysis revealed that the frequency of soup intake was significantly and inversely associated with plasma leptin concentration. These results indicate that soup intake is negatively correlated with obesity-related parameters such as BMI, waist circumference, waist-to-hip ratio, and plasma leptin concentration, suggesting that soup intake may reduce the risk of obesity in Japanese adults.

Chapter 5 - 5-Hydroxytryptamine (5-HT; serotonin) system is the major neurotransmitter system of interest in research on anorexia nervosa (AN). The AN patients show extreme dieting weight loss, hyperactivity, depression, obsession and loss of impulse control. Pharmacological studies show that manipulations that tend to increase brain serotonin functions are anorexiogenic. The hypothesis of suppression of appetite through excessive release of 5-HT to receptors is not supported by data on subjects with clinical symptoms of AN as cerebrospinal fluid (CSF) levels of 5-hydroxyindoleacetic acid (5-HIAA), a major metabolite of 5-HT, are reduced in AN patients and returned to normal in recovered patients. Loss of appetite in AN may simply follow self imposed dieting and diet restriction (DR). The hypothalamus is believed to be the site of the brain transducing satiety signals of serotonin. Studies on animal models show that acute starvation although increases brain serotonin metabolism but excessive DR over a period of few weeks decreased 5-HT metabolism and synthesis in the brain and hypothalamus and elicited hyperactivity. Based upon these finding animal models of DR-induced AN and activity based AN have been developed. This article highlights some of the important investigations on serotonin neurotransmission in animal models of AN. It focuses particularly on the role of serotonin in the regulation of appetite, activity and mood to understand ways in which DR-induced changes of brain serotonin may account for behavioral changes observed in AN patients with a hope that information contained herein would stimulate relevant research on AN for more rational and successful prevention/treatment of this tragic often fatal disease.

Chapter 6 - The purpose of this research is to identify and to valuate how healthy is the diet of some different groups of older and aging consumers living in Spain and to provide some actions, if any, to correct misbehaviors in food intake. Some variables affecting the diet as age, income, location and education are revisited. A large sample of older consumers' food expenditures is statistically treated using secondary data collected by the Spanish National Institute of Statistics by means of multivariate analysis techniques. Different levels of healthy diet are found regarding the consumers demographics.

Chapter 7 - Couples who had been dating exclusively for one year or longer were recruited to participate in the study from a public, east coast university. A total of 72 individuals (36 couples) completed a food related decision-making task first independently and then jointly. Participants completed a demographic questionnaire to gather information on gender, age, ethnicity, length of relationship, number of children, and living arrangements. Also, the Evaluation and Nurturing Relationship Issues, Communication and Happiness (ENRICH) Martial Satisfaction Scale (EMS) was modified for dating couples and administered. This scale has two subscales, which measure relationship satisfaction and idealistic thoughts about the relationship.

Hypotheses for the current study were partially supported. First, relationship satisfaction and idealistic thoughts were significantly related to likelihood ratings for eating at specific restaurants. One possible explanation for the current findings is that higher relationship satisfaction scores and lower idealistic thoughts are exhibited by couples who are more comfortable in their respective relationships and have set realistic expectations. Thus, these couples are more likely to demonstrate food preferences when making their likelihood ratings. On the contrary, couples who do not experience these same levels of satisfaction or feel an increased pressure to be the perfect couple, may be less likely to show preferences in their food ratings. Results also indicated that the levels of relationship satisfaction and idealistic thinking did not differ by the joint decision-making strategy of the couple. These results are surprising in that these measures were related to overall joint likelihood ratings. A larger sample of couples utilizing similar decision-making strategies may reveal differences on these measures.

The current study is not without limitations. As previously mentioned, the sample size could be increased to raise the power of the study. Secondly, the researcher was present as the couples were making joint decisions which may have influenced interactions and finally, not all of the couples were members of the clusters demonstrating common decision-making strategies. Although this study provides initial information on relationship measures and food decisions, additional research is needed. In particular, research directed at how couples make decisions about fast food is warranted given its popularity and health risks. Future research is also needed to explore how the stage of the romantic relationship influences food decisions and relationship domains.

Chapter 8 - The most common pathological form of anorexia is seen as part of the anorexia-cachexia syndrome. The anorexia-cachexia syndrome results in a devastating degree of body wasting that worsens quality of life and survival for patients suffering from already dire and restrictive diseases such as cancer, chronic kidney disease and chronic heart failure. The common features of anorexia-cachexia in these disease states and the common feature of systemic inflammation suggest shared pathophysiologic roots of cachexia in these conditions. However, previous attempts to treat anorexia-cachexia via anti-inflammatory interventions and multiple other means have not proven effective, and no unifying treatment has emerged that is effective in treating anorexia-cachexia in multiple disease states. Basic science investigations have revealed that inflammation-induced activation of the central melanocortin system is one likely means of producing anorexia and lean body wasting in this syndrome. Similarly, basic science approaches to blocking melanocortin activity appeared promising by demonstrating improvement of food intake and weight retention in anorexia-cachexia, though unfortunately data regarding human treatment is still lacking. Finally, a new treatment approach via administration of ghrelin or ghrelin agonists appears to be a promising means of treatment, as suggested by both basic science and early human experiments, though much more investigation is needed. The hope of all investigators and clinicians in the field is that successful treatment of the symptoms of anorexia-cachexia will lead to an improvement in quality of life and survival among all patients suffering from this disease.

Chapter 9 - The alarming increase of child obesity in many parts of the world suggests that children consume more energy than they need [1]. Insights into how children regulate their food intake will enable health professionals and parents to develop strategies to improve the balance between energy intake and energy expenditure.

From a biological point of view food intake is regulated by demand. When there is a shortage of energy, food intake needs to be increased. When there is enough energy consumed, food intake needs to be limited or terminated. The increase of obesity in the past decades clearly shows a mismatch between energy intake and energy expenditure in an obeseogenic environment [2]. It has been suggested that the human body is better able to protect itself from energy deprivation, than it is from over consumption of energy [3]. It has been argued that humans' body and brain is not able to handle today's food environment, where an overflow of highly palatable foods are available and easy accessible without severe hunting or gathering efforts [4].

The current chapter will provide a brief overview of the scientific evidence regarding children's ability to effectively regulate their energy intake, leading to a long-term energy balance. Furthermore, it will be discussed how portion size, energy density and parental control interfere with children's ability to effectively regulate their energy intake.

Chapter 10 - The regulation of energy balance and body weight is under the influence of complex neural, metabolic and genetic interactions. Despite this, obesity is now a global epidemic associated with significant morbidity and mortality in adults and ill health in children. Thus the effective management of obesity has become an important clinical issue. To date there are very few approaches to weight management effective in the long term. This contrasts with disorders such as anorexia and bulimia nervosa which also appear in part to be phenomena of the modern environment and equally difficult to treat. This review will focus on the mechanisms of body weight regulation and the effect of plants or plant extracts (phytochemicals) on these mechanisms. As phytochemicals are often not single compounds but rather a mixture of different unrelated molecules, their mechanism of action usually targets several systems. In addition, since some cellular receptors tend to be widely distributed, sometimes a single molecule can have a widespread effect. This chapter will attempt to describe the main phytochemicals that have been suggested to affect the homeostatic mechanisms that regulate, and some non-homeostatic system that influence, body weight. The in vitro, pre-clinical and clinical data will be summarised and scientific evidence will be reviewed.

Chapter 11 - Ghrelin is the endogenous ligand for the growth hormone secretagogue receptor. Ghrelin is a peptide of 28 amino acids possessing an uncommon octanoyl moiety on the serine in position 3, which is crucial for its biological activity. Ghrelin is predominantly produced and secreted into the blood stream by the endocrine X/A like cells of the stomach mucosa. Besides, it is also expressed in other tissues like duodenum, jejunum, ileum, colon, lung, heart, pancreas, kidney, testis, pituitary and hypothalamus. Some of the major biological actions of ghrelin are the secretion of growth hormone, the stimulation of appetite and food intake, the regulation of gastric motility and acid secretion and the modulation of the endocrine and exocrine pancreatic functions. Ghrelin is an orexigenic peptide involved in the short-term regulation of appetite and food intake. The plasma ghrelin levels increase before meal and decrease strongly during the postprandial phase. Long-term body weight is also regulated by ghrelin, since it induces adiposity. The purpose of this chapter is to provide updated information on ghrelin, the role of ghrelin in the control of appetite, as well as the potential clinical applications of ghrelin agonists and antagonists in certain physio-pathological conditions.

In: Appetite: Regulation, Role in Disease and Control
Editor: Steven R. Mitchell, pp. 1-28
ISBN 978-1-61209-842-5
© 2011 Nova Science Publishers, Inc.

Chapter 1

APPETITE REGULATION IN EARLY CHILDHOOD: THE IMPACT OF PARENTING BEHAVIOURS AND CHILD TEMPERAMENT

Faye Powell, Claire Farrow,
Emma Haycraft and Caroline Meyer

Loughborough University Centre for Research into Eating Disorders, School of Sport, Exercise and Health Sciences, Loughborough University, UK

ABSTRACT

The ability to appropriately regulate appetite appears to be intrinsic from birth. However as children develop and become socialised, problems with the control and regulation of appetite are commonplace, as evidenced by the high prevalence of overweight and obesity in later childhood and adulthood. This chapter explores different theories of appetite regulation and discusses the various eating behaviour traits which have been identified during early childhood. Although there are several aspects of parenting behaviour that may contribute to a child's appetite regulation, or lack of regulation, this chapter focuses on the impact of the feeding practices that parents employ, and the feeding environment that parents provide when parenting their children, in influencing children's eating behaviours, appetite and weight. This chapter also explores the literature on child temperament and its contribution to eating behaviour and appetite regulation. Although the literatures on parenting influence and child temperament have been poorly integrated in relation to early child eating, some speculative suggestions are made about how these two aspects of behaviour may interact together to influence the regulation and control of appetite in young children.

INTRODUCTION

Appetite regulation is part of a feedback system that controls an individual's energy balance. It involves a complex interplay of hunger and satiety signals modulated by appetite centres in the hypothalamus and brain stem, and hormonal signals of energy status released by the gut and the periphery (Druce and Bloom, 2006). Appetite influences energy balance and weight regulation through its effect on energy intake (Finlayson, Halford, King and Blundell, 2007) as it affects frequency, volume, choice and termination of eating episodes. The worsening global obesity epidemic has prompted an increase in the level of research about appetite regulation, as researchers attempt to understand the mechanisms responsible for human energy intake. Of particular concern is the increased prevalence of overweight and obesity among children and adolescents (Lobstein, Baur and Uauy, 2004), raising alarm about future trends for cardiovascular disease, diabetes and cancer (e.g., Maziak, Ward and Stockton, 2008; Sorof, Poffenbarger, Franko, Bernard, and Portman, 2002).

Debates about the causes of obesity are at the forefront of research and government agendas. Obesity occurs when energy intake remains higher than energy expenditure for an extended period of time (British Nutrition Foundation, 1999). Changes to the gene pool are unlikely to explain the increased global prevalence of obesity and, in the absence of such changes, diet and exercise appear the most likely candidates to explain increases in fat mass (Goran and Treuth, 2001). A daily imbalance between intake and expenditure of just 2%, if it is sustained over time, can promote overweight in growing children (Goran and Treuth, 2001). However, whilst it is agreed that the energy intake of children who are overweight exceeds their energy expenditure (Viana, Sinde and Saxton, 2008), less is known about the specific behaviours involved in weight gain. There is huge variability in population weight, and the mechanisms that cause some people to eat beyond their metabolic requirements and gain weight remains poorly understood (Carnell and Wardle, 2008a). Understanding the controls of energy intake within and beyond individual meals is an important priority as it may provide markers for overconsumption in children. This chapter will explore theories of appetite regulation and aims to elucidate some of the underlying behaviour traits that might contribute to differences in energy intake and weight status across children.

Whilst between 5% and 25% of weight variance has been attributed to genetic influences (Bouchard, Despres and Tremblay, 1991; Rayussin and Swinburn, 1992), the increasing prevalence of obesity suggests that environmental factors, such as the home environment and parental influence, are of particular importance (e.g., Carnell and Wardle, 2008a; McGarvey et al., 2004). Parents constitute one of the strongest influences on child development (Bugental and Goodnow, 1998), shaping children's eating environments and creating home environments that promote certain behaviours and social norms (Birch and Fisher, 1998; Rhee, 2008). Therefore, although many factors may contribute to an individual's eating behaviour appetite regulation and weight status, this chapter will discuss the impact of a broad range of parental factors. This incorporates the feeding environment that parents provide, parents' own eating behaviour and the feeding practices and styles that parents employ during food-based interactions with their children.

Interest in parental influences has also sparked interest into the feeding interactions between parents and their children, with research exploring the contribution of the child as well as the caregiver in the development of children's eating behaviour, appetite and weight (e.g., Agras, Hammer, McNicholas and Kraemer, 2004; Anderssen, Wold and Torsheim, 2006). Children are not merely passive responders to parental influences; feeding is a dynamic bidirectional process where children contribute substantially to the feeding interaction (Satter, 1986). Therefore this chapter also explores the literature on child temperament and its contribution to feeding interactions and the development of children's eating behaviour and appetite regulation.

This chapter will focus on early childhood as it represents a critical period where eating behaviours are becoming established and embedded (Kelder et al., 1994). Research has indicated that whilst very young children appear to be able to self-regulate their energy intake quite successfully, this self-regulation is less operational in older children (McConahy, Smicklas-Wright, Mitchell and Picciano, 2002). The pre-school years have been identified as a time when children's innate ability to self-regulate energy intake seems to diminish and eating is no longer depletion driven but is influenced by a variety of environmental factors (e.g., Rolls, Engell and Birch, 2000). Therefore, identifying factors that may impact on children's eating behaviours, appetite regulation and weight status during early childhood, before traits become engrained, is likely to be beneficial.

THEORIES OF APPETITE REGULATION

Despite huge rises in obesity levels over recent decades there is large variability in population weight and the mechanisms that cause some people to eat beyond their metabolic requirements and gain weight remains poorly understood (Carnell and Wardle, 2008a). Understanding the regulation of eating reflects a complex phenomenon as it is influenced by the integration of physical, psychological, genetic and environmental signals (Temple, Chappel, Shalik, Volcy and Epstein, 2008). Whilst there is no doubt that food intake is partially under homeostatic control, with hormonal and neural signals being critical to the regulation of intake (see, Woods, Schwartz, Baskin and Seeley, 2000), what is increasingly questioned is the importance of homeostatic regulation in the development of obesity and overweight (e.g., Lowe and Butryn, 2007; Lowe and Levine, 2005; Pinel, Assanand and Lehman, 2000). Within our modern food-rich environments, the effect of sensory and external stimulation on food intake has drawn attention to the hedonic dimensions of appetite, whereby external factors may have an overriding influence over our internal satiety cues.

Various different theories of appetite regulation have emerged over the decades and whilst our understanding of the physiological and homeostatic mechanisms underpinning appetite has greatly advanced (e.g., Schwartz, Woods, Seeley and Baskin, 2000), there is growing interest in the psychosocial and environmental influences on appetite regulation. Externality theory, a longstanding idea put forward by Schachter (1968), is based on the assumption that internal state is irrelevant to eating in overweight individuals and that instead, external, food-relevant cues trigger eating. Such cues could be the palatability of food or any aspect of the environment which signals palatable food, such as sight or smell of food, or learned associative factors such as time of day (Schachter, 1971). Schacter's work, along with various behavioural studies conducted in the 1960's and 1970's (e.g., Nisbett, 1972), highlighted that people who are obese may display a cluster of 'risky' appetite-related traits which people who are normal-weight do not. Although Schachter's theory was increasingly criticised because effects were weak and findings could not always be replicated (Rodin, 1981), recent rejuvenation of interest in this area has provided increasing support for these ideas (e.g., Jansen et al., 2003; Temple et al., 2008).

Twenty-first century food environments provide ample opportunities for over-consumption, yet despite common characteristics within the nutritional environment there are notable individual differences between children in their energy intake and adiposity (Jolliffe,

2004; Romon, Duhamel, Collinet and Weill, 2005; Wardle and Boniface, 2008). This has raised questions about whether there may be individual differences in children's susceptibility to the obesogenic environment and their capacity to regulate energy intake (e.g., Carnell and Wardle, 2008a). The 'Behavioural Susceptibility Theory' has been proposed by Carnell and Wardle (2008a) and it suggests that substantial individual differences in population weight may be due to differing susceptibility to the obesogenic environment which, in turn, may be explained by variations in appetitive traits or eating behaviours. It is conceived as a continuum explaining variation across the spectrum of weight (Carnell and Wardle, 2008b).

Appetitive traits are clusters of behaviours related either to satiety responsiveness or hyper-responsiveness to food cues (Carnell, Haworth, Plomin and Wardle, 2008). These behaviours include poor caloric compensation after a preload of food (Faith et al., 2004), eating in the absence of hunger (Fisher and Birch, 2002), a lack of deceleration of eating during a meal (Barkeling, Ekman and Rossner, 1992), enhanced salivation at the presentation of food (Epstein, Paluch and Coleman, 1996), and a higher reinforcing value of food (Saelens and Epstein, 1996); behaviours which will be expanded on later in the chapter. These behaviours have been observed in both children and adults who are overweight (e.g., Barkeling et al., 1992; Epstein et al., 1992) and preliminary research suggests that individuals' eating behaviour traits may influence energy intake, energy balance and body weight (Carnell and Wardle, 2008a), highlighting eating behaviour as a potentially modifiable predictor of weight gain in childhood. Associations have also been found between food approach behaviours (such as responsiveness to food, enjoyment of food and emotional overeating) and overweight in children, and between food avoidance behaviour (such as slowness in eating and good satiety responsiveness) and lower weights (e.g., Carnell and Wardle, 2008a, 2008b; Viana et al., 2008; Webber et al., 2009).

These theories suggest that external and environmental factors may exert a greater influence on appetite regulation and energy intake than homeostatic controls in some individuals. It is therefore essential to ascertain why some children seem able to successfully self-regulate their energy intake and maintain a stable, healthy weight yet others do not. Research investigating the behavioural correlates of obesity has begun to identify a variety of eating behaviour traits that may influence individuals' susceptibility to the obesogenic environment. These will be discussed in further detail in the following section.

APPETITIVE TRAITS IN CHILDREN

Recent research considering the behavioural correlates of obesity has identified a variety of eating behaviour traits in children and adults who are overweight or obese (Blundell et al., 2005; Carnell and Wardle, 2008a, 2008b). In line with Schachter's ideas, behavioural studies have shown that obese children have lower responsiveness to internal satiety signals (Fisher et al., 2007; Moens and Braet, 2007), and are more sensitive to external food cues (Jansen et al., 2003) than children with healthy weights. If such behavioural traits can be consistently linked to overconsumption, then they provide areas for potential modification and may be used to inform interventions to reduce overeating and thus obesity. The following section will discuss the roles of satiety responsiveness and hyper responsiveness to external cues and their relations with eating behaviours, appetite regulation and weight gain in early childhood.

SATIETY RESPONSIVENESS

Both within the adult and paediatric literature there is evidence that variations in satiety responsiveness may explain variations in energy intake and therefore adiposity. Satiation and satiety collectively inhibit food intake (Blundell and Rodgers, 1991) and are essential to successful appetite regulation. Satiety can be defined as "the effects of a food or meal after eating has ended" (Kral and Rolls, 2004, p. 132), whereby intake is inhibited after termination of a meal (Blundell and Rodgers, 1991). Satiety responsiveness reflects a sensitive response to internal satiety cues, and thus an efficient monitoring of energy intake, that protects against over-consumption (Viana et al., 2008).

Satiety responsiveness is often measured by assessing the effect of a preload on subsequent eating (Kral and Rolls, 2004). By comparing food intake after preloads of differing energy content, it is possible to calculate a compensation index (COMPX score), to assess how well individuals can compensate for higher or lower energy preloads (Cecil et al., 2005). An individual who is responsive to internal satiety cues will adjust their intake at a subsequent meal according to the energy content of the pre-load (Carnell and Wardle, 2008a), with a COMPX score of 100% reflecting perfect compensation (Cecil et al., 2005). Of particular importance in terms of obesity prevention is research which has suggested that a child's body weight status is related to self-regulation, with higher levels of adiposity being associated with poorer compensation (e.g., Johnson and Birch, 1994). However results are not conclusive, for example, Faith et al. (2004) failed to find a relationship between compensation and weight in a sample of 64 children aged 3-7 years.

Within the paediatric literature exploring satiety responsiveness, age appears to be an important factor, with evidence for a developmental shift in children's satiety responsiveness. Whilst very young children appear to be able to self-regulate their energy intake quite successfully this seems to be less operational in older children (McConahy, Smicklas-Wright, Mitchell and Picciano, 2002). One study found that after 6 weeks, infants who were fed more concentrated milk decreased their intake in volume to consume the same amount of energy as the control group who were given less concentrated milk (Fomon, Filer, Thomas, Anderson and Nelson, 1975). Preschool children also appear to be sensitive to the energy density of foods and pre-load snacks (Cecil et al., 2005) and have been found to achieve COMPX scores between 50% (Birch and Fisher, 2000) and 80% (Hetherington, Wood and Lyburn, 2000). However, older children are less effective at compensating for high-energy snacks and have been shown to have COMPX scores of just 20% (Hetherington et al., 2000). In addition, whilst younger children have been found to be better able to discriminate between high energy and low energy preloads, children rarely compensate accurately after the additional calories consumed through a preload or snack, thus contributing to a positive energy balance (e.g., Cecil et al., 2005).

Individual differences in appetite regulation are also often very prominent and research is striving to provide a comprehensive understanding of what predicts children's ability to self-regulate their appetites. It is not only important to detect appetitive traits such as a lower sensitivity to internal hunger and satiety cues, but also to discover the factors that relate to and predict the ability to regulate our appetites. An understanding of the complex interplay of factors that influence appetite could have far reaching implications for preventing the development of obesity. Such an understanding could be used to target interventions to prevent obesity in children with appetitive traits that place them at risk of weight gain. For instance, research with young children (aged 3–4 years) has shown that, with some training, including teaching children to focus on internal cues of hunger and satiety, the compensation index can be increased from 23% to 65% (Johnson, 2000). If we can understand and improve the controls of appetite and energy intake, appetite regulation could be utilised as a means to prevent obesity. In addition, satiety responsiveness tested within the preload paradigm has been found to be stable from childhood into adulthood (Zandstra, Mathey, Graaf, and van Staveren, 2000), highlighting the importance of focusing on its development within childhood. Some of the factors that may contribute to children's satiety responsiveness and self regulation will be discussed later.

HYPER-RESPONSIVENESS TO EXTERNAL CUES AND EATING IN THE ABSENCE OF HUNGER

As suggested by the increased prevalence of obesity worldwide, it seems that food consumption occurs for reasons other than acute energy deprivation and an increasing proportion of human food consumption appears to be driven by pleasure and the effect of sensory and external stimulation, not just by the need for calories (Brownell and Horgen, 2003). To explore the influence of these external factors on appetite regulation, research has investigated whether responses to these external influences vary between overweight and healthy individuals (e.g., Epstein et al, 1996; Jansen et al., 2003; Temple et al., 2008) and obese individuals have been found to have stronger appetitive responses to external cues than normal weight individuals (Epstein et al., 1996). Such behaviours included over-responsiveness to external food cues such as taste and smell (Jansen et al., 2003), overeating in response to emotional arousal (e.g., Slochower, 1976), finding food to have a high reinforcing value (Temple et al., 2008) and eating too fast thereby outpacing the onset of satiety during the course of the meal (Barkling et al., 1992), which can lead to eating in the absence of physiological hunger.

Eating in the absence of hunger (EAH) is a form of eating disinhibition initially described by Fisher and Birch (1999). It has been identified as one of the behavioural pathways implicated in the aetiology of childhood obesity (Birch, Fisher and Davison, 2003; Faith et al., 2006) and is indicative of a poor ability to self regulate energy intake. Within the EAH experimental paradigm, children consume ad libitum from a protocol meal in the laboratory setting, after which they rate themselves as feeling hungry, half-full, or full using age-appropriate silhouette scales. Immediately afterwards, children consume ad libitum from a variety of snack foods that vary in macronutrient content and taste properties. Consumption of the snack foods after rating oneself as full is indicative of eating in the absence of hunger, and variation in this consumption can be measured. Notable variability in this trait has been found and a number of studies have now shown that, compared with lean children, children who are overweight or obese show greater intake of palatable snack foods in the absence of hunger (Birch and Fisher, 2000; Butte, Cai, Cole and Wilson, 2007; Fisher et al., 2007). This suggests that the presence of food overwhelms the opposing satiety signals which may be weaker or absent in obese individuals. In addition, Jansen et al., (2003) observed greater energy intake in obese or overweight, but not normal weight, individuals following exposure to the smell of palatable foods. This suggests that food consumption may be initiated and influenced by a range of environmental cues, effecting individuals ability to effectively self-regulate their energy intake. Such a behaviour trait can be referred to as food cue responsiveness (Carnell and Wardle, 2008a, 2008b), which in essence represents an over-responsive meal initiation system, whereby eating episodes may occur in response to the hedonic properties of food and not homeostatic hunger.

Another eating behaviour that has been identified as reflecting eating in the absence of physiological hunger is emotional eating. The normal response to emotional arousal is loss of appetite, followed by a decrease in food intake (Larsen, van Strein, Eisinga and Engeles, 2006). However, some individuals respond to emotional arousal by enlarging their food intake, thereby emotionally over-eating. Research with adults has suggested that individuals who are overweight display higher levels of emotional eating than normal weight controls (e.g., Van Strien, Frijters, Bergers and Defares, 1986). There has been less research conducted in child populations, however, emotional eating has been associated with elevated BMI (Braet and Van Strein, 1997; Webber et al., 2009) and levels of emotional eating have been found to differ between obese children and adolescents and their normal weight counterparts (e.g., Scnoek, Van Strein, Janssens and Engels, 2007). Another study has found evidence that emotional eating is related to greater caloric intake of sweet and salty foods in adolescence (Braet and Van Strein, 1997), suggesting it may play a role in affecting children's ability to regulate their energy intake.

Eating rate has also been linked to appetite regulation whereby a fast rate of eating and a lack of deceleration has been linked to poor self-regulation of energy intake and also to overweight (Carnell and Wardle, 2008b). In an observational study of 6 year old children at school mealtimes, obese children ate faster, took more bites and chewed each bite fewer times compared to children with healthy weights (Drabman et al., 1979). Similarly, in a laboratory study using a computerised eating monitor, obese 11 year olds were found to eat faster over two lunchtime meals and showed no deceleration towards the end of the meal, despite describing themselves as having less motivation to eat before lunch than normal weight children (Barkeling et al., 1992).

It is essential to ascertain why some children seem able to successfully self-regulate their energy intake and maintain a stable, healthy weight yet others seem to gradually become more responsive to external cues and drivers to eat. It seems that the challenge to discover the underlying behaviours that might contribute to differences in appetite regulation and weight status across children is becoming clearer, however less is known about the factors implicated in the development of these eating behaviours. If these factors could be better elucidated then the implications for intervention and prevention are potentially colossal. Through the next section of this chapter some of the potential influences on children's ability to self-regulate their appetites will be discussed.

INFLUENCES ON THE DEVELOPMENT OF APPETITE REGULATION

Although genetic factors are undoubtedly implicated in the development of appetite regulation and children's emerging eating behaviours (e.g., Bouchard et al., 1991) the increasing prevalence of obesity suggests that environmental factors, such as the home environment and parental influence, are of particular importance (e.g., Carnell and Wardle, 2008a; McGarvey et al., 2004). Interest in the feeding interactions of parents and their children has led to research exploring the contribution of the child and the caregiver in the development of children's eating behaviour, appetite and weight. As feeding is a dynamic bidirectional process, it is likely that both children and their caregivers will influence children's emerging eating behaviours, preferences and attitudes. Therefore this section will focus on the contribution of the parent and the child in the feeding process and the development of eating behaviours and appetite regulation.

PARENTAL INFLUENCES

Parents are generally believed to constitute one of the strongest socialising agents for children (e.g., Baumrind, 1993; Bugental and Goodnow, 1998) and are believed to play a role in influencing their children's health behaviours (Anderssen, Wold and Torsheim, 2006). Parents influence their children through the use of specific parenting practices and by modelling specific behaviours and attitudes, which creates a home environment that promotes certain behaviours, expectations, beliefs, and social norms (Rhee, 2008). Due to this overarching influence, parents play an important role in the prevention and treatment of childhood overweight (Rhee, 2008), and parents of young children are now often the focus of public health interventions designed to reduce the prevalence of childhood obesity (Clark, Goyder, Bissell, Blank and Peters, 2007).

Research examining the influence of parents on childhood overweight has expanded in recent years (e.g., Moens, Braet, and Soetens, 2007; Zeller et al., 2007) and we have begun to understand the potential scope of parental influence on the development and treatment of childhood overweight. Parents are likely to influence children's eating behaviours and intake patterns through the feeding environment they provide and foods they make available to the child, their own eating behaviours, preferences and attitudes, and the parenting and feeding practices they employ. This section will therefore focus on the contribution of these parental factors to the development of children's eating behaviours and appetite regulation.

THE IMPACT OF THE FEEDING ENVIRONMENT ON APPETITE REGULATION

Parents create a home environment that promotes certain behaviours, expectations, beliefs, and social norms (Rhee, 2008) and are therefore central in shaping children's eating environments and the development of eating preferences and behaviours (Birch and Fisher, 1998). Particularly during early childhood, parental choices within the immediate home environment about the type, volume and frequency of eating episodes are likely to influence children's emerging ability to self-regulate their energy intakes. Children's self-regulation can be challenged by external food cues, such as availability of highly palatable foods (Wilson, 2000), numerous opportunities to snack in the absence of hunger (Fisher and Birch, 2002; Jahns, Siega-Riz and Popkin, 2001) and portion size (Neilson and Popkin, 2003), which can override internal satiety signals. The ways in which environmental influences within the home contribute to children's emerging ability to self regulate and weight status will now be discussed.

As indicated by the growing prevalence of global obesity, it seems that food consumption occurs for reasons other than acute energy deprivation and an increasing proportion of human food consumption appears to be driven by pleasure. For instance, the availability and palatability of foods in the home can have a major effect on whether the foods will be desired and consumed (Blundell and Finlayson, 2004) and an individual's level of current caloric repletion can become relatively unimportant. The consumption of highly palatable foods has been linked to food hedonics and subjective reward experience which are likely to be powerful motivators for intake (Carnell and Wardle, 2008b; Epstein et al., 2007).

Food hedonics is the subjective pleasure derived from food (Cabanac, 1985) and the reinforcing value of food refers to how much someone is motivated to obtain food (Epstein et al., 2007). Given the opportunity to consume foods that are high or low in hedonic value, individuals will generally choose to consume foods that they find palatable and this has been considered to be a determinant of energy consumption or the amount of food consumed within a meal (Drewnowski and Hann, 1999). The reinforcing value of food has also been found to influence energy intake, whereby high levels of food reinforcement are related to greater energy intake (Epstein et al., 2007). In addition, obese adults, who are likely to have higher energy intake than non-obese adults, have been found to find food more reinforcing than their slimmer counterparts (Epstein et al., 2007; Temple et al., 2007). This research suggests that if children are over exposed to highly palatable foods within their feeding environment, that this exposure may challenge their ability to respond to internal feelings of hunger and satiety and may instead teach them to respond to the hedonic properties of food.

Portion size, which is often determined by caregivers, reflects another important environmental factor that influences both energy intake and appetite regulation (e.g., McConahy, Smicklas-Wright, Birch and Picciano, 2002; Mrdjenovic and Levitsky, 2005). For example, numerous cross-sectional survey studies have reported positive associations between average food portions consumed and energy intake in children ranging from 6 months to 5 years (e.g., Fox, Devaney, Reidy Razafindrakoto and Ziegler, 2006; McConahy et al., 2002; McConahy et al., 2004). In a study of 2-5 year olds, portion size, frequency of eating and number of foods consumed were positively related to total energy intake, suggesting that these could be important predictors of energy intake as children transition from toddler to preschool years (McConahy et al., 2004). Similar results were found in a study of 4-6 year olds in which a strong positive correlation was observed between serving size and consumption over a 5-7 day period (Mrdjenovic and Levitsky, 2005). Rolls et al., (2000) observed a 60% increase in energy intake between large and small portion conditions (77g vs 123g) in 4-5 year olds, although no effect of portion size on intake was observed in 2-3 year old children.

The work of Rolls et al., (2000) and other studies in both controlled and natural everyday environments (e.g., Birch and Fisher, 1998; Shea, Stein, Basch, Contento and Zybert, 1992), provide evidence of a developmental shift in children's susceptibility to portion size. It has been demonstrated that whilst infants and young children have an innate ability to self-regulate energy intake, with intake being driven primarily by responses to hunger and satiety cues (e.g., Birch and Fisher, 1998), by 3 or 4 years old, eating is no longer depletion driven but is influenced by a variety of environmental factors (e.g., Rolls et al., 2000). It is possible that during the preschool period children's increased responsiveness to the environmental cues may emerge as a factor that contributes to overweight; in children who have learned to be responsive to environmental cues, very large portion sizes may elicit over-eating and thus promote the development of overweight (Rolls et al., 2000).

Recent studies have also begun to examine the effect of the energy density of foods on satiation and satiety (e.g., Bell and Rolls, 2001; Kral, Roe and Rolls, 2004) and results have shown that the energy density of a diet can directly influence energy intake (e.g., Bell and Rolls, 2001; Stubbs, Johnstone, O'Reilly, Barton and Reid, 1998). In addition, there is evidence that energy density combined with volume of a first course or meal act together to significantly affect satiety and total energy intake in a meal (Rolls, Roe and Meengs, 2003). Overall findings in this area suggest that adults eat a similar amount of food day to day irrespective of energy density, and that the consumption of high energy dense foods typically results in an increase in energy intake (Kral and Rolls, 2004). Although less research has been carried out in young children, recent studies investigating the effects of energy density on satiation and satiety among young children have found similar results to those in adults. For instance, Leahy, Birch and Rolls (2008) found that when the energy density of the primary component of a main meal (macaroni and cheese) was reduced by 30%, 2 to 5 year olds consumed 25% fewer calories. Similarly, a study of 5-6 year olds found that after increasing the energy density of a macaroni and cheese by 40% energy consumed increased by 33% (Fisher, Liu, Birch and Rolls, 2007). Collectively these findings suggest that energy density of a meal may affect children's ability to recognise internal feelings of satiety and satiation, therefore promoting the risk of overconsumption.

Unsurprisingly given the evident impact of these environmental cues, an important component of programs to prevent obesity and poor appetite regulation in young children is modifying the aforementioned environmental cues that can lead to positive energy balance (Epstein et al., 2001). Environmental factors such as the home milieu and parental influence are evidently highly important (McGarvey et al., 2004), yet the influence of parents stretches far beyond the food they make available in the home. With parents being such influential socialising agents for children (e.g., Baumrind, 1993; Bugental and Goodnow, 1998) it is likely that parents' eating behaviours and attitudes are also influential in the emergence of children's own eating behaviours (Nicklas et al., 2001). In line with Social Learning Theory (e.g., Bandura, 1977), some research has highlighted the role of observational learning and modelling in the development of a child's eating habits and behaviours (e.g., Contento et al., 1993; Olivera et al., 1992). The social contexts of the feeding environment, including the attitudes of and interactions with parents, are very important and therefore research has looked at associations between obesogenic eating behaviours and poor appetite regulation amongst children and their caregivers.

Disinhibited parental eating has been associated with lower child satiety responsiveness (Birch and Sullivan, 1991), eating in the absence of hunger (Cutting, Fisher, Grimm-Thomas and Birch, 1999; Francis, Ventura, Marini and Birch, 2007) and higher child body fat (Hood et al., 2000). Although there is evidence for the genetic transmission of disinhibited eating (e.g., de Castro and Lilenfield, 2005; Provencher et al., 2005), one study found 40% of the variance in disinhibited eating behaviour to be explained by a shared environmental component (de Castro and Lilenfield, 2005). Hood et al. (2000) suggest that this association may be mediated by direct parental role modelling of unhealthy eating behaviours, or through other indirect behavioural consequences that influence a child's innate regulation of dietary intake (Hood et al., 2000). Evidence seems to suggest that the family environment is particularly important and that these disinhibited eating behaviours are predominantly learned (Faith et al., 2007; Moens and Braet, 2007; Provencher et al., 2005). Support for this conception is provided by a recent longitudinal study which found that although mothers' disinhibited eating was not related to daughters' disinhibited eating style (eating in the absence of hunger; EAH) when daughters were 5 to 7 years old, it was related to girls' EAH at ages 9 to 13 years (Francis et al., 2007). It seems likely that disinhibited eating is a behavioural phenotype that may emerge during childhood as a result of environmental exposure, whereby parental displays of disinhibited eating can promote subsequent disinhibited eating in their children (Francis et al., 2007).

Parents of young children are key targets for interventions intended to reduce the prevalence of obesity in children (Clark et al., 2007). Increasing healthy eating behaviours in families and thus providing healthy role models has been suggested to be an important step in improving child diet. For example, research suggests that if obese parents reduce access to low-nutrient dense foods available in the family environment, model healthier eating and activity habits, and share positive food-related family experiences that reinforce eating high-nutrient dense foods, the parents may reduce the risk of their child becoming obese (Epstein et al., 2001).

Research has also explored the impact of parental eating psychopathology upon the child's relationship with food. Whilst maternal eating psychopathology has been associated with the presence and persistence of feeding problems in childhood and children's poor self regulation of food intake (Ammaniti, Ambruzzi, Lucarelli, Cimino and D'Olimpio, 2004; Blissett, Meyer and Haycraft, 2007; Stein, Woolley and McPherson 1999), much of the research assessing the associations between maternal eating psychopathology and overconsumption in young children has focused on how parents' eating attitudes impact on their child feeding practices, which in turn may influence children's eating behaviour and weight. For instance, a parent is more likely to constrain and control a child within a domain that is of high importance to them (Goodnow, Knight and Cashmore, 1985) and parents' own child-irrelevant social values and concerns about a given domain can elevate concern and constraint in parenting (Costanzo and Woody, 1985). Mothers' preoccupation with their own weight and eating has been linked to higher restriction of daughters' food intake (Francis and Birch, 2005) and both mothers and fathers with non-clinical levels of eating psychopathology have been shown to be more controlling over their children's eating (Blissett, Meyer and Haycraft, 2006). These controlling feeding practices have been associated with negative outcomes, overconsumption and weight gain in children (e.g., Birch, Fisher and Davison, 2003; Klesges, Klegses, Eck and Shelton, 1991) and appear to play an important role in the development of effective self-regulation in children. The impact of these feeding practices on children's eating behaviour will now be discussed.

THE IMPACT OF PARENTAL FEEDING PRACTICES ON CHILD APPETITE REGULATION

In recent years, the influence that parents can have on their children's dietary behaviour through food-related parenting practices has received particular attention (Kremers, Brug, de

Vries and Engles, 2003), and parents' child-feeding practices have been identified as a contributory environmental factor in childhood obesity (Birch and Fisher, 1998). Feeding practices are the specific strategies that parents use in an attempt to maintain or modify their child's eating style and diet (Ventura and Birch, 2008). Although parents may use child-feeding behaviours with the positive intention of modifying children's dietary intake (Klesges et al., 1991), research has suggested that overly controlling feeding practices, which may interfere with children's internal hunger and satiety cues, can be unintentionally detrimental by actually promoting overeating in young children (Fisher and Birch, 1998).

A variety of parental feeding practices have been linked to an increased risk of overeating. These include encouraging or pressuring a child to eat beyond satiety (Birch, McPhee, Shoba, Steinberg, and Krehbiel, 1987), restricting the amount and type of food a child can eat (Birch, Fisher and Davison, 2003) and using food as a reward for a behaviour (Birch et al., 1987). A central idea within the parental feeding practices literature is that parents who exert high levels of control over their child's eating may unintentionally effect their children's ability to regulate their appetites by encouraging them to eat according to external rather than internal hunger cues (e.g., Savage, Fisher and Birch, 2007), such as the time of day or amount of food left on a plate (Johnson, 2000). For instance, adult prompts to eat increase the likelihood that children will eat (Klesges et al., 1983), but can over-ride their own fullness as a guide to terminate eating (Birch et al., 1987). In addition pressuring children to eat foods that are 'good for them' has been associated with lower preference for that food (Batsell et al., 2002) and lower fruit and vegetable intake (Galloway, Fiorito, Lee, and Birch, 2005), which are likely to influence children's food choices and their ability to effectively regulate their energy intake.

Restrictive feeding practices may also discourage adequate self-control of eating by increasing children's preference for restricted foods and desire to eat them when available (Birch and Fisher, 2000; Fisher and Birch, 1996), suggesting that these restrictive feeding practices may be implicated in the etiology of disinhibited eating (Birch and Fisher, 2000; Fisher and Birch, 1999). Given our current obesogenic eating environment there is concern about whether restrictive feeding practices may inadvertently teach children to ignore their own hunger and fullness when placed in eating environments where palatable, previously restricted foods are readily available (Birch et al., 2003). In support of this idea, highly restrictive feeding practices have been associated with eating in the absence of hunger and overweight among young girls (Birch and Fisher, 2000; Fisher and Birch, 2002).

There has been some discrepancy among the literature as to the degree of negative impact that excessive control has on child eating behaviour and weight (Montgomery, Jackson, Kelly and Reilly, 2006), and some studies have also found favourable associations between these feeding practices and child food intake (e.g., Brown and Ogden, 2004; Zabinski et al., 2006) and links with lower child fat mass (Spruijt-Metz, Cohen, Birch and Goran, 2006). However, longitudinal research suggests that highly restrictive feeding practices have been most consistently associated with child weight gain (Clark et al., 2007) and less controlling practices, such as monitoring unhealthy snack intake, have been associated with slower weight gain (Faith et al., 2004).

Within the literature on feeding practices, the focus has been primarily on the use of control and there is very little research examining a broader range of child feeding practices, despite evidence that other feeding strategies influence children's eating (Orrell-Valente et al., 2007). However, interest is growing in dimensions of parental feeding practices which reflect parents' use of food to direct and manipulate behaviour, rather than only feeding their children in response to hunger and satiety, such as using food as a reward and to regulate emotions (Musher-Eizenman and Holub, 2007). For example, it is possible that if food is used for comfort, a child may develop a pattern of responding to emotional arousal with food intake (Bruch, 1973) and it has been proposed that the feeding practices employed by parents may unintentionally cause children to use food to address emotional arousal (Carper et al., 2000; Van Strein and Bazelier, 2007). If parents use food to regulate their child's emotional states, they may unintentionally 'teach' their child to respond to emotional states by eating thus leading to the development of emotional eating. Support for this premise is evident within a recent study that found maternal use of food to regulate emotions to be associated with cookie consumption in the absence of hunger (Blissett, Haycraft and Farrow, 2010). Carrying out further research which encompasses a broader range of parenting practices is essential to better elucidate how they may influence children's emerging eating behaviours and appetite regulation.

THE IMPACT OF PARENTING STYLE ON CHILD APPETITE REGULATION

Parenting style is another aspect of parenting that has been explored in relation to parents' child-feeding practices with research suggesting that parents' feeding practices are broadly linked with their parenting styles (Blissett and Haycraft, 2008; Hughes, Power, Fisher, Mueller, and Nicklas, 2005). There are strong conceptual reasons to expect that parenting style should be related to the management of children's health behaviours (Kitzmann, Dalton III and Buscemi, 2008), and empirical evidence suggests that an authoritative parenting style promotes more positive health behaviours in children (Tinsley, Markey, Ericksen, Ortiz, and Kwasman, 2002). In fact, parenting styles have been found to predict children's BMI (Rhee, Lumeng, Appugliese, Kaciroti and Bradley, 2006), healthier eating (Kremers, et al., 2003; Patrick, Nikolas, Hughes, Morales, 2005) and also physical activity level (Schmitz et al., 2002).

The construct of parenting style is used to capture normal variations in parents' attempts to control and socialise their children (Baumrind, 1991), and parenting styles are conceptualised as descriptions of how parents vary on the dimensions of warmth and nurturance versus control (Darling and Steinberg, 1993). They tend to be categorised into authoritative, authoritarian and permissive styles and reflect different naturally occurring patterns of parental values, practices and behaviours (Baumrind, 1991). Authoritative parents balance clear, high parental demands with emotional responsiveness, warmth and recognition of child autonomy (Baumrind, 1991). Authoritarian parents, however, are highly demanding and over-controlling and are also emotionally cold and unresponsive (Baumrind, 1991). Permissive parents impose little control, either through overly indulgent or neglectful and emotionally cold parenting (Baumrind, 1991).

Authoritative parenting has been consistently demonstrated to be associated with positive outcomes in children across many domains and has been identified as the most effective parental child-feeding modality (Kremers et al., 2003). However, the authoritarian style, where children are raised in a strict environment lacking in emotional responsiveness, has been associated with controlling feeding practices such as pressure to eat (Duke, Bryson, Hammer, and Agras, 2004; Hughes et al., 2005),) and an increased risk of childhood overweight (Rhee et al., 2006). It seems that authoritative parenting provides the structure and support needed for children to internalise and maintain positive behaviours, whereas non-authoritative parenting may interfere with children's ability to learn self-regulation (Grolnick and Farkas, 2002) including the self-regulation of eating (Davison and Birch, 2001). These ideas link back to early psychosomatic theory, where it was suggested that early life experiences characterised by a lack of parental regard for, and response to, children's real needs were implicated in the development of a lack of awareness of internal states and hunger cues in children (Bruch, 1973).

However, results are not conclusive and some researchers have not found support for the links between parenting style and feeding practices with child BMI (e.g., Brann and Skinner, 2005), highlighting the need for further research. In addition, the focus has largely been on authoritarian directives, such as rewards, punishment and restriction (e.g., Johnson and Birch, 1993) whereas very little research has evaluated authoritative feeding, which encompasses behaviours such as encouragement, reasoning, rationales and praise (Hughes et al., 2005). Extending research to investigate authoritative, child-responsive feeding strategies in addition to overt control of feeding is likely to further illuminate the role of parental feeding in the development of child appetite. More research is needed, as despite the discrepancies, parenting styles and practices represent potentially powerful influences on the development of children's eating behaviours and appetite regulation.

Whilst parents represent an essential influence on children's emerging eating behaviours through all of the aforementioned avenues, children are not merely passive responders to parental influences (Carnell and Wardle, 2008a). Feeding is a dynamic bidirectional process and children significantly contribute to the feeding interaction (Cabanac, 1987). It is important to remember that although parenting can influence children's eating and weight, individual child characteristics are likely to influence parenting and the way in which parents interact with their child. For example, parents have reported using different feeding practices in response to different characteristics between siblings (e.g., Brann and Skinner, 2005; Farrow, Galloway and Fraser, 2009). In addition, inherent child characteristics such as personality or temperament are also likely to directly influence children's eating behaviours and susceptibility to the obesogenic environment. There has therefore been a growing interest in individual difference variables that influence food intake (Franken and Muris, 2005) and recent developments have increased awareness of the impact that child temperament may have on eating behaviour (e.g., Agras et al., 2004; Pulkki-Raback et al., 2005). The following section will discuss the contribution of temperamental dimensions such as emotionally and impulsivity to children's eating behaviours and will suggest how temperament traits may influence children's eating behaviours or moderate the effects of the obesogenic environment on individuals' appetite regulation.

CHILD TEMPERAMENT AND ITS CONTRIBUTION TO APPETITE REGULATION

Temperament refers to individual differences in a person's emotional reactivity and regulation (Goldsmith et al., 1987) and has been defined as "personal characteristics that are biologically based, are evident from birth onwards, are consistent across situations and have some degree of stability" (Schaffer, 2006, p.70). There are a wide variety of temperaments which a child may convey and evidence has suggested that individual differences in temperamental characteristics may influence children's eating behaviour, either directly or through their influence on parenting (Thomas and Chess, 1987). Several dimensions of temperament are associated with variations in children's eating behaviours such as impulsive (Hetherington, 2007), difficult and demanding (Hagekull, Bohlin and Rydell, 1997; Lindberg, Bohlin, Hagekull and Thrunstorm, 1994), emotional (Agras et al., 2004), and shy and unsociable temperaments (Pliner and Loewen, 1997).

Impulsivity is the tendency to respond instantaneously to external or internal cues, without thinking about the consequences (Gray, 1987). Features of impulsivity include disinhibited and thrill-seeking behaviours (Flory et al., 2006) and it is characterised by a preference for small, immediate rewards (Hetherington, 2007). The Reinforcement Sensitivity Theory developed by Gray (1987) is one of the leading biological based models of personality and is useful in explaining individual differences in food consumption through differences in impulsivity. This theory suggests that there are two systems that control individuals' approach and avoidance behaviours: the Behavioural Activation System (BAS), which controls approach behaviours and is activated in the presence of a reward, guiding the individual towards appetitive stimuli; and, a Behavioural Inhibition System (BIS) which controls anxiety-based avoidance behaviours and inhibits responses in order to avoid punishment (Gray 1987). Impulsivity represents a lack of inhibitory control, and this may be attributed to heightened sensitivity to reward (Hetherington, 2007). Overeating may be characterised by an overdeveloped BAS, which may explain the exaggerated 'approach' response to food cues seen in some children, or it may be caused by an under developed BIS, as evidenced by an inability to resist situational cues to over-consume foods (Hetherington, 2007). Therefore individual differences in impulsivity or sensitivity reward may make some people more vulnerable to over-eating and weight gain than others.

So far, few studies have investigated the link between sensitivity to reward and relative body weight. However, initial evidence has suggested that individual difference variables, such as impulsivity, are associated with food intake (Kane, Loxton, Staiger, and Dawe, 2004; Nasser, Gluck, and Geliebter, 2004), relative body weight (Faith, Flint, Fairburn, Goodwin, and Allison, 2001), and obesity (Ryden et al., 2003). For example, people who are obese have been found to be more impulsive than people who are lean (e.g., Davis, Strachan, and Berkson, 2004; Ryden et al., 2003) and it has been suggested that impulsive people may be less able to retain control over eating behaviour (Nedderkoorn et al., 2007). For instance, it has been proposed that impulsive children seek immediate gratification and are less able to inhibit their responses making them more vulnerable to the temptation of tasty food (Nekerdoorn et al., 2007). In fact obese children have been found to overeat after exposure to tasty food, indicating that they are sensitive to the temptation of tasty food (Jansen et al., 2003). Reward sensitivity corresponds with a heightened sensitivity to unconditioned and conditioned rewarding stimuli (Dawe, Gullo and Loxton, 2004) and it seems that it may be an important individual difference in identifying those most vulnerable to overeating and weight gain.

A more wilful or difficult temperament, characterised by irritability, emotionality, slow adaptability and intensity (Hagekull et al., 1997), has also been associated with both overeating and weight gain (e.g., Niegel, Ystorm and Vollrath, 2007) as well as with feeding problems and underweight (e.g., Hagekull et al., 1997). This suggests that this temperament profile may affect children's ability to regulate their appetites, putting them at risk of maladaptive eating behaviours. Infants with difficult temperaments have shown more rapid weight gain up to the age of 3½, when compared with infants who do not display such patterns (Darlington and Wright, 2006; Niegel et al., 2007) and such temperament attributes in early childhood have also been associated with overweight in later childhood (Niegel et al., 2007). Similarly links have been found between an emotional child temperament and overweight (Agras et al., 2004; Darlington and Wright, 2006). Children with persistent tantrums over food during their first two years of life combined with a highly emotional temperament have been found to have elevated risk of becoming overweight than those children without that temperament profile (Agras et al., 2004) and child emotionality has been linked to overweight in adulthood even after controlling for multiple recognised risk factors, such as birth weight and parental body mass index (Pulkki-Raback et al., 2005).

Explanations for these links remain unclear, however it could be hypothesised that children with a more difficult temperament may show heightened emotional reactivity within feeding interactions or be more difficult and demanding in terms of their food preferences and mealtime behaviour. Differences in children's emotional reactivity, persistence and wilfulness are likely to influence the parenting process within the feeding context (Bates, Pettit, Dodge and Ridge, 1988; Rothbart, 1989). Such traits can evoke negative feelings, insensitivity and coercive feeding by parents and dyadic feeding interactions may then be characterised by little reciprocity, more conflict and struggles for control (Chatoor, 1989; Chatoor and Egan, 1983). As previous sections of the chapter have highlighted, such feeding practices can be detrimental to children's emerging eating behaviours, with coercion and feeding for emotion regulation being associated with children's over-consumption and poor appetite regulation (E.g., Blissett, Haycraft and Farrow, 2010; Savage, Fisher and Birch, 2007). Similarly, a more difficult or emotional child temperament may also influence how parents interact with and respond to behaviours outside the context of mealtimes. Parents of children who are harder to manage or sooth may feel they need to implement strategies such as using food as a reward or to regulate mood and emotional states, which may in turn interrupt and interfere with children's hunger and satiety cues.

There is some promising evidence for the mediatory role of temperament in the interaction between other factors and child weight and eating. For example, Agras et al. (2004) found, during a prospective study of 150 children from birth to 9 years of age, that child temperament mediated the association between parent and child overweight. The influence of child temperament in the pathway to overweight strongly differed dependent on parental overweight. For the thinner parent, the highest incidence of childhood obesity was found in children who had persistent tantrums over food, perhaps suggesting that this behaviour leads parents to implement reactive overfeeding of the child. For the overweight parent, showing low concern about their child's thinness combined with a highly emotional child temperament was associated with the greatest risk of child overweight or obesity (Agras et al., 2004). Further research is essential to see how child temperament interacts with other factors, not only to influence weight, but more specifically the development of children's eating behaviours and appetite regulation.

SUMMARY AND FUTURE DIRECTIONS

A comprehensive understanding of controls of energy intake in children and the regulation of children's appetites is essential. This chapter has explored theories of appetite regulation and elucidated some of the underlying behaviour traits that might contribute to differences in children's energy intake and appetite regulation. It has also highlighted the contribution of environmental, parental and individual difference factors, in the development of children's eating behaviour traits, appetite regulation and weight status.

Understanding the regulation of eating reflects a complex phenomenon as it is influenced by the integration of physical, psychological, social, genetic and environmental factors (e.g., Bouchard, Despres and Tremblay, 1991; Lowe and Butryn, 2007; Pinel, Assanand and Lehman, 2000; Schwartz et al., 2000; Temple et al., 2008). However, given the increased global prevalence of obesity, this chapter has highlighted how an increasing proportion of human food consumption appears to be driven by the effect of sensory, external and environmental stimulation, not just by the need for calories (e.g., Brownell and Horgen, 2003; Carnell and Wardle, 2008a; Schachter, 1968). Despite this there is huge variability in population weight and researchers have sought to discover the mechanisms that cause some people to eat more than their metabolic requirements and to gain weight when others do not. It has been suggested that individuals may differ in their susceptibility to the obesogenic environment, which may be explained by variations in appetitive traits or eating behaviours (e.g., Carnell and Wardle, 2008a, 2008b). Investigation into the behavioural correlates of obesity has identified a variety of eating behaviour traits that may be implicated in overconsumption and susceptibility to weight gain (e.g., Faith et al., 2004; Fisher and Birch, 2002; Saelens and Epstein, 1996). In particular this chapter has highlighted how individual differences in satiety responsiveness and responsiveness to external cues impact children's ability to regulate their energy intake (e.g., Cecil et al., 2005; Fisher and Birch, 1999; Fisher et al., 2007; Jansen et al., 2003; Hetherington et al., 2000).

Not only is it important to ascertain if certain eating styles can be consistently associated with childhood obesity and appetite regulation in community samples, but a focus on the factors that may be implicated in the development of these eating behaviour traits in young children is essential, particularly given evidence that early eating behaviours show stability into adolescence and adulthood (Ashcroft, Semmler, Carnell, Van Jaarsveld, and Wardle, 2008). Whilst genetic influences cannot be ignored (Bouchard, Despres and Tremblay, 1991; Rayussin and Swinburn, 1992), environmental factors, such as the home environment and parental influence, seem to be particularly important (e.g., Carnell and Wardle, 2008a; McGarvey et al., 2004). Parents influence children's eating behaviours through the foods they make available to the child and the feeding environment they provide (e.g., Blundell and Finlayson, 2004; Kral and Rolls, 2004; McConnahy et al., 2004), modelling their eating behaviours, preferences and attitudes (e.g., Francis et al., 2007; Hood et al., 2000), and through their parenting style (e.g., Tinsley et al., 2002) and the feeding practices they employ (e.g., Birch et al., 2003; Clark et al., 2007).

Children's self-regulation can be challenged by environmental influences within the home, such as the availability of highly palatable foods (Wilson, 2000), numerous opportunities to snack in the absence of hunger (Fisher and Birch, 2002; Jahns, Siega-Riz and Popkin, 2001), and portion size (Neilson and Popkin, 2003); all of which can override internal satiety signals. Parents also represent influential socialising agents for children (e.g., Baumrind, 1993; Bugental and Goodnow, 1998) and research has highlighted the role of observational learning and modelling of parents' eating behaviours and attitudes in the development of a child's eating habits and behaviours (e.g., Contento et al., 1993; Francis et al., 2007; Hood et al., 2000; Nicklas et al., 2001; Olivera et al., 1992). It has been suggested that reducing access to low-nutrient dense foods available in the family environment, modelling healthier eating and sharing positive food-related family experiences are important steps in improving child diet and preventing weight gain (Epstein et al., 2001) and the parents of young children are now frequently targeted in public health interventions aimed at reducing the prevalence of childhood obesity (Clark et al., 2007).

In addition, this chapter has highlighted that parents' use of controlling feeding practices, despite often being used with the positive intention of modifying children's dietary intake (Klesges et al., 1991), may interfere with children's internal hunger and satiety cues and can therefore be unintentionally detrimental by actually promoting overeating in young children (Fisher and Birch, 1998). Whilst other feeding practices, such using food as a reward or to regulate emotions were touched upon (e.g., Blissett, Haycraft and Farrow, 2010), this area is under-researched within the literature, highlighting that further investigation is essential. In addition, research exploring the impact of more positive and adaptive feeding practices, such as encouraging balance and varied food intake (Musher-Eizenman and Holub, 2007), could provide a better understanding of how to promote more successful feeding interactions and prevent negative feeding outcomes.

Ventura and Birch (2008), in their recent review, also highlight the need to look at mediational effects when investigating the effect of parental influences. They argue "logically parenting cannot have direct effects on child weight.....the influence of parenting on child weight must be mediated by effects of parenting on child eating (or other child behaviors)" (pp. 14-15). This highlights the need for research which looks at how children's eating behaviour traits interact with other factors, such as parental eating behaviours and the feeding practices that parents employ, to influence child weight. Assuming that parents' child-feeding practices are modifiable and are directly related to children's eating behaviours and childhood obesity, then they present potentially important avenues for interventions to prevent paediatric obesity to be focussed on. Parents could be targeted for education programmes to improve thier knowledge of adaptive feeding strategies and healthy home environments, which may be directly transferrable to child eating.

Whilst parents clearly represent an essential influence on children's emerging eating behaviours, children are not merely passive responders to parental influences (Carnell and Wardle, 2008a). Feeding is a dynamic bidirectional process and this chapter has evaluated the significant contribution of child temperament to both the feeding interactions of parents and their children (Brann and Skinner, 2005; Cabanac, 1987; Farrow, Galloway and Fraser, 2009) and the emergence of children's eating preferences, behaviours and appetites (e.g., Agras et al., 2004; Franken and Muris, 2005; Pulkki-Raback et al., 2005). However, a better understanding of the role of individual differences in temperament, personality and behavioural traits in the development of appetite regulation and eating behaviour is essential as it may allow health professionals to identify children in early childhood who may be at risk for weight gain or future problems with appetite regulation.

Although the literatures on parenting influence and child temperament have been poorly integrated in relation to early child eating, it is likely that a complex relationship exists between parent and child factors, which interact together to influence children's emerging eating behaviours. Initial findings described by Agras et al. (2004) provide promising evidence for the mediatory role of temperament in the pathway to overweight, however, further research is essential to see how child temperament interacts with other factors, not only to influence weight, but more specifically the development of children's eating behaviours and appetite regulation.

In addition, one of the widespread limitations within the research field is that evidence of the link between parent and child factors and child eating is largely cross-sectional. Future research should seek to utilise longitudinal designs to investigate whether parental factors, such as feeding practices, precede and predict the development of eating behaviour traits that reflect poor satiety responsiveness or whether these practices are used in response to eating behaviours and changes in weight. Given that eating behaviour traits have been shown to be relatively stable throughout childhood and into adulthood (Ashcroft et al., 2008), a focus on the early years should be maintained, as this is a critical period when eating preferences, attitudes and behaviours are becoming established, and when they may become embedded (Kelder et al., 1994). Future research is needed to further examine the unique and interactive contribution of parental and child factors, to better integrate knowledge and to provide further insight into the complex mechanisms involved in developmental of children's eating behaviour, appetite regulation and weight status.

REFERENCES

Agras, W. S., Hammer, L. D., McNicholas, F., and Kraemer, H. C. (2004). Risk factors for childhood overweight: A prospective study from birth to 9.5 years. *The Journal of Pediatrics, 145*(1), 20-25.

Ammaniti, M., Ambruzzi, A. M., Lucarelli, L., Cimino, S., and D'Olimpio, F. (2004). Malnutrition and dysfunctional mother-child feeding interactions: Clinical assessment and research implications. *Journal of the American College of Nutrition*, 23, 259–271.

Anderssen, N., Wold, B., and Torsheim, T. (2006). Are parental health habits transmitted to their children? An eight year longitudinal study of physical activity in adolescents and their parents. *Journal of Adolescence,* 29 (4), 513-524.

Ashcroft, J., Semmler, C., Carnell, S., van Jaarsveld, C. H. M., and Wardle, J. (2008). Continuity and stability of eating behaviour traits in children. *European Journal of Clinical Nutrition,* 62, 985–990.

Bates, J. E., Pettit, G. S., Dodge, K. A., and Ridge, B. (1988). The interaction of temperamental resistance to control and restrictive parenting in the development of externalizing behavior. *Developmental Psychology*, 34, 982–995.

Batsell, R. W., Brown, A. S., Ansfield, M. E., and Paschall, G. Y. (2002). You will eat all of that: A retrospective analysis of forced consumption episodes, *Appetite,* 38(3),211–219.

Bandura, A. (1977) *Social Learning Theory.* Englewood Cliffs, NJ: Prentice-Hall.

Barkeling, B., Ekman, S., and Rössner, S. (1992). Eating behaviour in obese and normal weight 11-year-old children. *International Journal of Obesity Related Metabolic Disorders, 16*(5), 355-360.

Baumrind, D. (1991). The influence of parenting style on adolescent competence and substance use. *Journal of Early Adolescence, 11(1),* 56-95.

Baumrind, D. (1993). The average expectable environment is not good enough: A response to Scarr. *Child Development,* 64(5), 1299–1317.

Bell, E. A., and Rolls, B. J. (2001). Energy density of foods affects energy intake across multiple levels of fat content in lean and obese women. *American Journal of Clinical Nutrition,* 73(6),1010-1018.

Birch, L. L., and Fisher, J. O. (1998). Development of eating behaviors among children and adolescents. *Pediatrics, 101*(3), 539.

Birch, L.L., and Fisher, J. O. (2000). Mothers' child-feeding practices influence daughters' eating and weight. *American Journal of Clinical Nutrition,* 71(5), 1054-1061.

Birch, L. L., Fisher, J. O., and Davison, K. K. (2003). Learning to overeat: Maternal use of restrictive feeding practices promotes girls' eating in the absence of hunger. *The American Journal of Clinical Nutrition, 78*(2), 215-220.

Birch, L., McPhee, L., Shoba, B., Steinberg, L,. and Krehbiel, R. (1987). "Clean up your plate": effects of child feeding practices on the conditioning of meal size. *Learning and Motivation, 18*(3), 301–317.

Blissett, J., and Haycraft, E. (2008). Are parenting style and controlling feeding practices related? *Appetite, 50,* 477-485.

Blissett, J., Haycraft, E., and Farrow, C. (2010) Inducing preschool children's emotional eating: relations with parental feeding practices. *American Journal of Clinical Nutrition,* 92, 359-365.

Blissett, J., Meyer, C., and Haycraft, E. (2006). Maternal and paternal controlling feeding practices with male and female children. *Appetite,* 47(2), 212-219.

Blissett, J., Meyer, C., and Haycraft, E. (2007). Maternal mental health and child feeding problems in a non-clinical group. *Eating Behaviours,* 8, 311–318.

Blundell, J. E., and Finlayson, G. (2004). Is susceptibility to weight gain characterized by homeostatic or hedonic risk factors for overconsumption? Physiology and Behavior, 82, 21–25.

Blundell, J., and Rogers, P. (1991). Hunger, hedonics, and the control of satiation and satiety. *Chemical Senses, 4,* 127-148.

Blundell, J. E., Stubbs, R. J., Golding, C., Croden, F., Alam, R., Whybrow, S., et al. (2005). Resistance and susceptibility to weight gain: Individual variability in response to a high-fat diet. *Physiology and Behaviour, 86*(5), 614-622.

Bouchard, C., Despres, J. P., and Tremblay, A. (1991). Genetics of obesity and human energy metabolism. *Proceedings of Nutrition Society,* 50, 139–147.

Braet, C., and Van Strein, T. (1986). Assessment of emotional, externally induced and restrained eating behaviour in nine to twelve-year-old obese and non-obese children, *Behaviour Research and Therapy, 35*(9), 863-873.

Brann, L. S., and Skinner, J. D. (2005). More controlling child-feeding practices are found among parents of boys with an average body mass index compared with parents of boys with a high body mass index. *Journal of the American Dietetic Association*, 105, 1411–1416.

British Nutrition Foundation. (1999). *Obesity: The Report of the British Nutrition Foundation Task Force.* (pp 37-38) Oxford: Blackwell Science.

Brown, R., and Ogden, J. (2004). Children's eating attitudes and behaviour: a study of the modelling and control theories of parental *influence, Health Education Research*, 19(3), 261-271.

Brownell, L.D., and Horgan, K. B. (2003) *Food fight: The inside story of the food industry, America's obesity crisis and what we can do about it*, New York: McGraw Hill.

Bruch, H. (1973). *Hunger awareness and individuation.* In: H. Bruch. (Ed.) Eating disorders: obesity, anorexia nervosa, and the person within. (pp. 44– 65). New York: Basic Books, Inc.

Bugental, D. B., and Goodnow, J. J. (1998). Socialization processes. In: I. W. Damon. (Ed.) *Handbook of Child Psychology.* (5th ed., pp. 389–462). New York: Wiley.

Butte, N. F., Cai, G., Cole, S. A., and Wilson, T. A. (2007). *Metabolic and behavioral predictors of weight gain in Hispanic children: the Viva la Familia Study. American Journal of Clinical Nutrition,* 85(6), 1478-1485.

Cabanac, M. (1985). Preferring for pleasure. *American Journal of Clinical Nutrition, 42,*1151–1155.

Carper, J. L., Fisher, J. O., and Birch, L. L. (2000). Young girls' emerging dietary restraint and disinhibition are related to parental control in child feeding. *Appetite, 35,* 121–129.

Carnell, S., Haworth, C. M. A., Plomin, R., and Wardle, J. (2008). Genetic influence on appetite in children. *International Journal of Obesity, 32*(10), 1468-1473.

Carnell, S., and Wardle, J. (2008a). Appetite and adiposity in children: Evidence for a behavioral susceptibility theory of obesity. *American Journal of Clinical Nutrition, 88*(1), 22-29.

Carnell, S., and Wardle, J. (2008b). Appetitive traits and child obesity: Measurement, origins and implications for intervention. *Proceedings of the Nutrition Society, 67,* 343-355.

Cecil, J. E., Palmer, C. N. A., Wrieden, W., Murrie, I., Bolton-Smith, C., Watt, P., et al. (2005). Energy intakes of children after preloads: Adjustment, not compensation. *American Journal of Clinical Nutrition, 82*(2), 302-308.

Chatoor, I. (1989). Infantile anorexia nervosa: A developmental disorder of separation and individuation. *Journal of the American Academy of Psychoanalysis, 17,* 43–64.

Chatoor, I., and Egan, J. (1983). Nonorganic failure to thrive and dwarfism due to food refusal: A separation disorder. *Journal of the American Academy of Child Psychiatry, 22,* 294–301.

Clark, H. R., Goyder, E., Bissell, P., Blank, L., and Peters, J. (2007). How do parents' child-feeding behaviours influence child weight? Implications for childhood obesity policy, *Journal of Public Health*, 29,(2),132–141.

Contento, I.R., Basch, C., Shea, S., Gutin, B., Zybert, P., Michela, J.L., and Rips, J. (1993). Relationship of mothers' food choice criteria to food intake of pre-school children: identication of family subgroups. *Health Education Quarterly, 20,* 243-259.

Costanzo, P. R., and Woody, E. Z., (1985). Domain specific parenting styles and their impact on the child's development of particular deviance: The example of obesity proneness. *Journal of Social and Clinical Psychology*, 3(4), 425-445.

Cutting, T. M., Fisher, J. O., Grimm-Thomas,K., and Birch, L. L. (1999). Like mother, like daughter: familial patterns of overweight are mediated by mothers' dietary disinhibition. American Journal of Clinical Nutrition, 69, 608–13.

Darling, N., and Steinberg, L. (1993). Parenting style as context: An integrative model. *Psychological Bulletin, 113*(3), 487-496.

Darlington, A. S., and Wright, C. M. (2006). The influence of temperament on weight gain in early infancy. *Journal of Developmental and Behavioral Pediatrics, 27,* 329–335.

Davis, C., Strachan, S., and Berkson, M. (2004). Sensitivity to reward: Implications for overeating and overweight. *Appetite, 42*(2), 131-138.

Davison, K. K., and Birch, L. L. (2001). Childhood overweight: a contextual model and recommendations for future research, *Obesity Reviews, 2(*3),158-171.

Dawe, S., Gullo, M. J., and Loxton, N. J. (2004). Reward drive and rash impulsiviness as dimensions of impulsivity: Implications for substance misuse. Addictive Behaviors, 29, 1389–1405.

de Castro, J. A., and Lilenfeld, L. R. R. (2005). Influence of heredity on dietary restraint, disinhibition, and perceived hunger in humans, *Nutrition,* 21, 446 –55.

Drabman, R. S., Cordua, G. D., Hammer, D., Jarvie, G. J., and Horton, W. (1979). Developmental trends in eating rates of normal and overweight preschool children. *Child Development,50(1)*, 211-216.

Drewnowski, A., and Hann, C. (1999). Food preferences and reported frequencies of food consumption as predictors of current diet in young women. *American Journal of Clinical Nutrition, 70,* 28–36.

Druce, M., and Bloom, S. R. (2006). The Regulation of Appetite. *Archives of Disease in Childhood,* 91,183-187.

Duke, R. E., Bryson, S., Hammer, L. D., and Agras, W. S. (2004). The relationship between parental factors at infancy and parent-reported control over children's eating at age 7. *Appetite*, 43, 247–252.

Epstein, L. H., Leddy, J. J., Temple, J. L., and Faith, M. S. (2007). Food reinforcement and eating: A multilevel analysis. *Psychological Bulletin, 133*(5), 884.

Epstein, L. H., Paluch, R., and Coleman, K. J. (1996). Differences in Salivation to Repeated Food Cues in Obese and Nonobese Women. *Psychosomatic Medicine,58,*160-164 .

Faith, M. S., Berkowitz, R. I., Stallings, V. A., Kerns, J., Storey, M., and Stunkard, A. J. (2006). Eating in the absence of hunger: A genetic marker for childhood obesity in prepubertal boys? *Obesity, 14*(1), 131-138.

Faith, M. S., Flint, J., Fairburn, C., Goodwin, G. M., and Allison, D. B. (2001). Gender Differences in the Relationship between Personality Dimensions and Relative Body Weight *Obesity Research* 9, 647–65.

Faith, M.S., Keller, K. L., Johnson, S. J., Pietrobelli, A., Matz, P. E., Must, S., Jorge, M. A., Cooperberg, J., Heymsfield, S. B., and Allison, D. B. (2004). Familial aggregation of energy intake in children. *American Journal of Clinical Nutrition, 79*(5), 844-850.

Farrow, C.V., Galloway, A. T., and Fraser, K. (2009). Sibling eating behaviours and differential child feeding practices reported by parents, Appetite, 52, 307–312.

Fisher, J. O., and Birch, L. L. (1999). Restricting access to palatable foods affects children's behavioral response, food selection, and intake. *American Journal of Clinical Nutrition*, 69, 1264–1272.

Fisher, J. O., and Birch, L. L. (2002). Eating in the absence of hunger and overweight in girls from 5 to 7 y of age. *American Journal of Clinical Nutrition*, 76(1), 226-231.

Fisher, J. O., Cai, G., Jaramillo, S. J., Cole, S. A., Comuzzie, A. G., and Butte, N. F. (2007). Heritability of hyperphagic eating behavior and appetite-related hormones among hispanic children. *Obesity Research*, 15(6), 1484- 1495.

Fisher, J. O., Liu, Y., Birch, L. L., and Rolls, B. J. (2007). Effects of portion size and energy density on young children's intake at a meal. *American Journal of Clinical Nutrition*, 86, 174 –179.

Finlayson, G., Halford, J. C. G., King, N. A., and Blundell, J. E. (2007). *The Regulation of Food Intake in Humans.* In: T, Matthias (Ed) *Obesitext - The Source.* Endotext.com.

Flory, J. D., Harvey, P.D., Mitropolou, V., et al. (2006) Dispositional impulsivity in normal and abnormal samples. *Journal of Psychiatric Research,40*, 438–447.

Fomon, S. J., Filmer, L. J., Thomas, L. N., Anderson, T. A., and Nelson, S. E. (1975). Influence of formula concentration on caloric intake and growth of normal infants. *Acta Pediatrica*, 64(2),172-181.

Fox, M. K., Devaney, B., Reidy, K., Razafindrakoto, M. S., and Ziegler, P. (2006). Relationship between Portion Size and Energy Intake among Infants and Toddlers: Evidence of Self-Regulation. *Journal of the American Dietetic Association,106(1),177-183.*

Francis, L. A., and Birch, L. L. (2005). Maternal influences on daughters restrained eating behaviour. *Health Psychology*, 24(6), 548-554.

Francis, L. A., Ventura, A. K., Marini, M., and Birch, L. L. (2007). Parent Overweight Predicts Daughters' Increase in BMI and Disinhibited Overeating from 5 to 13 Years, *Obesity,15*(6),1445-1553.

Franken, I. H. A., and Muris, P. (2005). Individual differences in reward sensitivity are related to food craving and relative body weight in healthy women. *Appetite, 45*(2), 198-201.

Galloway, A. T., Fiorito, L., Lee, Y., and Birch, L. L. (2005). Parental Pressure, Dietary Patterns, and Weight Status among Girls Who Are "Picky Eaters", Journal of American Dietic Association, 105(4), 541-548.

Goldsmith, H. H., Buss, A.H., Plomin, R., Rothbart, M. K., Thomas, A., and Chess, S. (1987). What is temperament? Four approaches. *Child Development*, 58, 505-529.

Goodnow, J. J., Knight, R., and Cashmore, J. (1985). Adult social cognition: Implications of parents' ideas for approaches to development. In M. Perlmutter (Ed.), *Social cognition: Minnesota symposia on child development* (Vol 18, pp. 287-324). Hillsdale, NJ: Erlbaum.

Goran, M. I., and Treuth, M. S. (2001). Energy expenditure, physical activity and obesity in children. *Pediatric Clinics of North America*, 48(4), 931-953

Gray, J. A. (1987). *The psychology of fear and stress.* Cambridge: Cambridge University Press.

Grolnick, W. S., and Farkas, M. (2002). Parenting and the development of children's self-regulation. In M. H. Bornstein (Ed.), *Handbook of parenting: Vol. 5. Practical issues in parenting* (2nd ed., pp. 89–110). Mahwah, NJ: Lawrence Erlbaum Associates.

Hagekull, B., Bohlin, G. and Rydell, A, M. (1997) Maternal Sensitivity, Infant Temperament, and the Development of Early Feeding Problems. *Infant Mental Health Journal*, 18(1) 92–106.

Hetherington, M. (2007). Individual differences in the drive to overeat. *Nutrition Bulletin, 32*, 14-21.

Hetherington, M. M., Wood, C., and Lyburn, S. C. (2000). Response to energy dilution in the short term: evidence of nutritional wisdom in young children? *Nutritional Neuroscience, 3*, 321–329.

Hood, M. Y., Moore, L. L., Ramamurti, S. A., Singer, M., Cupples, L. A., and Ellison, R. C. (2000). Parental eating attitudes and the development of obesity in children. The Framingham Children's Study. *International Journal of Obesity Related Metabolic Disorders, 24*(10), 1319-1325.

Hughes, S. O., Power, T. G., Fisher, J. O., Mueller, S., and Nicklas, T. A. (2005). Revisiting a neglected construct: Parenting styles in a child feeding context. *Appetite*, 44, 83–92.

Jahns, L., Siega-Riz, A. M., and Popkin, B. M. (2001). The increasing prevalence of snacking among American children from 1977 to 1996. *The Journal of Pediatrics, 138*, 493-498.

Jansen, A., Theunissen, N., Slechten, K., Nederkoorn, C., Boon, B., Mulkens, S., et al. (2003). Overweight children overeat after exposure to food cues. *Eating Behaviors, 4*, 197-209.

Johnson, S. L. (2000). Improving preschoolers' self-regulation of energy intake. *Pediatrics, 106*, 1429-1435.

Johnson, S. L., and Birch, L. L. (1994). Parents' and children's adiposity and eating style. *Pediatrics, 94*(5), 653-661.

Jolliffe, D. (2004). Extent of overweight among US children and adolescents from 1971 to 2000. International Journal of Obesity Related Metabolic Disorders, 28, 4–9.

Kane, T. A., Loxton, N. J., Staiger, P. K., and Dawe, S. (2004). Does the tendency to act impulsively underlie binge eating and alcohol use problems? An empirical investigation. *Personality and Individual Differences, 36*(1), 83-94.

Kelder, S.H., Perry, C.L., Klepp, K. I. and Lytle, L.L. (1994). Longitudinal tracking of adolescent smoking, physical activity and food choice behaviours. *American Journal of Public Health, 84,* 1121–1126.

Kitzmann, K. M., Dalton III, W. T., and Buscemi, J. (2008). Beyond Parenting Practices: Family Context and the Treatment of Pediatric Obesity. *Family Relation,* 57(1), 13-23.

Klesges, R.C., Klesges, L. M., Eck, L. H., and Shelton, M. L. (1995). A longitudinal analysis of accelerated weight gain in preschool children. *Pediatrics,* 95, 126–130.

Kral, T. V. E., Roe, L. S., and Rolls, B. J. (2004). Combined effects of energy density and portion size on energy intake in women. American Journal of Clinical Nutrition, 79(6), 962-968.

Kral, T. V. E., and Rolls, B. J. (2004). Energy density and portion size: Their independent and combined effects on energy intake. *Physiology and Behavior, 82*(1), 131-138.

Kremers, S. P., Brug, J., de Vries, H., and Engels, R. C. M. E. (2003). Parenting style and adolescent fruit consumption. *Appetite,* 41, 43–50.

Larsen, J. K., van Strein, T., Eisinga, R., and Engeles, R. C. M. E. (2006). Gender Differences in the association between alexithymia and emotional eating in obese individuals. *Journal of Psychosomatic Research, 60*(3), 237-243.

Leahy, K. E., Birch, L. L., and Rolls, B. J. (2008). Reducing the Energy Density of an

Entrée Decreases Children's Energy Intake at Lunch. *Journal of the American Dietetic Association, 108(1)*, 41-48.

Lindberg, L., Bohlin, G., Hagekull, B., and Thunström, M. (1994). Early food refusal: Infant and family characteristics. *Infant Mental Health Journal, 15,* 262–277.

Lobstein T, Baur L. and Uauy, R. (2004). Obesity in children and young people: a crisis in public health. *Obesity Reviews,* 5(1), 4-85.

Lowe, M. R., and Butryn, M. L. (2007). Hedonic hunger: A new dimension of appetite? Physiology and Behaviour, 91(4), 432-439.

Lowe, M. R., and Levine, A. S. (2005). Eating motives and the controversy over dieting: Eating less than needed versus less than wanted. *Obesity Research, 13*(5), 797-806.

Marchi, M., and Cohen, P. (1990). Early childhood eating behaviors and adolescent eating disorders. *Journal of American Academy of Child and Adolescent Psychiatry, 29,* 112–117.

Maziak, W., Ward, K. D., and Stockton, M. B. (2008). Childhood obesity: are we missing the big picture? *Obesity Reviews,* 9(1), 35-42.

McConahy, K. L., Smiciklas-Wright, H., Birch, L. L., Mitchell, D. C., and Picciano, M. F. (2002). Food portions are positively related to energy intake and body weight in early childhood. *The Journal of Pediatrics, 140*(3), 340-347.

McConahy, K. L., Smiciklas-Wright, H., Mitchell, D. C., and Picciano, M. F. (2002). Portion size of common foods predicts energy intake among preschool-aged children. *Journal of the American Dietetic Association,*104(6), 975-979.

McGarvey, E., Keller, A., Forrester, M., Williams, E., Seward, D., and Suttle, D. E. (2004). Feasibility and Benefits of a Parent-Focused Preschool Child Obesity Intervention *American Journal of Public Health*, 94(9)1490-1495.

Moens, E., and Braet, C. (2007). Predictors of disinhibited eating in children with and without overweight. *Behaviour Research and Therapy, 45(6)*, 1357-1368.

Moens, E., Braet, C., and Soetens, B. (2007). Observation of family functioning at mealtime: A comparison between families of children with and without overweight. *Journal of Pediatric Psychology, 32,* 52-63.

Montgomery, C., Jackson, D. M., Kelly, L. A., and Reilly, J. J. (2006). Parental feeding style, energy intake and weight status in young Scottish children. *British Journal of Nutrition,* 96, 1149–1153.

Mrdjenovic, G., and Levitsky, D. A. (2005). Children eat what they are served: the imprecise regulation of energy intake. *Appetite, 44*(3), 273-282.

Musher-Eizenman, D., and Holub, S. (2007). Comprehensive Feeding Practices Questionnaire: Validation of a New Measure of Parental Feeding Practices. *Journal of Pediatric Psychology, 32,* 960-972.

Nasser, J. A., Gluck, M. E., and Geliebter, A. (2004). Impulsivity and test meal intake in obese binge eating women. *Appetite, 43*(3), 303-307.

Nederkoorn, C., Jansen, E., Mulkens, S., and Jansen, A. (2007). Impulsivity predicts treatment outcome in obese children. *Behaviour Research and Therapy, 45*(5), 1071-1075.

Nicklas, T., Baranowski, T., Baranowski, J., Cullen, K., Rittenberg, L., and Olvera, N. (2001). Family and child-care provider influences on preschool children's fruit, juice, and vegetable consumption. *Nutrition Reviews,*59(7), 224–35.

Niegel, S., Ystrom, E., and Vollrath, M. E. (2007). Is difficult temperament related to overweight and rapid early weight gain in infants? A prospective cohort study. *Journal of Developmental and Behavioral Pediatrics, 28,* 462–466.

Nielson, S. J., and Popkin, B. M. (2003). Patterns and trends in food portion sizes, 1977–1998. The Journal of the American medical Association, *289,* 450-453.

Nisbett, R. E. (1972) Hunger, obesity, and the ventromedial hypothalamus. *Psychological Review, 79,* 433–453.

Nguyen-Rodriguez, S.T., Chou, C. P., Unger, J. B., and Spruijt-Metz, D. (2008). BMI as a moderator of perceived stress and emotional eating in adolescents. *Eating Behaviours, 9,* 238–246.

Olivera, S.A., Ellison, R.C., Moore, L.L., Gillman, M.W., Garrahie, E.J., and Singer, M.R. (1992) Parent-child relationships in nutrient intake: the Framingham Children's Study. American Journal of Clinical Nutrition, 56, 593-598.

Orrell-Valente, J. K., Hill, L. G., Brechwald, W. A., Dodge, K. A., Pettit, G. S., and Bates, J. E. (2007) Just three more bites": An observational analysis of parents' socialization of children's eating at mealtime. *Appetite*, 34(1), 37-45

Pinel, J. P. J., Assanand, S., and Lehman, D. R. (2000). Hunger, eating, and ill health. *American Psychologist, 55*(10), 1105-1116.

Pliner, P. and Loewen, R. E. (1997) Temperament and Food Neophobia in Children and their Mothers, *Appetite*, 28(3), 239-254.

Provencher, V., Perusse, L., Bouchard, L., Drapeau, V., Bouchard, C., Rice, T., et al., (2005). Familial resemblance in eating behaviors in men and women from the Quebec Family Study. *Obesity Research,* 13, 1624 –1629.

Pulkki-Raback, L., Elovainio, M., Kivimaki, M., and Raitakari, O. (2005). Temperament in childhood predicts body mass in adulthood: the cardiovascular risk in young finns study. *Health Psychology*, 24, 307–315.

Ravussin, E., Swinburn, B. A. (1992). Pathophysiology of obesity. *Lancet,* 340, 404–408.

Rhee, K. (2008). Parenting Style, and Family Functioning, Childhood Overweight and the Relationship between Parent Behaviors. *The ANNALS of the American Academy of Political and Social Science,* 615(1), 11-37.

Rhee, K, E., Lumeng, J. C., Appugliese, D. P., Kaciroti, N., and Bradley, R. H. (2006). Parenting styles and overweight status in first grade. *Pediatrics*, 117, 2047-2054.

Rodin, J. (1981). Current status of the internal-external hypothesis for obesity: What went wrong? *American Psychologist,* 36(4), 361-372.

Rolls, B. J., Engell, D., and Birch, L. L. (2000). Serving portion size influences 5-year-old but not 3-year-old children's food intakes. *Journal of the American Dietetic Association, 100*(2), 232-234.

Romon, M., Duhamel, A., Collinet, N., and Weill, J. (2005). Influence of social class on time trends in BMI distribution in 5-year-old French children from 1989 to 1999. International *Journal of Obesity Related Metabolic Disorders*, 29, 54–59.

Rothbart, M. K. (1989). Temperament and development. In: G. A. Kohnstamm., J. E. Bates., and M. K. Rothbart. (Eds.). *Temperament in Childhood.* Chichester, England: Wiley

Ryden, A., Sullivan, M., Torgerson, J., Karlsson, J., Lindroos, A., and Taft, C. (2003). Severe obesity and personality: A comparative controlled study of personality traits. *International Journal of Obesity, 27*(12), 1534-1540.

Saelens, B. E., and Epstein, L. H. (1996). Reinforcing value of food in obese and non-obese women, *Appetite, 27*(1), 41-50.

Satter, E. M. (1986). The feeding relationship. *Journal of the American Dietetic Association, 86,* 352–356.

Savage, J. S., Fisher, J. O., and Birch, L. L. (2007). Parental influence on eating behavior: Conception to adolescence. *The Journal of Law, Medicine and Ethics, 35*(1), 22.

Schachter, S. (1968). Obesity and eating. Internal and external cues differentially affect the eating behavior of obese and normal subjects. *Science, 161,* 751-756.

Schachter, S. (1971). Some extraordinary facts about obese humans and rats. *American Psychologist, 26,* 129-144.

Schaffer, H.R. (2006). *Key concepts in developmental psychology*. London, United Kingdom: Sage Publications.

Schmitz, K. H., Lytle, L. A., Phillips, G. A., Murray, D. M., Birnbaum, A. S., and Kubik, M. Y. (2002). Psychosocial correlates of physical activity and sedentary leisure habits in young adolescents: The Teens Eating for Energy and Nutrition at School study. *Preventative Medicine,* 34, 266-278.

Schwartz, M. W., Woods, S. C., Porte, D., Seeley, R. J., and Baskin, D. G. (2000). Central nervous system control of food intake. *Nature,* 404, 661-671.

Scnoek, H. M., Van Strein, T., Janssens, J. M., Engels, R.C., (2007). Emotional, external. Restrained eating and overweight in Dutch adolescents. *Scandinavian Journal of Psychology, 48,* 23-32.

Shea, S., Stein, A. D., Basch, C. E., Contento, I. R., Zybert, P. (1992). Variability and Self-regulation of Energy Intake in Young Children in Their Everyday Environment. *Pediatrics, 90(4), 524-546.*

Slochower, J. (1976). Emotional labeling and overeating in obese and normal weight individuals. *Psychosomatic Medicine, 38*(2), 131-139.

Sorof, J., Poffenbarger, T., Franko, K., Bernard, L., and Portman, R. (2002). Isolated systolic hypertension, obesity and hyperkinetic homodynamic states in children. *Journal of Pediatrics*, 140, 660-666.

Spruijt-Metz, D., Chaoyang, L., Cohen, E., Birch, L., and Goran, M. (2006). Longitudinal influence of mother's child-feeding practices on adiposity in children. *The Journal of Pediatrics,* 148(3), 314-320.

Stein, A., Woolley, H., and McPherson, K. (1999) Conflict between mothers with eating disorders and their infants during mealtimes. *British Journal of Psychiatry, 175,* 455–461.

Stubbs, R. J., Johnstone, A. M., O'Reilly, L. M., Barton, K., and Reid, C. (1998). The effect of covertly manipulating the energy density of mixed diets on ad libitum food intake in 'pseudo free-living' humans. *International Journal of Obesity Related Metabolic Disorders,* 22(10), 980-987.

Temple, J. L., Giacomelli, A. M., Roemmich, J. N., and Epstein, L. H. (2007). Overweight children habituate slower than non-overweight children to food. *Physiology and Behavior, 91*(2-3), 250-254.

Temple, J. L., Chappel, A., Shalik, J., Volcy, S., and Epstein, L. H. (2008). Daily consumption of individual snack foods decreases their reinforcing value. *Eating Behaviors, 9*(3), 267-276.

Thomas, A. and Chess, S. (1977) *Temperament and Development*. New York, NY: Brunner/Mazel.

Tinsley, B. J., Markey, C. N., Ericksen, A. J., Ortiz, R. V., and Kwasman, A. (2002). Health promotion for parents. In M. H. Bornstein (Ed.), *Handbook of parenting: Vol. 5. Practical issues in parenting* (2nd ed., pp.311–328). Mahwah, NJ: Lawrence Erlbaum Associates.

Van Strien, T., and Bazelier, F. G. (2007). Perceived parental control of food intake is related to external, restrained and emotional eating in 7-12-year-old boys and girls. *Appetite, 49,* 618–625.

Van Strien, T., Frijters, J.E.R., Bergers, G.P.A., and Defares, P.B. (1986). The Dutch Eating Behaviour Questionnaire (DEBQ) for assessment of emotional, external and restrained eating behaviour. *International Journal of Eating Disorders,* 5, 295–313.

Van Strien, T., and Oosterveld, P. (2008) The children's DEBQ for assessment of restrained, emotional, and external eating in 7- to 12-year-old children. *International Journal of Eating Disorders, 41,* 72–81.

Ventura, A. K., and Birch, L. L. (2008). Does parenting affect children's eating and weight status? *International Journal of Behavioral Nutrition and Physical Activity,* 5, 15-27.

Viana, V., Sinde, S., and Saxton, J. C., (2008). Children's Eating Behaviour Questionnaire: associations with BMI in Portuguese children. *British Journal of Nutrition,* 100, 445-450.

Wardle, J., and Boniface, D. (2008). Changes in the distributions of body mass index and waist circumference in the adult population of England, 1993/1994 to 2002/2003. *International Journal of Obesity, 32,* 527–532.

Webber, L., Hill, C., Saxton, J., Van Jaarsveld, C. H. M., and Wardle, J. (2009). Eating Behaviour and weight in children. *International Journal of Obesity*, 33, 21–28.

Wilson, J. F. (2000). Preschool children maintain intake of other foods at a meal including sugared chocolate milk. *Appetite, 16,* 61-67.

Woods, S. C., Schwartz, M. W., Baskin, D. G., and Seeley, R. J. (2000) Food Intake and the regulation of body weight. *Annual Review of Psychology, 51,* 255-277.

Zabinski, M. F., Daly, T., Gregory, R. D., Norman, J., Rupp, J. W., Calfas, J. K., Sallis, J. F., and Patrick, K. (2006). Psychosocial Correlates of Fruit, Vegetable, and Dietary Fat Intake among Adolescent Boys and Girls. *Journal of the American Dietetic Association*, 106 (6), 814–821.

Zandstra, E. H., Mathey, M. F., Graaf, C., and van Staveren, W. A. (2000). Short-term regulation of food intake in children, young adults and the elderly. *European Journal of Clinical Nutrition, 54,* 239-246.

Zeller, M, H., Reiter-Purtill, J, Modi, A. C., Gutzwiller, J., Vannatta, K and Davies, W, H. (2007). Controlled study of critical parent and family factors in the obesigenic environment. *Obesity,* 15, 126-136.

In: Appetite: Regulation, Role in Disease and Control
Editor: Steven R. Mitchell, pp. 29-53
ISBN 978-1-61209-842-5
© 2011 Nova Science Publishers, Inc.

Chapter 2

ROLE OF APPETITE CONTROL IN METABOLIC DISEASE CONDITIONS

Stephen D. Anton[*], Pamela J. Dubyak[‡] and Kelly M. Naugle[≠]
University of Florida, Gainesville, Florida, U.S.A

OVERVIEW

Excessive caloric intake is a significant health concern in the United States and in industrialized countries around the world (Ogden, et al., 2006). Today, individuals are consuming significantly more food than in previous years. Epidemiological studies indicate that per capita energy intake increased by approximately 300 kcal per day from 1985 to 2000, after having remained fairly constant for the previous 75 years (Finkelstein, Ruhm, & Kosa, 2005). If an individual's energy expenditure remained constant, a daily increase in energy intake of 300 calories would result in a weight gain of two to three pounds per month. Many studies suggest, however, that individuals are much more sedentary today than in previous years (Hill, Wyatt, Reed, & Peters, 2003). Thus, rates of weight gain may be even greater than this estimate. In line with this, there has been a substantial increase in body weight across all segments of the U.S. population over the past few decades (Ogden, et al., 2006). Current estimates indicate that approximately 66% of the U.S. adult population is overweight or obese; an estimate that is 20% greater than 30 years ago (Ogden, Yanovski, Carroll, & Flegal, 2007).

The increasing rates of obesity are of significant concern because overweight and obese individuals are at increased risk for a number of deleterious health conditions, such as cancer, diabetes and heart disease (Kenchaiah, et al., 2002; Key, Allen, Spencer, & Travis, 2002; J.

---

[*] Department of Aging and Geriatric Research, Department of Clinical and Health Psychology, University of Florida, Gainesville, Florida, U.S.A, Address: 210 E Mowry Rd., ARRC, Bldg. 210, Phone: 352-273-7514, Fax: 352-273-5920, Email: santon@aging.ufl.edu

[‡] Department of Clinical and Health Psychology, University of Florida, Gainesville, Florida, U.S.A. , Address: HPNP, 101 S. Newell Drive, Suite 4101, Gainesville, FL 32610, Phone: 352 273-5234, Fax: 352 273-5109, Email: pdubyak@phhp.ufl.edu

[≠] Department of Aging and Geriatric Research, University of Florida, Gainesville. Address: 210 E Mowry Rd., ARRC, Bldg. 210, Phone: 352-294-5230, Fax: 352-273-5920, Email: kgamble@aging.ufl.edu

Roth, Qiang, Marban, Redelt, & Lowell, 2004). Moreover, recent evidence suggests adiposity is associated with accelerated aging (Das, Gabriely, & Barzilai, 2004; Kloting & Bluher, 2005). Against the backdrop of the increasing obesity epidemic, research over the past sixty years has documented the benefits of caloric restriction (CR) for increasing longevity and delaying the onset of age-related diseases in numerous species (Roth, Ingram, & Joseph, 2007). Preliminary reports suggest that CR may also have beneficial effects in primates (Bodkin, Alexander, Ortmeyer, Johnson, & Hansen, 2003; Kayo, Allison, Weindruch, & Prolla, 2001) and humans (Heilbronn, et al., 2006).

Although it is currently unknown if all humans benefit from adopting a CR lifestyle, extensive research has shown that overweight and obese individuals receive numerous health benefits following weight loss achieved through CR (Goldstein, 1992). Long-term compliance to conventional weight loss programs, however, is notoriously poor (Scheen, 2008), possibly due to internal feedback systems that defend against body weight change by signaling the body to increase food intake and decrease energy expenditure in response to caloric restriction. Additionally, our current environment, which consists of a variety of low-cost, high-calorie palatable foods, has been termed "toxic" and "obesigenic," because it can promote excessive food intake (Hill, et al., 2003).

This chapter will discuss the role excessive food intake has in contributing to today's most prominent health conditions, as well as the role that appetite control has in promoting health and wellness. We will also review the emerging role that postprandial states have on appetite control, body weight and fat metabolism, as well as discuss treatment approaches that facilitate appetite control.

HEALTH BENEFITS OF CALORIE CONTROL

The extant research indicates that short and long-term caloric control has beneficial effects on short-lived organisms, nonhuman primates and overweight humans. Prolonged caloric restriction has been found to extend the average and maximal life-span in numerous species (Weindruch, Walford, Fligiel, & Guthrie, 1986), as well as delay the onset of age-associated disease conditions such as cancer and diabetes (Weindruch, Naylor, Goldstein, & Walford, 1988; Weindruch & Walford, 1982) in rodents and in nonhuman primates (Colman, et al., 2009). More recently, CR has been shown to improve several cardiac risk factors (Eilat-Adar, Eldar, & Goldbourt, 2005; Fontana, et al., 2007; Klein, et al., 2004; Lefevre, et al., 2009), improve mitochondrial function (Civitarese, et al., 2007) and reduce DNA damage (Heilbronn, et al., 2006) in overweight and obese humans. While this chapter cannot provide an extensive review of the numerous studies documenting the health benefits of calorie control, the below sections will briefly review key findings from both animal and human studies during the past two decades.

Animal Studies

Key early studies in rodents revealed the potential of CR to increase longevity. For example, Weindruch and colleagues found that mice with 55-65% calorie restricted diets started after weaning exhibited 35-65% greater mean and maximal lifespan than mice eating a non-purified ad libitum diet (Weindruch, et al., 1986). Additionally, mice with moderate caloric restriction (20-40%) starting in middle-aged adulthood demonstrate on average a 10-20% increase in mean and maximal life span (Weindruch & Walford, 1982). Several different mechanisms may account for the increased longevity in response to caloric restriction. For example, aging is characterized by an exponential increase of oxidatively damaged proteins, and CR in mice down regulates the expression of genes involved in oxidative stress and ameliorates oxidative damage in several different tissues (Lee, Klopp, Weindruch, & Prolla, 1999; Sohal, Ku, Agarwal, Forster, & Lal, 1994). Furthermore, CR using nutrient enriched diets in long lived strains of mice inhibits spontaneous lymphoma and lowers the incidence of cancer and tumors (Weindruch & Walford, 1982).

Nonhuman primates and humans share striking anatomical, physiological and behavioral similarities. As such, nonhuman primate studies have the potential to provide novel insights into the beneficial effects of prolonged caloric restriction on disease patterns and aging. Colman and colleagues recently conducted an elegant 20-year longitudinal study examining the effects of caloric restriction on resistance to illness and mortality in rhesus monkeys (Colman, et al., 2009). Compared to a control group, moderate caloric restriction (~30%) significantly reduced body weight and body fat mass, and decreased the incidence of diabetes, cancer, neoplasia and cardiovascular disease. Accordingly, the control group had three times the rate of death from age-related causes relative to the CR group. Furthermore, CR reduced age-associated atrophy in subcortical brain regions integral to motor function and certain aspects of executive function.

Many other studies have also shown that caloric restriction reduces the pathological effects of aging in nonhuman primates. For example, a caloric restricted diet for 12-17 years attenuated brain iron accumulation and preserved motor function in older rhesus monkeys (Kastman, et al., 2010). Furthermore, prolonged caloric restriction in rhesus monkeys has been shown to enhance glucoregulatory health (Gresl, et al., 2001) and attenuate sarcopenia (Colman, Beasley, Allison, & Weindruch, 2008). Collectively, animal research indicates that CR extends lifespan in rodents and delays age-related disease conditions in nonhuman primate species. However, it is important to note that dietary restriction paradigms in most animal studies compare free-feeding animals (i.e., usually leading to overconsumption) to calorie restricted animals. Therefore, the results of studies to date likely represent the effects of calorie restriction versus overconsumption, rather than calorie restriction versus weight maintenance diets.

Human Studies

Numerous studies have demonstrated a variety of health benefits of a caloric restricted diet in overweight and obese humans. Substantial evidence has shown that CR is associated with significant reductions in body weight, whole body fat mass and visceral and subcutaneous abdominal adipose tissue in overweight and obese humans (Racette, et al., 2006; Weiss, et al., 2006). Moreover, prolonged CR in obese patients with type 2 diabetes mellitus improves myocardial function as indicated by decreased heart rate and cardiac output and reduced left ventricular mass, which are predictive of cardiovascular morbidity and mortality (Hammer, et al., 2008). Weight loss induced by CR also improves cardiovascular disease risk factors and lowers coronary heart disease event rates in obese individuals (Eilat-Adar, et al., 2005; Klein, et al., 2004).

Caloric restriction also improves health in non-obese individuals. For example, the comparison of cardiac performance in middle-aged individuals practicing caloric restriction for 6.5 (± 4.6) years to individuals consuming Western diets revealed that long-term CR improves diastolic function by lowering systemic blood pressure and decreasing systemic inflammation and myocardial fibrosis (Meyer, et al., 2006). Weight loss induced by one year of CR also improves glucose tolerance and insulin action in non-obese sedentary middle-aged men and women, thereby presumably lowering the risk of type 2 diabetes (Weiss, et al., 2006). Finally, CR without malnutrition (i.e., CR at 25% for 6 months) also improves mitochondrial function in young to middle-aged overweight adults as demonstrated by reduced DNA damage and increased expression of genes encoding proteins involved in mitochondrial function (Civitarese, et al., 2007).

A multi-site human randomized control study, called the CALERIE study, recently revealed beneficial effects of caloric restriction on biomarkers of aging and cardiovascular disease risk factors in humans (Heilbronn, et al., 2006). Heilbronn and colleagues examined the effects of 6 months of CR on biomarkers of aging and oxidative stress in overweight, non-obese individuals (Heilbronn, et al., 2006). Participants were randomized into one of the following four groups: weight maintenance diet, 25% CR diet, 12.5% CR diet plus 12.5% increase in energy expenditure by exercise, and a very low calorie diet (890 kcal/d until 15% weight reduction, followed by weight maintenance diet). The results revealed favorable effects of CR on two biomarkers of aging, as evidenced by decreased fasting insulin levels in all the intervention groups and reduced core body temperatures in the calorie restricted and calorie restricted plus exercise groups. Additionally, all intervention groups demonstrated significant reduction in oxidative DNA damage.

Also part of the CALERIE study, Fontana and colleagues conducted a 1-year controlled trial to determine the effects of a 20% CR diet or an exercise intervention (i.e., 20% increase in energy expenditure) on coronary heart disease risk factors in middle-aged lean and overweight men and women (Fontana, et al., 2007). The results showed that both interventions had beneficial effects on most major coronary heart disease risk factors, including body fat mass, plasma LDL cholesterol, total cholesterol/HDL ratio, C-reactive proteins and blood pressure (Fontana, et al., 2007; Lefevre, et al., 2009). Research with humans suggests that calorie restriction has multiple beneficial effects that may improve the aging process. However, longer-duration studies are needed to determine whether these favorable effects are sustained. Long-term controlled studies (15-20 years) investigating the effect of CR on aging may be impossible to conduct in humans; however, recent findings from trials involving primates suggest that long-term CR may have profound effects on human health and longevity. To further explore this possibility, the CALERIE research program has recently developed an intricate protocol designed to determine whether 2 years of sustained CR results in beneficial effects similar to those observed in animal studies (Rochon, et al., 2010). Specifically, the research team will examine the influence of a 25% reduction of ad libitum energy intake in nonobese, middle-aged men and women (21-50 years) for 2 years on markers of aging, cardiovascular risk markers, insulin sensitivity and secretion, immune function, neuroendocrine function, quality of life and cognitive function. Importantly, this study will provide data concerning the effects of CR beyond the initial weight loss phase; thereby exploring for the first time whether CR effects become stable or whether the early effects found in previous studies are transitory.

HEALTH CONDITIONS RELATED TO EXCESSIVE CALORIC INTAKE

Several of today's most prominent health problems are related to excessive caloric intake including obesity, type 2 diabetes and cardiovascular disease. In the sections below, we describe the role excessive caloric intake has in promoting the development of these chronic disease conditions and associated health consequences.

Obesity

Obesity is the second leading cause of preventable death in the United States (Stein & Colditz, 2004) and is associated with five of the ten leading causes of death including cardiovascular disease, type 2 diabetes and certain cancers (Jakicic, et al., 2001; Mokdad, et al., 2003; U.S. Department of Health and Human Services, 2000). The prevalence of obesity (defined as a Body Mass Index [BMI] of 30 kg/m^2 or greater) has increased dramatically in the United States and across the world in the past several decades (Ogden, et al., 2006; World Health Organization, 1998). According to the National Health and Nutrition Examination Survey [NHANES], about one-third of Americans are overweight (BMI between 25 and 29.9) and one-third are obese (BMI $\geq$ 30; Flegal, Carroll, Ogden, & Curtin, 2010). As previously noted, NHANES indicate that individuals eat about 300 calories more today than they did in the 1980s (Finkelstein, et al., 2005). In addition, there has been a dramatic increase in portion sizes and availability of high calorie items in the last several decades (Finkelstein, et al., 2005; Hill, Wyatt, & Melanson, 2000; Hill, et al., 2003).

Although excessive caloric intake may not be the sole cause of the obesity epidemic, numerous studies have demonstrated a strong causal link between excessive caloric intake and weight gain (Cohen, Sturm, Lara, Gilbert, & Gee, 2010; Rosenheck, 2008). For example, in an overfeeding experiment in which 23 men were provided a surplus of 353 MJ (843,123 calories) over 100 days, body weight increased in direct proportion to the increased caloric intake. In addition, the researchers noted that two-thirds of the excess calories were stored as fat (Tremblay, Despres, Theriault, Fournier, & Bouchard, 1992). Dallosso and James found similar results in their fat over-feeding study in which they increased the caloric intake of eight men by 50% for one week (Dallosso & James, 1984). During the overfeeding week, there was a significant increase in body weight from 69.42 kg to 70.64 with all participants gaining weight.

Type 2 Diabetes

Type 2 diabetes is a serious metabolic disorder characterized by high blood glucose levels in combination with insulin resistance and/or deficiency (Centers for Disease Control and Prevention, 2007). If left untreated, it can have a number of major medical consequences and ultimately result in death. In line with the increase in obesity rates, the prevalence of type 2 diabetes has dramatically increased over the past few decades. In children, adolescents and young adults, there has been a 33% increase in the incidence and prevalence of type 2 diabetes in the last ten years (Kaufman, 2002). In 2007 the prevalence of type 2 diabetes in adults in the United States was estimated to be over 21 million (National Institute of Diabetes and Digestive and Kidney Diseases, 2007). Current estimates suggest that the number of adults with diabetes will increase from 135 million in 1995 to 300 million in 2025 (King, Aubert, & Herman, 1998). This statistic is alarming, because approximately 90% of diabetes' cases are type 2 diabetes (National Institute of Diabetes and Digestive and Kidney Diseases, 2007).

Excessive caloric intake appears to be a strong contributor to the increasing prevalence of type 2 diabetes. For example, consumption of high calorie meals full of processed carbohydrates and saturated fats, which are staples in the Western diet, can lead to exaggerated elevations in blood glucose (Ceriello, et al., 2005; Lastra, Dhuper, Johnson, & Sowers, 2010; Poirier, et al., 2006). In a study by Ceriello and colleagues, the researchers had 20 participants with type 2 diabetes eat three different meals (a high fat meal, 75 g glucose alone, and a high-fat meal plus glucose; Ceriello, et al., 2005). The high-fat meal and glucose alone meal produced a decrease in endothelial function and an increase in nitrotyrosine, C-reactive protein, intercellular adhesion molecule-1 and interleukin-6 (Ceriello, et al., 2005). When the high fat and glucose meals were combined, the results were even more pronounced (Ceriello, et al., 2005). These findings suggest a mechanism through which excessive food consumption at meals may contribute to the development of hypertriglyceridemia and hyperglycemia and ultimately adversely affect endothelial function and systemic inflammation levels (Ceriello, et al., 2005).

In contrast, caloric restriction may significantly reduce an individual's risk for type 2 diabetes. For example, Kelley and colleagues examined the impact of CR on changes in insulin sensitivity and secretion in adults with type 2 diabetes and obesity after: (1) 7 days of a baseline maintenance diet,(2) 7 days of CR (800 kcal/day), (3) 2 months of a weight maintenance diet, and (4) 7 days of CR (800 kcal/day). Following the first seven days of CR, fasting plasma glucose was significantly decreased and insulin sensitivity and secretion were increased (Kelley, et al., 1993). Interestingly, only after participants lost approximately 12 kg did each variable improve further, suggesting that one week of caloric restriction mimics the results of two months of weight loss on the metabolic regulation system (Kelley, et al., 1993). Specifically, in these participants, the seven days of CR produced half of the overall improvement in insulin sensitivity and insulin secretion of that found after a 12 kg weight loss (Kelley, et al., 1993).

In another recent study, researchers examined the effect of a low-carbohydrate diet on blood glucose levels in obese individuals with type 2 diabetes (Boden, Sargrad, Homko, Mozzoli, & Stein, 2005). Participants maintained their usual diets for seven days and then consumed a low-carbohydrate diet (21 grams/day) with no fat or protein restrictions for 14 days (Boden, et al., 2005). While on the low-carbohydrate diet, participants' daily caloric intake decreased from 3111 to 2164, and they lost approximately 1.65 kg (Boden, et al., 2005). During this two-week study, participants' 24-hour glucose profiles improved, mean hemogloblin A_{1c} decreased from 7.3% to 6.8 % ($P < 0.01$), insulin sensitivity improved by

75%, mean plasma triglyceride levels decreased by 35% and mean cholesterol levels decreased by 10% (Boden, et al., 2005).

Cardiovascular Disease

Cardiovascular disease (CVD) is a major public health concern for men and women in the United States. Approximately 35% of women and 38% of men in the U.S. have some form of cardiovascular disease, which includes coronary heart disease, stroke, heart failure and related risk factors (Lloyd-Jones, et al., 2010). Furthermore, CVD is the number one cause of death in the United States, accounting for 37% of all deaths (Rosamond, et al., 2007). The American Heart Association has estimated that if all major forms of CVD were eliminated, the average life expectancy would increase by approximately seven years (Rosamond, et al., 2007).

Numerous studies have shown that excessive caloric intake increases a number of risk factors for cardiovascular disease (CVD), such as high blood cholesterol levels, diabetes, overweight and high blood pressure (Finkelstein & Strombotne, 2004; Frazao, 2009). For example, Jakulj and colleagues revealed that the consumption of a high caloric/fat meal compared to a low-fat meal resulted in greater systolic and diastolic blood pressure and total peripheral resistance following two standard laboratory stressors (Jakulj, et al., 2007). Furthermore, Straznicky and colleagues showed that a high fat diet (i.e., 41% of total calories as fat) compared to a low fat diet (i.e., 23% of total calories as fat) consumed for 2 weeks leads to exaggerated cardiovascular reactivity in healthy individuals, marked by increased blood pressure, cholesterol and heart rate (Straznicky, Louis, McGrade, & Howes, 1993). Similarly, Vogel et al. reported that a single meal high in saturated fat impairs flow-mediated vasoactivity of the brachial artery up to 50% for 4 hours post consumption (Vogel, Corretti, & Plotnick, 1997). Moreover, evidence suggests that insulin resistance exists not only in skeletal muscle, adipose tissue and liver, but also in cardiovascular tissues where it contributes to the development of CVD.

EFFECT OF POST-PRANDIAL METABOLIC STATES ON HEALTH

The hormonal changes following a meal can play a significant role in influencing hunger and satiety levels, as well as fat metabolism for a number of hours. Food consumption at each meal can have profound effects on post-prandial (post-meal) metabolic processes and either promotes fat deposition or fat oxidation. Excessive food intake at a single meal can lead to a number of unhealthy metabolic and hormonal changes that simultaneously promote fat deposition and appetite dysregulation. These changes generally last for 4 – 6 hours but may occur for even longer time periods following large meals (O'Keefe, Gheewala, & O'Keefe, 2008). Given that most individuals spend 18 to 20 hours per day in the post-prandial state, the effect postprandial states have on health and wellness has emerged as an important topic for study. In the sections below, we review the latest research findings on the effects that post-prandial states have on appetite (hunger and satiety levels), body weight regulation and fat metabolism.

Effect of Post-Prandial States on Appetite

Following a high calorie meal, a large amount of nutrients enters the bloodstream, which raises plasma glucose, triglycerides and other pro-inflammatory chemicals above basal (or resting) levels. The rise in plasma glucose and other nutrients then generates signals that are relayed to the brain (Friedman, 1998). The brain has the important function of sensing signals from the periphery and limiting meal size to allow for optimal circulation and storage of energy-rich nutrients (Woods & Ramsay, 2007). Unfortunately, in our current environment of energy-dense, highly palatable foods, it is easy to consume an excess of nutrients (calories) at meals before the natural satiety signals can prevent further intake.

It is ironic, but consuming large portions of food at one time does not appear to increase satiety and may actually increase hunger levels over time. Large meals lead to abnormally high increases in post-prandial glucose. In response to these elevations in glucose, the body secretes large amounts of insulin and other counter-regulatory hormones to lower blood glucose levels in an attempt to return to homeostasis (healthy metabolic state). At first, this process may work well but if it is repeated, a state of reactive hypoglycemia can occur which can stimulate hunger since food intake is elicited when blood glucose levels decline quickly (Langhans, 1996). When an individual repeatedly eats in response to low glucose levels, this can lead to excess caloric consumption and ultimately weight gain (Langhans, 1996). Thus, large meals may not only trigger the body to store body fat but can also dysregulate glucose homeostasis, setting up a viscous weight gain cycle. Moreover, the degree of post-prandial dysregulation appears to be closely related to caloric intake at subsequent meals (Arora & McFarlane, 2005).

In line with this, a number of studies indicate that participants do not compensate by eating less following consumption of large meals or snacks before meals. For example, participants who consumed progressively larger portion sizes of a snack food (i.e., potato chips) prior to a dinner meal consumed significantly more calories (143 kcal) in the largest portion condition compared to the smallest portion condition (i.e., Rolls, Roe, Kral, Meengs, & Wall, 2004). Another study found that consumption of preloads an hour and a half before testing did not influence the amount consumed in the following meal (Rolls, et al., 1991). A more recent study found that participants who consumed pre-meal snacks sweetened with sucrose that contained 203 more kcal than pre-meal snacks sweetened with either aspartame or stevia, did not eat fewer calories at subsequent lunch and dinner meals (Anton, et al., 2010). Findings such as these suggest that eating behavior and specifically food intake at meals is not strongly related to previous caloric intake, at least in the short-term.

Other recent studies suggest that individuals do not compensate for large portion sizes by eating less, even over extended time periods. For example, when given larger than normal portion sizes throughout the day, both normal and overweight individuals were found to consume substantially more calories everyday over an 11 day period (Rolls, Roe, & Meengs, 2007). Specifically, participants in this study increased their caloric intake by approximately 423 kcal each day during this 11 day period, resulting in calorie intakes that exceeded energy requirements. If this eating pattern were continued for long time periods, significant weight gain would occur.

Larger portion sizes at meals have also been shown to significantly influence appetite, as well as glucose and insulin concentrations (Barton, Beigg, Macdonald, & Allison, 2000; Cluskey & Dunton, 1999; Melanson, et al., 1998). For example, in a study involving healthy, normal-weight older women, circulating glucose and insulin were assessed over a 5 hour period after the consumption of the following test meals: 0 (fasting), 250 kcal (snack-size meal), 500 kcal (small meal), 1,000 kcal (large meal). Compared to fasting and the snack-size meal, the participants showed exaggerated responses, and a delayed return to pre-meal glucose and insulin concentrations following the larger meals (Melanson, et al., 1998). Thus, findings from studies conducted to date suggest two things: (1) Large portion sizes do not increase satiety levels as would be expected (Ello-Martin, Ledikwe, & Rolls, 2005), and (2) excessive intake of calories at meals can override normal appetite regulating mechanisms.

Effect of Post-Prandial States on Body Weight

Emerging research suggests that weight gain or loss occurs on a *per meal basis*, as opposed to a total calorie (per day) basis (Berg, et al., 2009; Furnes, Tommeras, Arum, Zhao, & Chen, 2008; Furnes, Zhao, & Chen, 2009). Within this new paradigm, the physiological changes that occur following each meal appear to play a critical role in weight management. In support of this new paradigm, the two dietary factors that have been associated with the sharp rise in obesity observed over the past few decades include (1) higher energy intakes at meals due to larger portion sizes and (2) increased consumption of energy-dense foods (Hill & Peters, 1998; Poston & Foreyt, 1999).

Recent studies further demonstrate the importance of food intake at each meal in contributing to weight gain or loss. For example, a high fat diet was found to produce weight gain and lead to obesity only among animals whose eating behavior was characterized by larger but less frequent meals (Furnes, et al., 2009). Importantly, body weight gain was not associated with either total caloric intake or energy expenditure but was directly related to caloric intake at meals. In a previous study, the same research team performed gastric bypass surgery on a set of animals and found that although these animals lost large amounts of weight, their total calorie intake did not change. Rather, the animals who received gastric bypass surgery were observed to eat more frequent meals during the daytime and to consume smaller meals during the nighttime compared with age-matched controls (Furnes, et al., 2008). In an even more recent study, animals that received Roux-en-Y gastric bypass surgery were found to significantly reduce the portion size of each meal and not eat at a high enough frequency to compensate for the reduced caloric intake at meals (Zheng, et al., 2009). Thus, smaller, more frequent meals appeared to increase satiety and decrease hunger levels despite the animals reducing their total caloric intake (Zheng, et al., 2009).

Emerging research suggests consumption of smaller portion sizes at meals also assists with weight management in humans. For example, a recently published study involving 3,610 Swedish men and women found that obesity was not associated with total caloric intake but was significantly related to larger self-reported portion sizes of main meals, as well as eating meals in the later part of the day (Berg, et al., 2009). Although this study was cross-sectional in nature, the findings suggest that the portion size and timing of each meal may be critical variables that influence body weight gain or loss. Additionally, observations of obese individuals who receive bariatric surgery indicate that the decrease in food intake following surgery is due to significantly reduced meal size that isn't compensated by increased meal frequency (Sugerman, et al., 1992). Noteworthy, the patients in this study lost 60% of their excess weight at 5 years and over half of their excess weight at 8 and 9 years on average.

Because gastric bypass surgery is currently the *only* effective treatment for producing long-term weight loss, it can provide a model of the type of eating behavior patterns needed to achieve and sustain weight loss.

Collectively, studies suggest that the metabolic and hormonal changes that occur following each meal can promote weight gain or loss. Said more poignantly, excessive food ingestion during short time periods appears to be damaging to the body because it leads to an unhealthy metabolic shift that promotes body fat/weight gain. Thus, food intake at each meal can directly affect the body's metabolic state, which can play a critical role in body weight regulation.

Role of Post-Prandial Metabolic States on Fat Metabolism

For many individuals, the amount of food eaten at meals exceeds the amount of calories the body needs for energy (Woods, 2009). Excess caloric and carbohydrate consumption at meals leads to elevations in postprandial plasma glucose levels, and these elevations can directly stimulate fat accumulation through a number of mechanisms. First, high glucose levels can promote fat accumulation by being glycolytically converted to acetyl-CoA, a necessary precursor in the creation of fatty acids. Second, elevated post-prandial glucose concentrations may increase lipogenesis (i.e., process by which acetyl-CoA is converted to fat) by stimulating the release of insulin and inhibiting the release of glucagon from the pancreas (Henquin, 2000; Randle, Garland, Hales, & Newsholme, 1963). Insulin and glucagon exert opposing effects on acetyl-CoA caroxylase (ACC), the enzyme responsible for producing malonyl-CoA from acetyl-CoA in fatty acid biosynthesis (Ruderman, Saha, Vavvas, & Witters, 1999; Winder & Hardie, 1999). Insulin activates ACC by promoting its dephosphorylation, whereas glucagon deactivates ACC by promoting ACC phosphorylation. Thus, elevated levels of insulin in combination with decreased levels of glucagon ultimately lead to an overall increase in malonyl-CoA, a substrate required for lipogenesis. Additionally, intracellular malonyl-CoA directly inhibits mitochondrial carnitine palmitoyltransferase 1 (CPT-1), the enzyme which transports long-chain fatty acids across the mitochondrial membrane (McGarry, 2002; McGarry & Brown, 1997). Hence, elevated glucose concentrations stimulate fatty acid synthesis, while simultaneously inhibiting fat oxidation.

Elevated glucose levels can also induce the expression of lipogenic genes, and thereby increase rates of fatty acid synthesis and accumulation. For example, one long-term animal model study examined substrate utilization over 6 hours post-prandially during a 32-week dietary intervention (Brand-Miller, Holt, Pawlak, & McMillan, 2002). One group of rats was fed a high carbohydrate diet based on foods that promote a high glycemic response (high GI) and another group was fed a diet including carbohydrates that promote a low glycemic response (low GI). Across the 32-week intervention, the high GI group demonstrated a marked reduction in whole body fat oxidation and significant weight gain. Moreover, the high GI group exhibited increased expression of lipogenic enzymes such as ACC mRNA, and a decrease in the expression of enzymes involved in fat oxidation, such as CPT-1. Thus, a chronic high GI diet not only decreases fat oxidation acutely, but can also lead to changes in lipogenic enzyme expression which reduce the potential for fat oxidation.

As one of the functions of insulin secretion is to suppress the release of free fatty acids from adipose tissue and thereby inhibit fat oxidation (i.e., fat burning), the release of insulin in response to high glucose levels would promote fat accumulation and storage. When insulin and glucose levels are high, glucose, rather than fatty acids, is utilized as a fuel source in skeletal muscle. Conversely, when plasma glucose and insulin concentrations are low (typically 3-4 hours after a meal), fatty acids naturally become the major fuel for skeletal muscle (Frayn, 2003). Thus, fat oxidation is increased when glucose and insulin levels are low and decreased when glucose and insulin levels are elevated, which occurs following excess food consumption at meals. As noted above, exaggerated post-prandial glucose and lipid levels can trigger a biochemical cascade that leads to elevated insulin secretion, excessive sympathetic activity and impaired fatty acid oxidation. Because unhealthy metabolic states can increase hunger levels (Arora & McFarlane, 2005), this can elevate risk of these unhealthy post-prandial physiological states being repeated multiple times each day.

TREATMENT APPROACHES THAT FACILITATE APPETITE CONTROL

In the section below, we discuss emerging strategies individuals can utilize to achieve a state of "Post-Prandial Wellness," which occurs when the post-absorptive processes produce satiety and enhance metabolic and hormonal signals that encourage the body to increase fat oxidation (i.e., use body fat for energy). Therapies that change the pre and post-prandial states of overweight individuals to be similar to that of normal weight individuals should be effective in improving appetite and food intake regulation, which would ultimately result in sustained weight loss. We also discuss general approaches to facilitate healthy caloric intake, as well as program components that may facilitate long-term behavior change and subsequently sustain weight loss.

Dietary Strategies to Promote Post-Prandial Wellness and Healthy Caloric Intake

There are a number of dietary strategies that can increase satiety levels and promote healthy caloric intake including a low fat diet, foods high in water content, and consumption of lean sources of protein . In a review of the literature, Rolls and Bell (Rolls & Bell, 2000) noted that a diet low in energy density, such as the Mediterranean and Okinawan diets, can lead to a reduced caloric intake while still satisfying hunger and meeting nutritional needs. These types of diets, which usually include foods high in water content, complex carbohydrates, lean protein, and antioxidants, have been found to have a number of health benefits and may also produce a state of postprandial wellness (Lichtenstein, et al., 2006). In one randomized-controlled study, participants were placed on a low-fat diet, a Mediterranean diet and given one liter of virgin oil per week, or a Mediterranean diet and given 30 grams per day of nuts (Fito, et al., 2007). After the 3-month intervention, LDL levels significantly decreased among participants assigned to the Mediterranean Diet plus virgin oil dietary condition (−10.6 U/L [−14.2 to −6.1]) and Mediterranean Diet plus nuts dietary condition (−7.3 U/L [−11.2 to −3.3]), but not in the low-fat diet condition (Fito, et al., 2007). In addition, participants in the two Mediterranean diets experienced a clinically significant reduction in systolic blood pressure and fasting glucose (Fito, et al., 2007). Some researchers have speculated that these diets with a focus on fresh, unprocessed foods are ideal for our bodies, because they resemble the diets humans had as hunter-gatherers and are still genetically adapted for them (O'Keefe Jr. & Cordain, 2004).

One reason that the Mediterranean and Okinawan diets may promote post-prandial wellness is that they incorporate carbohydrates with large quantities of water including fruits and vegetables, while limiting dry, energy dense carbohydrates, such as crackers and pretzels. These water-filled food items can increase satiety by increasing food volume (Rolls & Bell, 2000). For example, in a study by Rolls and colleagues (Rolls, et al., 1998), normal-weight men were given milk of the same energy content but of different volumes. The authors found a positive relationship between the volume of the drinks and the participant's ratings of hunger and fullness (Rolls, et al., 1998). These types of diets also encourage consuming carbohydrates which are high in fiber and have a low glycemic index in order to increase satiety. This is due to "ideal" carbohydrates causing a lower increase in post-prandial glucose and triglyceride levels than "less ideal" carbohydrates such as many processed foods (Jenkins, et al., 2008). In addition to maintaining glucose levels, dietary fiber and ideal carbohydrates aid at slowing digestion, which can facilitate feelings of fullness (Rolls & Bell, 2000). This low glycemic index also lowers the risk for cardiovascular disease and type 2 diabetes (Lichtenstein, et al., 2006). For example, in a 9-year study by Beulens and colleagues (Beulens, et al., 2007) the researchers examined the rates of cardiovascular disease in a prospective cohort of Dutch women. The authors found that women who consumed a diet with a high glycemic index, especially those who were overweight, were at an increased risk for cardiovascular disease (Beulens, et al., 2007).

Another component of these diets is lean protein, which can curb excessive caloric intake and improve nutrition. Lean protein can reduce post-prandial glucose levels and increase satiety due to the protein's impact on gastrointestinal satiety signals and levels of circulating metabolites and hormones, including amino acids, glucose and insulin (O'Keefe, et al., 2008; Uhe, Collier, & O'Dea, 1992). In addition, one study found that protein increases the basal metabolic rate due to its thermogenic effect and thereby expends additional calories (Arora & McFarlane, 2005). In another study (Nilsson, Holst, & Bjorck, 2007), participants who consumed a drink with whey protein versus a reference drink experienced a lower post-prandial blood glucose area under the curve (56% reduction) and an increase in insulin secretion (60% increase). A combination of ideal carbohydrates, specifically soluble fiber with protein, can improve healthy eating while consuming a low energy diet because this combination allows an individual to feel satiated (Rolls & Bell, 2000).

Based on research findings described above, low energy density diets appear to be an effective dietary approach for decreasing caloric intake, while still satisfying hunger and meeting nutritional needs (Rolls & Bell, 2000). There are a number of behavioral strategies that individuals can use to facilitate adherence to a low energy diet including: (1) increasing consumption of foods with high fiber and water content including fruits, vegetables and soups, (2) limiting more energy-dense dry foods, such as crackers and pretzels, (3) selecting lean protein and low-fat dairy products, and (4) reading labels carefully in order to choose foods with fewer calories (Rolls & Bell, 2000).

Behavior Strategies to Facilitate Calorie Control

There are also a number of empirically supported behavior skills that can be utilized to facilitate adherence to a low calorie diet. Some of the key skills include goal setting, self-monitoring, stimulus control and problem solving. Below we briefly describe each of these skills and how they can be utilized to encourage adherence to CR.

Goal setting can help facilitate adherence to a CR regimen because it can provide individuals with specific achievable targets related to behavior change. For example, individuals are encouraged to create goals that are related to changing specific behaviors such as substituting diet soda for regular soda and eating celery and carrots in lieu of cookies for a snack (Van Dorsten & Lindley, 2008). Self-monitoring, or the recording of a specific behavior or data points such as daily caloric intake, is another key behavioral change tool that has been associated with improved adherence to CR regimens in numerous studies (Van Dorsten & Lindley, 2008). Stimulus control, which consists of modifying one's environment in order to decrease or increase a behavior, is a strategy or behavior skill individuals can use to create an environment that encourages healthy behaviors (Van Dorsten & Lindley, 2008). For example, an individual can modify his/her environment to discourage unhealthy eating behaviors (i.e., remove all candy from the house) and to encourage healthy eating behaviors (i.e., have fruits and vegetables readily accessible). Problem solving is another empirically supported behavioral change skill that individuals can use to overcome barriers they may encounter during the behavior change process. A five-stage problem solving model was designed by Perri and colleagues and includes: (1) orienting to the problem, (2) defining the problem, (3) generating possible solutions, (4) evaluating and choosing a solution, and (5) implementing and evaluating the solution (Perri, et al., 2001). These tools can help an individual maintain caloric restriction. Please see *Handbook of Obesity Treatment* edited by Thomas Wadden and Albert Stunkard for additional information on behavioral strategies individuals can utilize to sustain CR.

Emerging Role of Botanical Compounds

Botanicals represent important sources of potential new adjunctive therapies for obese and insulin resistant individuals and may enhance the effects of weight loss interventions by reducing hunger. Although there are a number of potential botanical compounds that may assist with appetite regulation, below we briefly review five compounds that appear to be highly promising based on recent research findings. These botanical compounds include Garcina Cambogia, Glucomannan, Propol Mannan, Pinolenic acid, and Stevia.

Garcina Cambogia, whose primary organic acid is (–)-Hydroxycitric acid (HCA), has been used for years to make food more filling (Mattes & Bormann, 2000). HCA has been found to reduce food intake in animals, and there is new data in human trials which suggests that this botanical can be used to supplement weight loss (Heymsfield, et al., 1998; Mattes & Bormann, 2000; Preuss, et al., 2004). In recent studies, HCA was found to significantly reduce food intake by approximately 15% from baseline levels (Preuss, et al., 2004; Westerterp-Plantenga & Kovacs, 2002). HCA may induce satiety by inhibiting malonylCoA formation (Watson, Fang, & Lowenstein, 1969), which would lead to increased carnitine transferase activity and result in decreased fat synthesis and increased fat oxidation (McCarty,

1994; Sullivan, Hamilton, Miller, & Wheatley, 1972). Consistent with this, HCA has been found to inhibit lipid droplet accumulation in fat cells (Kim, Kim, Kwon, & Park, 2004) and also induce leptin expression (Roy, et al., 2007).

Glucomannan is a water-soluble, fermentable dietary fiber, which may be more effective than other soluble fibers in promoting satiety due to its high viscosity. Glucomannan consists of a polysaccharide chain of beta-D glucose and beta-D mannose with attached acetyl groups in a molar ration of 1:1.6 with beta – 1, 4 linkages (Tye, 1991). Glucomannan holds significant promise for assisting with weight loss (Doi, 1995; Hopman, Houben, Speth, & Lamers, 1988). Based on a recent meta-analysis of 14 randomized controlled trials (mean study duration = 5.2 weeks), glucomannan was found to produce a small, but statistically significant reduction in weight (0.79 kg; Sood, Baker, & Coleman, 2008). Proposed mechanisms through which glucomannan may increase satiety include delayed gastric emptying (Burton-Freeman, 2000; Howarth, Saltzman, & Roberts, 2001), slowed food absorption in the small intestine producing smaller postprandial insulin surges (Vuksan, et al., 2001), accelerated delivery of food to the terminal ileum (McCarty, 2002) and increased levels of plasma cholecystokinin (Bourdon, et al., 1999).

Propol Mannan is a selected species among the Konjac Plant Family and is the most purified form of glucomannan. This fiber is unique in that it maintains its viscous structure throughout the digestive tract. By maintaining its viscous properties, Propol Mannan appears to be particularly effective in regulating or reducing appetite and may also assist with weight loss. In support of this, a number of recent studies have reported significant weight loss following use of Propol Mannan. For example, in one recent placebo-controlled study, participants taking 1 gram of Propol Mannan before meals lost an average of 5.5 pounds after eight weeks, whereas the body weight of participants in the placebo group did not change (Walsh, Yaghoubian, & Behforooz, 1984). In another recent study, participants who consumed Propol Mannan before meals lost 7.92 pounds, whereas weight did not change among participants in the placebo group (Biancardi, Palmiero, & Ghirardi, 1989). In both of these studies, participants also had significant reductions in blood lipid and glucose levels. Importantly, participants were not instructed to modify their diet in either of these studies.

Pinolenic acid, a triple-unsaturated fatty acid, is found exclusively in pine nut oil (genus Pinus). In a recent randomized, double-blind, placebo controlled trial, participants who received pinolenic acid rated their "desire to eat" 29% lower and their "prospective food consumption" 36% lower than participants in the placebo condition (Causey, 2006). Postprandial levels of CCK and GLP-1 were also significantly higher (60% and 25%, respectively) in participants receiving pinolenic acid versus placebo. In a recent study, Pasman and colleagues evaluated whether Korean pine nut free fatty acids (FFA) and triglycerides (TG) worked as an appetite suppressant (Pasman, et al., 2008). In this randomized, placebo-controlled, double-blind, cross-over trial, the authors found that the gut hormones cholecystokinin (CCK-8) and glucagon like peptide-I (GLP-I) were significantly higher in individuals who consumed the pine nut oil versus placebo (Pasman, et al., 2008). Specifically, over a four hour period, the total amount of plasma CCK-8 was 60% higher with the pine nut FFA and 22% higher with the pine nut TG than with placebo. In addition, GLP-I levels were 25% higher with pine nut FFA than with placebo.

Stevia, the common name for the extract stevioside from the leaves of *Stevia rebaudiana* Bertoni, is a natural, sweet-tasting, calorie-free botanical that may also be used as a sugar substitute or as an alternative to artificial sweeteners. Stevia has been found to increase insulin sensitivity in rodent models (Chang, Wu, Liu, & Cheng, 2005) and to have beneficial effects on blood glucose and insulin levels in humans (Curi, et al., 1986; Gregersen, Jeppesen, Holst, & Hermansen, 2004), which suggests it may have a role in food intake regulation. A recent study directly tested the effects of stevia, aspartame and sucrose on food intake, satiety and postprandial glucose and insulin levels. In this crossover study participants did not compensate by eating more at either their lunch or dinner meal when they consumed lower calorie preloads containing stevia or aspartame compared to when they consumed higher calorie preloads containing sucrose (Anton et al, 2010). In other words, even after a lower calorie preload, food intake at subsequent lunch and dinner meals was not increased and discretionary food intake did not differ between the conditions. In addition, stevia preloads reduced postprandial blood glucose and insulin levels compared to aspartame and sucrose preloads, which suggests stevia may assist with glucose regulation(Anton, et al., 2010).

RESEARCH IMPLICATIONS

There is now strong evidence that calorie control with adequate nutrition can protect individuals against obesity, CVD and Type 2 diabetes, which are leading causes of mortality and morbidity in the United States. Emerging literature also suggests that CRin humans results in the same metabolic and functional adaptations associated with extended longevity in calorie-restricted rodents and nonhuman primates. More research is needed, however, to demonstrate the efficacy of caloric control or restriction in promoting healthy aging and disease prevention among individuals at risk for obesity, type 2 diabetes and/or CVD.

While the benefits of CR have been demonstrated in overweight and obese individuals, most overweight individuals are unable to sustain the reduction in calorie intake needed for weight loss and weight loss maintenance. In addition to internal feedback mechanisms that signal the body to increase food intake and decrease energy expenditure in response to the weight reduced state, our current environment makes it extremely challenging to sustain a reduced calorie diet. Therefore, future research should focus on understanding the molecular, behavioral, psychological and environmental mechanisms underlying eating behavior, as well as their interactions. A greater understanding of these dynamic processes could facilitate the development of new interdisciplinary approaches designed to assist overweight individuals in adhering to a CR regimen over the long-term.

Promising future research directions in appetite control include the continued rigorous testing of behavioral change strategies that facilitate long-term change in dietary intake, the search for new pharmacological targets in the brain for appetite and weight control and the study of botanical compounds that may promote satiety. Additionally, a greater understanding of the exact molecular mechanisms that control feeding behavior could lead to the development of more effective pharmacological treatments. For example, studies have recently identified the AMPK cascade as having a critical role in appetite regulation; thus making it a promising new pharmacological target for the treatment of obesity. Finally, alternative therapeutic strategies, such as botanicals, represent a potential source of new adjunctive treatments for obesity.

CLINICAL IMPLICATIONS

There is accumulating evidence that specific types of low calorie diets in combination with behavioral strategies may encourage long-term calorie control. Unfortunately, there is also a large body of literature to indicate that maintaining this caloric restriction is extremely difficult. Research indicates that individuals who restrict their calories and lose weight within a behavioral weight management program typically regain two-thirds of the weight back within one year and almost all of the weight back in five years (Stern & Thomas, 1995; Wadden, Sternberg, Letizia, Stunkard, & Foster, 1989). A clinician looking to help a patient restrict his or her calories in a healthy and safe way can utilize many of the tools described in this chapter. Based on research findings over the past few decades, the following behavioral and dietary strategies can be used to promote calorie control:

- Low energy density diets that meet hunger and nutritional needs
- Small meals consumed consistently throughout the day
- Specific and achievable behavior change goals
- Self-monitoring logs to track progress
- Eating triggers should be identified and then modified to facilitate calorie control

Finally, if a clinician is looking for additional routes to help a patient with CR, there have been some exciting new developments in botanical research that suggests some compounds may assist with appetite regulation. Specifically, botanicals may represent a safe and helpful tool to aid in appetite control when individuals are restricting their caloric intake.

CONCLUSIONS AND FUTURE DIRECTIONS

Several of today's most prominent health problems are directly related to excessive caloric intake including obesity, type 2diabetes and cardiovascular disease. More specifically, obesity is the second leading cause of preventable death in the United States, and is associated with a number of chronic health conditions including cardiovascular disease, type 2 diabetes and certain cancer. The increasing prevalence and incidence of obesity and its associated negative health impact has increased the need for effective treatments. Overweight and obese individuals receive numerous health benefits following weight loss achieved through CR. Long-term weight loss, however, has proven to be very difficult for most individuals to achieve, possibly due to internal feedback systems that signal the body to increase food intake and decrease energy expenditure in response to reductions in caloric intake. An increased understanding of the biological changes associated with caloric restriction and exercise may reveal how natural compounds and/or pharmacotherapy can potentiate the effects of behavioral interventions.

Novel treatment approaches are urgently needed to assist overweight individuals in adhering to reduced calorie diets over the long-term. Botanicals represent an important and underexplored source of potential new therapies that may facilitate CR. Similar to pharmaceutical agents, these compounds would likely be most effectively used as adjunctive treatments in conjunction with hypocaloric diets and behavioral self management programs.

Given the increasing popularity of these products among overweight and obese individuals, studies are needed to examine their safety and efficacy.

REFERENCES

Anton, S. D., Martin, C. K., Han, H., Coulon, S., Cefalu, W. T., Geiselman, P., et al. (2010). Effects of stevia, aspartame, and sucrose on food intake, satiety, and postprandial glucose and insulin levels. *Appetite, 55*(1), 37-43.

Arora, S. K., & McFarlane, S. I. (2005). The case for low carbohydrate diets in diabetes management. *Nutrition & Metabolism, 2*, 16.

Barton, A. D., Beigg, C. L., Macdonald, I. A., & Allison, S. P. (2000). A recipe for improving food intakes in elderly hospitalized patients. *Clinical Nutrition, 19*(6), 451-454.

Berg, C., Lappas, G., Wolk, A., Strandhagen, E., Toren, K., Rosengren, A., et al. (2009). Eating patterns and portion size associated with obesity in a Swedish population. *Appetite, 52*(1), 21-26.

Beulens, J. W. J., de Bruijne, L. M., Stolk, R. P., Peeters, P. H. M., Bots, M. L., Grobbee, D. E., et al. (2007). High dietary glycemic load and glycemic index increase risk of cardiovascular disease among middle-aged women: A population-based follow-up study. *Journal of the American College of Cardiology, 50*(1), 14-21.

Biancardi, G., Palmiero, L., & Ghirardi, P. E. (1989). *Glucomannan in the treatment of overweight patients with osteoarthrosis* (Vol. 46). Belle Mead, NJ, ETATS-UNIS: Excerpta medica.

Boden, G., Sargrad, K., Homko, C., Mozzoli, M., & Stein, T. P. (2005). Effect of a low-carbohydrate diet on appetite, blood glucose levels, and insulin resistance in obese patients with type 2 diabetes. *Annals of Internal Medicine, 142*(6), 403-411.

Bodkin, N. L., Alexander, T. M., Ortmeyer, H. K., Johnson, E., & Hansen, B. C. (2003). Mortality and morbidity in laboratory-maintained rhesus monkeys and effects of long-term dietary restriction. *Journal of Gerontology, 58*(3), 212-219.

Bourdon, I., Yokoyama, W., Davis, P., Hudson, C., Backus, R., Richter, D., et al. (1999). Postprandial lipid, glucose, insulin, and cholecystokinin responses in men fed barley pasta enriched with beta-glucan. *American Journal of Clinical Nutrition, 69*(1), 55-63.

Brand-Miller, J. C., Holt, S. H., Pawlak, D. B., & McMillan, J. (2002). Glycemic index and obesity. *American Journal of Clinical Nutrition, 76*(1), 281S-285.

Burton-Freeman, B. (2000). Dietary fiber and energy regulation. *Journal of Nutrition, 130*(2S Suppl), 272S-275S.

Causey, J. L. (2006). *Korean pine nut fatty acids induce satiety- producing hormone release in overweight human volunteers*. Paper presented at the American Chemical Society National Meeting and Exposition.

Centers for Disease Control and Prevention (2007). Leading causes of death Retrieved October 19, 2010, 2010

Ceriello, A., Assaloni, R., Da Ros, R., Maier, A., Piconi, L., Quagliaro, L., et al. (2005). Effect of atorvastatin and irbesartan, alone and in combination, on postprandial endothelial dysfunction, oxidative stress, and inflammation in type 2 diabetic patients. *Circulation, 111*(19), 2518-2524.

Chang, J. C., Wu, M. C., Liu, I. M., & Cheng, J. T. (2005). Increase of insulin sensitivity by stevioside in fructose-rich chow-fed rats. *Hormone and Metabolic Research, 37*, 610-616.

Civitarese, A. E., Carling, S., Heilbronn, L. K., Hulver, M. H., Ukropcova, B., Deutsch, W. A., et al. (2007). Calorie restriction increases muscle mitochondrial biogenesis in healthy humans. *PLoS Medicine, 4*(3), e76.

Cluskey, M., & Dunton, N. (1999). Serving meals of reduced portion size did not improve appetite among elderly in a personal-care section of a long-term-care community. *Journal of the American Dietetic Association, 99*(6), 733-735.

Cohen, D. A., Sturm, R., Lara, M., Gilbert, M., & Gee, S. (2010). Discretionary calorie intake a priority for obesity prevention: Results of rapid participatory approaches in low-income US communities. *Journal of Public Health, 32*(3), 379-386.

Colman, R. J., Anderson, R. M., Johnson, S. C., Kastman, E. K., Kosmatka, K. J., Beasley, T. M., et al. (2009). Caloric restriction delays disease onset and mortality in rhesus monkeys. *Science, 325*(5937), 201-204.

Colman, R. J., Beasley, T. M., Allison, D. B., & Weindruch, R. (2008). Attenuation of sarcopenia by dietary restriction in rhesus monkeys. *The Journals of Gerontology Series A: Biological Sciences and Medical Sciences, 63*(6), 556-559.

Curi, R., Alvarez, M., Bazotte, R. B., Botion, L. M., Godoy, J. L., & Bracht, A. (1986). Effect of Stevia rebaudiana on glucose tolerance in normal adult humans. *Brazilian Journal of Medical and Biological Research, 19*, 771-774.

Dallosso, H. M., & James, W. P. T. (1984). Whole-body calorimetry studies in adult men. *British Journal of Nutrition, 52*(01), 49-64.

Das, M., Gabriely, I., & Barzilai, N. (2004). Caloric restriction, body fat and ageing in experimental models. *Obesity Reviews, 5*(1), 13-19.

Doi, K. (1995). Effect of konjac fibre (glucomannan) on glucose and lipids. *European Journal of Clinical Nutrition, 49 Suppl 3*, S190-197.

Eilat-Adar, S., Eldar, M., & Goldbourt, U. (2005). Association of intentional changes in body weight with coronary heart disease event rates in overweight subjects who have an additional coronary risk factor. *American Journal of Epidemiology, 161*(4), 352-358.

Ello-Martin, J. A., Ledikwe, J. H., & Rolls, B. J. (2005). The influence of food portion size and energy density on energy intake: Implications for weight management. *American Journal of Clinical Nutrition, 82*(1 Suppl), 236S-241S.

Finkelstein, E. A., Ruhm, C. J., & Kosa, K. M. (2005). Economic causes and consequences of obesity. *Annual Review of Public Health, 26*, 239-257.

Finkelstein, E. A., & Strombotne, K. L. (2004). The economics of obesity. *American Journal of Clinical Nutrition, 91*(5), 1520S-1524.

Fito, M., Guxens, M., Corella, D., Saez, G., Estruch, R., de la Torre, R., et al. (2007). Effect of a traditional Mediterranean diet on lipoprotein oxidation: A randomized controlled trial. *Archives of Internal Medicine, 167*(11), 1195-1203.

Flegal, K. M., Carroll, M. D., Ogden, C. L., & Curtin, L. R. (2010). Prevalence and trends in obesity among US adults, 1999-2008. *JAMA, 303*(3), 235-241.

Fontana, L., Villareal, D. T., Weiss, E., Racette, S. B., Steger-May, K., Klein, S., et al. (2007). Calorie restriction or exercise: Effects on coronary heart disease risk factors: A randomized, controlled trial. *American Journal of Physiology: Endocrinology and Metabolism, 293*(1), E197-202.

Frayn, K. N. (2003). The glucose-fatty acid cycle: A physiological perspective. *Biochemical Society Transactions, 31*(Pt 6), 1115-1119.

Frazao, E. (2009). Less-energy-dense diets of low-income women in California are associated with higher energy-adjusted costs but not with higher daily diet costs. *The American Journal of Clinical Nutrition, 90*(3), 701-.

Friedman, M. I. (1998). Fuel partitioning and food intake. *American Journal of Clinical Nutrition, 67*(3 Suppl), 513S-518S.

Furnes, M. W., Tommeras, K., Arum, C. J., Zhao, C. M., & Chen, D. (2008). Gastric bypass surgery causes body weight loss without reducing food intake in rats. *Obesity Surgery, 18*(4), 415-422.

Furnes, M. W., Zhao, C. M., & Chen, D. (2009). Development of obesity is associated with increased calories per meal rather than per day. A study of high-fat diet-induced obesity in young rats. *Obesity Surgery, 19*(10), 1430-1438.

Goldstein, D. J. (1992). Beneficial health effects of modest weight loss. *International Journal of Obesity, 16*(6), 397-415.

Gregersen, S., Jeppesen, P. B., Holst, J. J., & Hermansen, K. (2004). Antihyperglycemic effects of stevioside in type 2 diabetic subjects. *Metabolism, 53*, 73-76.

Gresl, T. A., Colman, R. J., Roecker, E. B., Havighurst, T. C., Huang, Z., Allison, D. B., et al. (2001). Dietary restriction and glucose regulation in aging rhesus monkeys: A follow-up report at 8.5 yr. *American Journal of Physiology: Endocrinology and Metabolism, 281*(4), E757-765.

Hammer, S., Snel, M., Lamb, H. J., Jazet, I. M., van der Meer, R. W., Pijl, H., et al. (2008). Prolonged caloric restriction in obese patients with type 2 diabetes mellitus decreases myocardial triglyceride content and improves myocardial function. *Journal of the American College of Cardiology, 52*(12), 1006-1012.

Heilbronn, L. K., de Jonge, L., Frisard, M. I., DeLany, J. P., Larson-Meyer, D. E., Rood, J., et al. (2006). Effect of 6-month calorie restriction on biomarkers of longevity, metabolic adaptation, and oxidative stress in overweight individuals: A randomized controlled trial. *JAMA, 295*(13), 1539-1548.

Heilbronn, L. K., de Jonge, L., Frisard, M. I., DeLany, J. P., Larson-Meyer, D. E., Rood, J., et al. (2006). Effect of 6-month calorie restriction on biomarkers of longevity, metabolic adaptation, and oxidative stress in overweight individuals: A randomized controlled trial. *JAMA, 295*(13), 1539-1548.

Henquin, J. C. (2000). Triggering and amplifying pathways of regulation of insulin secretion by glucose. *Diabetes, 49*(11), 1751-1760.

Heymsfield, S. B., Allison, D. B., Vasselli, J. R., Pietrobelli, A., Greenfield, D., & Nunez, C. (1998). Garcinia cambogia (hydroxycitric acid) as a potential antiobesity agent: A randomized controlled trial. *JAMA, 280*(18), 1596-1600.

Hill, J. O., & Peters, J. C. (1998). Environmental contributions to the obesity epidemic. *Science, 280*(5368), 1371-1374.

Hill, J. O., Wyatt, H. R., & Melanson, E. L. (2000). Genetic and environmental contributions to obesity. *Medical Clinics of North America, 84*(2), 333-346.

Hill, J. O., Wyatt, H. R., Reed, G. W., & Peters, J. C. (2003). Obesity and the environment: Where do we go from here? *Science, 299*(5608), 853-855.

Hopman, W. P., Houben, P. G., Speth, P. A., & Lamers, C. B. (1988). Glucomannan prevents postprandial hypoglycaemia in patients with previous gastric surgery. *Gut, 29*(7), 930-934.

Howarth, N. C., Saltzman, E., & Roberts, S. B. (2001). Dietary fiber and weight regulation. *Nutrition Reviews, 59*(5), 129-139.

Jakicic, J. M., Clark, K., Coleman, E., Donnelly, J. E., Foreyt, J., Melanson, E., et al. (2001). American College of Sports Medicine position stand: Appropriate intervention strategies for weight loss and prevention of weight regain for adults. *Medicine & Science in Sports & Exercise, 33*(12), 2145-2156.

Jakulj, F., Zernicke, K., Bacon, S. L., van Wielingen, L. E., Key, B. L., West, S. G., et al. (2007). A high-fat meal increases cardiovascular reactivity to psychological stress in healthy young adults. *Journal of Nutrition, 137*(4), 935-939.

Jenkins, D. J., Kendall, C. W., Faulkner, D. A., Kemp, T., Marchie, A., Nguyen, T. H., et al. (2008). Long-term effects of a plant-based dietary portfolio of cholesterol-lowering foods on blood pressure. *European Journal of Clinical Nutrition, 62*(6), 781-788.

Kastman, E. K., Willette, A. A., Coe, C. L., Bendlin, B. B., Kosmatka, K. J., McLaren, D. G., et al. (2010). A calorie-restricted diet decreases brain Iron accumulation and preserves motor performance in old rhesus monkeys. *The Journal of Neuroscience, 30*(23), 7940-7947.

Kaufman, F. R. (2002). Type 2 diabetes in children and young adults: A new epidemic. *Clinical Diabetes, 20*(4), 217-218.

Kayo, T., Allison, D. B., Weindruch, R., & Prolla, T. A. (2001). Influences of aging and caloric restriction on the transcriptional profile of skeletal muscle from rhesus monkeys. *Proceedings of the National Academy of Sciences, 98*(9), 5093-5098.

Kelley, D., Wing, R., Buonocore, C., Sturis, J., Polonsky, K., & Fitzsimmons, M. (1993). Relative effects of calorie restriction and weight loss in noninsulin- dependent diabetes mellitus. *Journal of Clinical Endocrinology & Metabolism, 77*(5), 1287-1293.

Kenchaiah, S., Evans, J. C., Levy, D., Wilson, P. W., Benjamin, E. J., Larson, M. G., et al. (2002). Obesity and the risk of heart failure. *New England Journal of Medicine, 347*(5), 305-313.

Key, T. J., Allen, N. E., Spencer, E. A., & Travis, R. C. (2002). The effect of diet on risk of cancer. *Lancet, 360*(9336), 861-868.

Kim, M. S., Kim, J. K., Kwon, D. Y., & Park, R. (2004). Anti-adipogenic effects of Garcinia extract on the lipid droplet accumulation and the expression of transcription factor. *Biofactors, 22*(1-4), 193-196.

King, H., Aubert, R. E., & Herman, W. H. (1998). Global burden of diabetes, 1995-2025: Prevalence, numerical estimates, and projections. *Diabetes Care, 21*(9), 1414-1431.

Klein, S., Burke, L. E., Bray, G. A., Blair, S., Allison, D. B., Pi-Sunyer, X., et al. (2004). Clinical implications of obesity with specific focus on cardiovascular disease: A statement for professionals from the American Heart Association Council on Nutrition, Physical Activity, and Metabolism: Endorsed by the American College of Cardiology Foundation. *Circulation, 110*(18), 2952-2967.

Kloting, N., & Bluher, M. (2005). Extended longevity and insulin signaling in adipose tissue. *Experimental Gerontology, 40*(11), 878-883.

Langhans, W. (1996). Metabolic and glucostatic control of feeding. *Proceedings of the Nutrition Society, 55*(1B), 497-515.

Lastra, G., Dhuper, S., Johnson, M. S., & Sowers, J. R. (2010). Salt, aldosterone, and insulin resistance: Impact on the cardiovascular system. *Nature Reviews Cardiology, 7*(10), 577-584.

Lee, C., Klopp, R. G., Weindruch, R., & Prolla, T. A. (1999). Gene expression profile of aging and its retardation by caloric restriction. *Science, 285*(5432), 1390-1393.

Lefevre, M., Redman, L. M., Heilbronn, L. K., Smith, J. V., Martin, C. K., Rood, J. C., et al. (2009). Caloric restriction alone and with exercise improves CVD risk in healthy non-obese individuals. *Atherosclerosis, 203*(1), 206-213.

Lichtenstein, A. H., Appel, L. J., Brands, M., Carnethon, M., Daniels, S., Franch, H. A., et al. (2006). Diet and lifestyle recommendations revision 2006: A scientific statement from the American Heart Association Nutrition Committee. *Circulation, 114*(1), 82-96.

Lloyd-Jones, D., Adams, R. J., Brown, T. M., Carnethon, M., Dai, S., De Simone, G., et al. (2010). Heart disease and stroke statistics--2010 update: A report from the American Heart Association. *Circulation, 121*(7), e46-215.

Mattes, R. D., & Bormann, L. (2000). Effects of (-)-hydroxycitric acid on appetitive variables. *Physiology & Behavior, 71*(1-2), 87-94.

McCarty, M. F. (1994). Promotion of hepatic lipid oxidation and gluconeogenesis as a strategy for appetite control. *Medical Hypotheses, 42*(4), 215-225.

McCarty, M. F. (2002). Glucomannan minimizes the postprandial insulin surge: A potential adjuvant for hepatothermic therapy. *Medical Hypotheses, 58*(6), 487-490.

McGarry, J. D. (2002). Banting lecture 2001. *Diabetes, 51*(1), 7-18.

McGarry, J. D., & Brown, N. F. (1997). The mitochondrial carnitine palmitoyltransferase system: From concept to molecular analysis. *European Journal of Biochemistry, 244*(1), 1-14.

Melanson, K. J., Greenberg, A. S., Ludwig, D. S., Saltzman, E., Dallal, G. E., & Roberts, S. B. (1998). Blood glucose and hormonal responses to small and large meals in healthy young and older women. *J Gerontol A Biol Sci Med Sci, 53*(4), B299-305.

Meyer, T. E., Kovács, S. J., Ehsani, A. A., Klein, S., Holloszy, J. O., & Fontana, L. (2006). Long-term caloric restriction ameliorates the decline in diastolic function in humans. *Journal of the American College of Cardiology, 47*(2), 398-402.

Mokdad, A. H., Ford, E. S., Bowman, B. A., Dietz, W. H., Vinicor, F., Bales, V. S., et al. (2003). Prevalence of obesity, diabetes, and obesity-related health risk factors, 2001. *Journal of the American Medical Association, 289*(1), 76-79.

National Institute of Diabetes and Digestive and Kidney Diseases (2007). National Diabetes Statistics Retrieved October 19, 2010, 2010

Nilsson, M., Holst, J. J., & Bjorck, I. M. E. (2007). Metabolic effects of amino acid mixtures and whey protein in healthy subjects: studies using glucose-equivalent drinks. *The American Journal of Clinical Nutrition, 85*(4), 996-1004.

O'Keefe, J. H., Gheewala, N. M., & O'Keefe, J. O. (2008). Dietary strategies for improving post-prandial glucose, lipids, inflammation, and cardiovascular health. *Journal of the American College of Cardiology, 51*(3), 249-255.

O'Keefe Jr., J. H., & Cordain, L. (2004). Cardiovascular disease resulting from a diet and lifestyle at odds with our Paleolithic genome: How to become a 21st-century hunter-gatherer. *Mayo Clinic Proceedings, 79*(1), 101-108.

Ogden, C. L., Carroll, M. D., Curtin, L. R., McDowell, M. A., Tabak, C. J., & Flegal, K. M. (2006). Prevalence of overweight and obesity in the United States, 1999-2004. *JAMA, 295*(13), 1549-1555.

Ogden, C. L., Yanovski, S. Z., Carroll, M. D., & Flegal, K. M. (2007). The Epidemiology of Obesity. *Gastroenterology, 132*(6), 2087-2102.

Pasman, W. J., Heimerikx, J., Rubingh, C. M., van den Berg, R., O'Shea, M., Gambelli, L., et al. (2008). The effect of Korean pine nut oil on in vitro CCK release, on appetite sensations and on gut hormones in post-menopausal overweight women. *Lipids in Health and Disease, 7*(10).

Perri, M. G., Nezu, A. M., McKelvey, W. F., Shermer, R. L., Renjilian, D. A., & Viegener, B. J. (2001). Relapse prevention training and problem-solving therapy in the long-term management of obesity. *Journal of Consulting and Clinical Psychology, 69*(4), 722-726.

Poirier, P., Giles, T. D., Bray, G. A., Hong, Y., Stern, J. S., Pi-Sunyer, F. X., et al. (2006). Obesity and cardiovascular disease: Pathophysiology, evaluation, and effect of weight loss: An update of the 1997 American Heart Association scientific statement on obesity and heart disease from the Obesity Committee of the Council on Nutrition, Physical Activity, and Metabolism. *Circulation, 113*(6), 898-918.

Poston, W. S., 2nd, & Foreyt, J. P. (1999). Obesity is an environmental issue. *Atherosclerosis, 146*(2), 201-209.

Preuss, H. G., Bagchi, D., Bagchi, M., Rao, C. V., Dey, D. K., & Satyanarayana, S. (2004). Effects of a natural extract of (-)-hydroxycitric acid (HCA-SX) and a combination of HCA-SX plus niacin-bound chromium and Gymnema sylvestre extract on weight loss. *Diabetes, Obesity and Metabolism, 6*(3), 171-180.

Racette, S. B., Weiss, E. P., Villareal, D. T., Arif, H., Steger-May, K., Schechtman, K. B., et al. (2006). One year of caloric restriction in humans: Feasibility and effects on body composition and abdominal adipose tissue. *The Journals of Gerontology Series A: Biological Sciences and Medical Sciences, 61*(9), 943-950.

Randle, P. J., Garland, P. B., Hales, C. N., & Newsholme, E. A. (1963). The glucose fatty-acid cycle: Its role in insulin sensitivity and the metabolic disturbances of diabetes mellitus. *Lancet, 1*(7285), 785-789.

Rochon, J., Bales, C. W., Ravussin, E., Redman, L. M., Holloszy, J. O., Racette, S. B., et al. (2010). Design and Conduct of the CALERIE Study: Comprehensive Assessment of the Long-term Effects of Reducing Intake of Energy. *The Journals of Gerontology Series A: Biological Sciences and Medical Sciences*.

Rolls, B. J., & Bell, E. A. (2000). Dietary approaches to the treatment of obesity. *Medical Clinics of North America, 84*(2), 401-418, vi.

Rolls, B. J., Castellanos, V. H., Halford, J. C., Kilara, A., Panyam, D., Pelkman, C. L., et al. (1998). Volume of food consumed affects satiety in men. *The American Journal of Clinical Nutrition, 67*(6), 1170-1177.

Rolls, B. J., Kim, S., McNelis, A. L., Fischman, M. W., Foltin, R. W., & Moran, T. H. (1991). Time course of effects of preloads high in fat or carbohydrate on food intake and hunger ratings in humans. *American Journal of Physiology, 260*(4 Pt 2), R756-763.

Rolls, B. J., Roe, L. S., Kral, T. V., Meengs, J. S., & Wall, D. E. (2004). Increasing the portion size of a packaged snack increases energy intake in men and women. *Appetite, 42*(1), 63-69.

Rolls, B. J., Roe, L. S., & Meengs, J. S. (2007). The effect of large portion sizes on energy intake is sustained for 11 days. *Obesity, 15*(6), 1535-1543.

Rosamond, W., Flegal, K., Friday, G., Furie, K., Go, A., Greenlund, K., et al. (2007). Heart disease and stroke statistics--2007 update: A report from the American Heart Association Statistics committee and Stroke Statistics subcommittee. *Circulation, 115*(5), e69-171.

Rosenheck, R. (2008). Fast food consumption and increased caloric intake: a systematic review of a trajectory towards weight gain and obesity risk. *Obesity Reviews, 9*(6), 535-547.

Roth, G., Ingram, D. K., & Joseph, J. A. (2007). Nutritional interventions in aging and age-associated diseases. *Annals of the New York Academy of Science, 1114*, 369-371.

Roth, J., Qiang, X., Marban, S. L., Redelt, H., & Lowell, B. C. (2004). The obesity pandemic: Where have we been and where are we going? *Obesity Research, 12 Suppl 2*, 88S-101S.

Roy, S., Shah, H., Rink, C., Khanna, S., Bagchi, D., Bagchi, M., et al. (2007). Transcriptome of primary adipocytes from obese women in response to a novel hydroxycitric acid-based dietary supplement. *DNA and Cell Biology, 26*(9), 627-639.

Ruderman, N. B., Saha, A. K., Vavvas, D., & Witters, L. A. (1999). Malonyl-CoA, fuel sensing, and insulin resistance. *American Journal of Physiology: Endocrinology and Metabolism, 276*(1), E1-18.

Scheen, A. J. (2008). The future of obesity: new drugs versus lifestyle interventions. *Expert Opinion on Investigational Drugs, 17*(3), 263-267.

Sohal, R. S., Ku, H.-H., Agarwal, S., Forster, M. J., & Lal, H. (1994). Oxidative damage, mitochondrial oxidant generation and antioxidant defenses during aging and in response to food restriction in the mouse. *Mechanisms of Ageing and Development, 74*(1-2), 121-133.

Sood, N., Baker, W. L., & Coleman, C. I. (2008). Effect of glucomannan on plasma lipid and glucose concentrations, body weight, and blood pressure: systematic review and meta-analysis. *American Journal of Clinical Nutrition, 88*(4), 1167-1175.

Stein, C. J., & Colditz, G. A. (2004). The epidemic of obesity. *Journal of Clinical Endocrinology & Metabolism, 89*(6), 2522-2525.

Stern, J. S., & Thomas, P. R. (1995). A commentary on weighing the options: Criteria for evaluating weight-management programs. *Obesity Research, 3*(6), 589-590.

Straznicky, N. E., Louis, W. J., McGrade, P., & Howes, L. G. (1993). The effects of dietary lipid modification on blood pressure, cardiovascular reactivity and sympathetic activity in man. *Journal of Hypertension, 11*(4), 427-437.

Sugerman, H. J., Kellum, J. M., Engle, K. M., Wolfe, L., Starkey, J. V., Birkenhauer, R., et al. (1992). Gastric bypass for treating severe obesity. *American Journal of Clinical Nutrition, 55*(2 Suppl), 560S-566S.

Sullivan, A. C., Hamilton, J. G., Miller, O. N., & Wheatley, V. R. (1972). Inhibition of lipogenesis in rat liver by (-)-hydroxycitrate. *Archives of Biochemistry and Biophysics, 150*(1), 183-190.

Tremblay, A., Despres, J., Theriault, G., Fournier, G., & Bouchard, C. (1992). Overfeeding and energy expenditure in humans. *The American Journal of Clinical Nutrition, 56*(5), 857-862.

Tye, R. (1991). Konjac flour: Properties and applications. *Food Technology, 45*, 11-16.

U.S. Department of Health and Human Services (2000). *Nutrition and overweight.*

Uhe, A. M., Collier, G. R., & O'Dea, K. (1992). A Comparison of the Effects of Beef, Chicken and Fish Protein on Satiety and Amino Acid Profiles in Lean Male Subjects. *The Journal of Nutrition, 122*(3), 467-472.

Van Dorsten, B., & Lindley, E. M. (2008). Cognitive and behavioral approaches in the treatment of obesity. *Endocrinology and Metabolism Clinics in North America, 37*(4), 905-922.

Vogel, M. D. R. A., Corretti, M. D. M. C., & Plotnick, M. D. G. D. (1997). Effect of a single high-fat meal on endothelial function in healthy subjects. *The American Journal of Cardiology, 79*(3), 350-354.

Vuksan, V., Sievenpiper, J. L., Xu, Z., Wong, E. Y., Jenkins, A. L., Beljan-Zdravkovic, U., et al. (2001). Konjac-Mannan and American ginsing: Emerging alternative therapies for type 2 diabetes mellitus. *Journal of the American College of Nutrition, 20*(5 Suppl), 370S-380S; discussion 381S-383S.

Wadden, T. A., Sternberg, J. A., Letizia, K. A., Stunkard, A. J., & Foster, G. D. (1989). Treatment of obesity by very low calorie diet, behavior therapy, and their combination: A five-year perspective. *International Journal of Obesity, 13 Supplement*, 239-246.

Walsh, D. E., Yaghoubian, V., & Behforooz, A. (1984). Effect of Glucomannan on obese patients: A clinical study. *International Journal of Obesity, 8*, 289-293.

Watson, J. A., Fang, M., & Lowenstein, J. M. (1969). Tricarballylate and hydroxycitrate: Substrate and inhibitor of ATP: Citrate oxaloacetate lyase. *Archives of Biochemistry and Biophysics, 135*(1), 209-217.

Weindruch, R., Naylor, P. H., Goldstein, A. L., & Walford, R. L. (1988). Influences of aging and dietary restriction on serum thymosin alpha 1 levels in mice. *Journal of Gerontology, 43*(2), B40-42.

Weindruch, R., & Walford, R. L. (1982). Dietary restriction in mice beginning at 1 year of age: Effect on life-span and spontaneous cancer incidence. *Science, 215*(4538), 1415-1418.

Weindruch, R., Walford, R. L., Fligiel, S., & Guthrie, D. (1986). The retardation of aging in mice by dietary restriction: Longevity, cancer, immunity and lifetime energy intake. *Journal of Nutrition, 116*(4), 641-654.

Weiss, E. P., Racette, S. B., Villareal, D. T., Fontana, L., Steger-May, K., Schechtman, K. B., et al. (2006). Improvements in glucose tolerance and insulin action induced by increasing energy expenditure or decreasing energy intake: a randomized controlled trial. *Am J Clin Nutr, 84*(5), 1033-1042.

Westerterp-Plantenga, M. S., & Kovacs, E. M. (2002). The effect of (-)-hydroxycitrate on energy intake and satiety in overweight humans. *International Journal of Obesity, 26*(6), 870-872.

Winder, W. W., & Hardie, D. G. (1999). AMP-activated protein kinase, a metabolic master switch: Possible roles in type 2 diabetes. *American Journal of Physiology: Endocrinology and Metabolism, 277*(1), E1-10.

Woods, S. C. (2009). The control of food intake: Behavioral versus molecular perspectives. *Cell Metabolism, 9*(6), 489-498.

Woods, S. C., & Ramsay, D. S. (2007). Homeostasis: Beyond Curt Richter. *Appetite, 49*(2), 388-398.

World Health Organization (1998). *Obesity: Preventing and Managing the Global Epidemic*. Geneva: World Health Organization.

Zheng, H., Shin, A. C., Lenard, N. R., Townsend, R. L., Patterson, L. M., Sigalet, D. L., et al. (2009). Meal patterns, satiety, and food choice in a rat model of Roux-en-Y gastric bypass surgery. *American Journal of Physiology: Regulatory, Integrative and Comparative Physiology, 297*(5), R1273-1282.

Chapter 3

APPETITE REGULATION AND ROLE OF APPETIZERS

K. S. Premavalli and D. D. Wadikar
Food Preservation Division, Defense Food Research Laboratory,
Siddhartha Nagar, Mysore, Karnataka, India

ABSTRACT

Appetite is a pleasant sensation of having urge for consuming food and appetite regulation, a multifaceted phenomenon is influenced by many factors such as food intake, energy expenditure, nutrition and active ingredients such as spices and passive components as polycarbohydrates. Apart from these harmones leptin and ghrelin have an impact on appetite regulation and altitude increase shows a profound effect on increased harmonal levels thereby reduced appetite. The natural appetisers with spices as an active component and their role on leptin levels thereby appetite regulation has been dealt in this chapter.

Appetite is a psycho-physiological phenomenon in living beings which can be referred to the urge for consuming food. In general, the food pattern, quantum of food, feeling of satiety and hunger, physiological body constitution, weather conditions have the influence on appetite. In fact, appetite phenomenonly possess three distinct phases i.e., appetite control, appetite suppression and appetite regulation which have an impact on physiological actions, body weight, as well as food intake, energy expenditure and the fitness of the digestive system. Appetite reflects the synchronous operation of events and processes at three levels, neural events trigger involving a behavioral response in the peripheral physiology, in turn the same is translated into brain neuro-chemical activity which represents the strength of motivation and willingness, to eat or refrain from eating. Besides these, the psychological events of craving for food, choice of sensations as well as behavioral operations of taking meals, snacks, energy products (Blundell and Halford, 1998) have a greater impact at the holistic level of food consumption and utilization by the body. Attitude and awareness towards healthy eating is also very important besides the motivation. Hearty et al., (2007) in their study on 1256 Irish adults by random sampling concluded that attitude and motivation towards eating healthily was related to measured dietary behavior and lifestyle.

Appetite is a pleasant sensation that causes a person to desire or anticipate food. Appetite reflects on physiological components through hormonal control, but also possesses psychological state for arriving at a decision. Appetite is often felt in mouth or palate depending more on odour or flavor and the pleasant memory of food. In fact, appetite is product specific, whereas appetite expression is human specific, however, the appetizing effect encompasses the product, appetite expression and its mode of measurement. The whole mechanism of operations in appetite expression covers various phases for giving the judgement. Firstly, the reaction of sensory attributes which is responsible to the food characteristics reflects the judgement on the quality of food. Secondly, the physiological responses from the gastro-intestinal tract generate signals reflecting the quantity of food consumed. Thirdly, the food utilization and absorption along with energy expenditure is obtained by metabolic information. Fourthly, the adipose tissue reserves influences the appetite through lipostatic signal. Fifthly, these signals reaches the brain network, processes, organizes the functional response. Thus, the food type and feeding behavior have a greater impact on appetite; physiological responses influences the appetite control while the brain network process play a greater role in appetite regulation, while, the appetite suppression is related to the satiety signals when the physiological events are triggered as responses for not eating the food or which suppresses urge to eat for a particular period of time. However, all these states of appetite are inter-related in the physiological events as well as psychological behavior. The potential use of olibra, an appetite suppressant in dairy products, fruit drinks, soups and chocolate mixes has been discussed by Heasman and Mellentin (1998). More than these aspects, these states of appetite are influenced by various nature related factors such as altitudes, oxygen availability, living temperatures, basic tastes perception of sensory organs as well as type of food for consumption.

1. APPETITE REGULATION

The appetite regulation is governed by three major aspects : Cognizance and psychological aspects; Physiological and metabolic factors and Harmonal and neurological reflections. The peripheral and cognitive factors which refer to sight, touch, aroma concept in memory, etc., specifies to the action of sensory attributes of humans at the instance of food memorization as well as food consumption. Thus, the *appetite, lack of appetite, appetite control* comes under appetite regulation and the appetizers have a great role to play in this phenomenon. In general, appetite regulation is more often related to obesity and thus involved mechanisms, harmonal changes, obesity related diseased conditions may be dealt in detail in some other chapter of the book. In this chapter, the functional aspects of appetite regulation in terms of type of food, nutrition, appetizing components and their behavior on hormonal changes have been emphasized. The oro-sensory stimulation plays an important role in appetite regulation. Food components, say, protein exerts greater suppressive effects while carbohydrates shows an immediate effect on subjective hunger and fat have a delayed effect. However, the energy density has a reversal phase, but energy intake is again related on metabolic and absorptive phases. Hlebowicz (2009) have reported that in glucostatic appetite regulation, cephalic phase digestion, gastric emptying and absorption influences the blood glucose response and satiety in healthy, non-obese overweight fasting subjects. Thus, the diet, nutrient factors, effects on physiology on appetite regulation is a complex phenomenon and a debatting issue.

1.1. Effect of Food and Nutrition

Food and nutrients consumption influences the human appetite through multiple feedbacks in terms of processes of food location, ingestion, digestion, absorption and metabolism. The major nutrients i.e., carbohydrates, proteins and fat not only contributes to energy intake but also leads to orosensory stimulation which may influence appetite and gastro-intestinal responses. High fat diet (Cunningham et al., 1991a) or high glucose diet in humans (Cunningham et al., 1991b) resulted in faster gastric emptying and it appears to be nutrient specific. Further, Cunningham (1998) research findings on sugar-fat varied diets reveal that sugar plays a role in appetite control and that reducing the sugar levels in the diet undermines appetite regulation. While Anderson (1995) opined that there is no evidence that sugar affects food intake. Poppit et al., (1998) in their study on effect of macronutrients preloads on appetite and energy intake in lean women found that protein has a differential short term satiating effect as compared to carbohydrates, fat and alcohol.

Cecil et al., (1999) showed that high carbohydrate and high fat soups oral administration suppresses the appetite ratings and reduces the meal intake. Hall et al., (2003) have emphasized the importance of protein type i.e., whey and casein on the appetite response in terms of satiety in a mixed meal. According to Stubbs et al (1996), high macronutrients based breakfast led to detectable changes in hunger, but was not of higher magnitude to have lunch even after 5 hrs which shows more a satiety feeling rather than appetizing. Camire and Blackmore (2007) have also discussed the role of breakfast foods in promoting satiety. High protein breakfasts leads to satiety while optimal amounts and type of carbohydrates result in appetite control, modification of foods delays fat digestion and coffee, tea being stimulants leads to reduced appetite. Ratliff et al (2009) have shown that carbohydrate restriction diet reduces the body weight while whole egg intake increased satiety. But, Park et al., (2007) have concluded that the high fat diet did not show significant changes in gastric motor functions. However, according to Little et al (2007) presence of the fat in the small intestine shows gastric emptying, stimulates the release of gastrointestinal harmones and suppresses appetite and energy intake. Marciani et al (2009) have shown the possibility of delay in satiety by stabilizing the intragastric distributions of fat emulsions against gastric acid environment. Cassady et al (2009) have reported on the effect of another fat source, almonds mastication which leads to suppressed hunger levels and declined insulin concentrations. Beasley et al., (2009) have reported that the diet rich in protein reduces self reported appetite as compared with diets rich in carbohydrates and unsaturated fat. The effect of bioactive peptides on appetite has been studied on 20 male and 32 female subjects of 18-35 years of age by Gustafson et al (2001), and concluded that bioactive peptide from milk has no influence on appetite. However, as per the study of Blundell and Naslund (1999) glucagon-like-peptide exerts a role on appetite control through the inhibition of gastric emptying. leRoux and Bloom (2005) have shown that peptide YY is important in everyday regulation of food intake thereby appetite control. Thus, the food and the nutrients fat, protein and carbohydrates do not exert a greater impact on appetite, but, to a very little extent carbohydrates play a role in appetite control, while protein and fat rather works in the opposite direction. Hence, any appetizer should be carbohydrate based with low protein and fat. Alcohol consumption in low quantities is known for stimulation leading to better digestion. Delin and Lee (1992) have declared from their study that consumption of alcoholic beverages acts as an adjunct in the diet and leads to proper digestion and absorption of food. While, Poppit et al., (1996) concluded that alcoholic beverages consumption in the diet result in overall increase in energy intake. Westertrep Planteg and Verweger (1999) have inferred that alcohol may increase appetite and stimulates food intake. Raben et al., (2003) have reported on the meals effect on appetite and concluded that intake of an alcohol rich meal stimulates energy expenditure but suppresses fat oxidation as compared to dense meals rich in protein carbohydrate and fat.

The poly-carbohydrates exert a positive role in many physiological actions such as prebiotics on gastro-intestinal reactions, dietary fibres in reduced absorption of sugar, reduction in cholesterol and elimination of constipation, etc., which will have an indirect role on appetite regulation. Prentice and Poppit (1996) emphasized the need to increase the intake of complex carbohydrates so that it will be effective in decreasing energy density and regulation of energy balance. Bosscher (2006) has discussed the potential of chicory derived inulin and oligofructosaccharide in appetite control and food intake which is mediated through harmones. While, ONeill (2008) has reviewed the inulin and oligofrcutose benefits in adolescents regarding the effects of appetite and satiety. Roberfroid (2007) has reported that inulin type fructans modulate the secretion of gastrointestinal peptides involved in appetite regulation as well as metabolism. Consumption of millet products in turn slowly digestible starch fraction present influences the satiety feeling because of longer transit time. Stubbs et al., (2008) has discussed the role of micronutrients, feeding behavior and weight control in humans and concluded that the macronutrients influence on appetite calls for a simple policy messages that consumers can understand rather than complicated messages of multifactors so that evidence of research cannot be easily understood.

Besides these, the micronutrients status especially dietary minerals influence the food intake. According to Beard (2008) in animal models studied on iron, iodine, selenium, zinc and copper, the deficiency of these reflects on the neural function, food intake and energy utilization. Zinc plays a role in appetite signals alterations in the periphery as well as at the hypothalamus that control food intake, but, in the case of other minerals, it is not so specific. In human system, Dorthy and Carolyn (2008) have reported that zinc deficiency reduces food intake, higher calcium may lead to reduced fat accumulation whereas on iron and iodine deficiency, clear evidences for reduced intake is not found. Thus, these minerals act as an anti-appetizer, however, depends on the levels. Thus, the effect of food and nutrients on the appetite regulations is more based on the food intake measurement which is one of the methods of rating appetite behavior.

1.2. Role of Spices

Spices are a key to the physiological system for the stimulative action leading to several health benefits. The various parts of plant are used as spices may be leaves, bark, buds, fruits, seeds, etc., which provide basic effects to impart flavor, colour and taste referring to pungency, bitterness and sweetness and also exerts anti-microbial, antioxidant, medicinal and nutritional effects. Besides these, the complex effect refers to increased appetite, flavor masking effect, improvement of texture and preservation of foods. Black pepper is the "King of Spices" is used for flavouring food. Over the years, the fact is well recognized that the spices possess digestive stimulant action besides the contribution for enhancing the taste and flavour of food. Ginger and turmeric as a spice and flavourant has been reviewed (Premavalli,

2005, 2007). The characteristic active components are responsible for flavouring or the taste of pungency, bitterness, sweetness. For example, ginger, black pepper, red peppers are hot pungent spices which has the main component of pungency as gingerol, piperine and capsaicin respectively. These compounds influence the stimulating action. The profile of common spices with the active components and beneficial properties are listed in Table 1.

Table 1. Common spices profile with active component and beneficial properties

Sl. No.	Common Name Spice/Condiment/Herb	Botanical Name	Parts Used	Active component	Beneficial Properties	Reference
1	Ajowan, (Bishop's Weed)	*Trachyspermum ammi*	Seeds	Thymol, carvacrol	Digestive, antiflatulant, thermogenic, stimulant, tonic	Warrier, 1989 Prajapati et al 2003
2	Anise	*Pimpinella anisum L*	Seeds	Anethale, methyl chavicol, limonene, anise aldehyde	Carminative, useful against nausea, indigestion and bloating	Nadkarni and Nadkarni 1976 Prajapati et al 2003
3	Asafoetida	*Ferula asafoetida*	Exudate gum	Hydroxyumbellipr enins, asafoetidin, ferocolicin, disulphides	Laxativ;e, anti-spasmodic, carminative and antiflatulant diuretic, expectorant	Nadkarni and Nadkarni 1976 Chopra et al, 1958 Prajapati et al 2003
4	Black Pepper	*Piper nigrum*	Seeds/Fruit	Piperine, caryophylene, α-pinene, phellandrene, myrcene, camphene	Carminative and laxative, remedy for dyspepsia, diarrhea, flatulence, nausea and vomiting	Chopra et al, 1958 Chelladurai, 1991 Warrier, 1989 Augusti, 1996 Kaweda et al, 1988
5	Cardamom	*Elettaria cardamonum*	Seeds/Fruit	Cineol, α-terpinyl acetate, limonene, sabinene myrcene	Antiemetic and stomachic appetite and digestion stimulant, carminative	Warrier, 1989 Prajapati et al 2003
6	Clove	*Eugenia caryophyllus/ aromatica* Kuntz	Dry flower	Eugenol, caryophylene, acetyl-eugenol	Gastric stimulant and carminative, useful in nausea, indigestion and dyspepsia, appetizer	Rama and Krishnamoorthy 1992, Prajapati et al 2003
7	Cinnamon	*Cinnamomum zeylanicum/v erum*	Tree bark	Cinnamaldehyde, eugenol, caryophylene and pinene	Carminative, astringent and stimulant; antiemetic, oil useful in anorexia and stomachalgia	Rama and Krishnamoorthy 1992, Prajapati et al 2003
8	Coriander	*Coriandrum sativum*	Seeds and leaves	Linalool, α, β-pinene, p-cymene, thymol, cineol	Stimulant and carminative, stomachic, digestive stimulant, Fruits are aromatic, thermogenic, stimulant, appetizing, useful in anorexia	Warrier, 1989 Prajapati et al 2003
9	Cumin	*Cuminum cyminum L*	Seeds	Cuminaldehyde, limonene phellandrene	Stimulant and carminative, stomachic and astringent, useful in dyspepsia and diarrhea	Nadkarni and Nadkarni 1976 Chopra et al, 1958
10	Fennel	*Foeniculum vulgare* Mill	Seed	Anethole, limonene, fenchone, α-pinene, camphene	Warming and appetizing carminative, aromatic, flavorant	Nadkarni and Nadkarni, 1976, Prajapati et al 2003
11	Fenugreek	*Trigonella foenum-gracum L*	Seed	Trigonelline	Carminative, tonic Appetite stimulant, diuretic, thermogenic	Nadkarni and Nadkarni 1976 Chopra et al, 1958 Warrier, 1989 Ramachandran and Ambasta, 1986

Table 1. (Continued)

Sl. No.	Common Name Spice/Condiment/Herb	Botanical Name	Parts Used	Active component	Beneficial Properties	Reference
12	Garlic	*Allium sativum*	Bulb (stem)	Diallyl disulfide and trisulfide, allyl propyl disulfide	Gastric stimulant, anti-flatulant carminative	Nadkarni and Nadkarni 1976 Augusti, 1996
13	Ginger	*Zingiber officinate*	Root	Gingerol, shaogol, linalool, zingerone	Remedy for dyspepsia, and indigestion stomachic, relieves stomach pain and nausea, antiemetic	Chopra et al, 1958 Warrier, 1989 Chelladurai, 1991 Kawada et al, 1988
14	Mint	*Mentha spicata*	Leaves/root	Carvone, dipentent, limonene, dihydrocarveol and its acetate	Carminative, stomachic, tonic antispasmodic	Nadkarni and Nadkarni 1976 Warrier, 1989 Thampi, 1991 Prajapati et al 2003
15	Mustard	*Brassica nigra*	Seeds	Allyl isothiocyanate	Useful in abdominal colic, vomiting; gastric stimulant	Chopra et al, 1958 Ramachandran and Ambasta 1986
16	Onion	*Allium cepa*	Bulb/Stem	Amino acids, phenolic acid	Aromatic, thermogenic, Carminative, stomachic, useful in flatulence, dysentery, vomiting.	Prajapati et al 2003
17	Red pepper (Red chilli)	*Capsicum annum* (Paprika) *Capsicum frutescens*	Fruit	Capsaicin, pyrazines, linalool, methyl salicylate, ocimene, hex-cis-3enol	Remedy for dyspepsia, stomachic and carminative digestive	Chopra et al, 1958, Chelladurai, 1991 Kawada et al, 1988, Prajapati et al 2003
18	Turmeric	*Curcuma longa* Linn	Root	Curcumin, turmerone, sesquiterpines, cineole, curcumene, zingiberene	Antiflatulant, stomachic, tonic, antacid and carminative; reduces pungency of food by increasing mucin content of gastric juice	Schneider et al, 1956 Bhavanishankar et al, 1985, Prajapati et al 2003
19	Nutmeg/Mace Lacy covering/aril of the nutmeg seed	*Myristica fragrans*	Seed	Myristin, α-pinene, eugenol, geraniol, limonene, terpineol sabinene, safrole, linalool	Digestive, antiflatulant, stimulant, carminative, useful in flatulence, stomach ache, nausea, vomiting	Prajapati et al 2003 Shastri 1962
20	All spice	*Pimento dioica*	Dried unripe mature fruits	Eugenol, thymol, cineole phellandrene, caryophylene	Digestive, antiseptic, carminative, stimulant	Krishnamoorthy 1969
21	Indian Borage	*Coleus amninicus/aromaticus*	Leaves	Thymol, carvacrol, α-pinene	Antiflatulant, digestive, remedy for cold and cough, appetizing, liver tonic, thermogenic	Prajapati et al 2003
22	Basil	*Ocimum basilicum* L	Leaves	Methyl chavicol (estragole), linalool and cineol, anithole	flavorant	Prajapati et al 2003
23	Bay leaves	*Laurus nobilis* L.	Leaves	Cineol, α-pinene, linalool, phellandrene, eugenol, borneol	Appetite stimulant, digestive, aromatic, useful in treating upper GI tract disorders	Prajapati et al 2003 Shastri 1962

The properties mainly refers to be a stimulant, aromatic, carminative, flavourant, digestive, antiflatulent and so on. Some of the spices such as cardamom, fennel, ginger etc. have also been reported as appetizing. Spices exhibits many functional processes for example, intensifies salivary flow, secretion of amylase, cleansing of oral cavity, help to check infections and caries, may help to protect the mucous membrane against thermic, mechanical and chemical irritation. Majority of the spices i.e., curcumin, capsaicin, ginger, fenugreek, onion, mint, cumin, fennel and ajowan in animal models have shown to stimulate pancreatic digestive enzymes lipase, amylase and proteases (Platel and Srinivasan, 2000). Glatzel (1968) has researched on the physiological aspects of active principles in spices and opined that spices contribute for many functional processes in the human system where pepper effects the salivary and gastric secretions while chilli influences the thrombosis. Bhat and Chandrashekara (1987) have reported that black pepper or the active principle peppirine stimulates the bile secretion. Further, Bryant and Green (1997) have reported on the perception of pungent sensations with the comparison of trigeminal nerves and non-trigeminal areas action. Hirasa and Takemasa (1998) have reported that red pepper promote lipid metabolism and induce body heat production. In rat studies, capsaicin when injected result in a release of neurotransmitter substance which activates the sympathetic nerves and enhances adrenal catecholamine, while piperine and zingerone showed relatively lower action. Platel and Srinivasan (2001) have reported that spices reduced the food transition time in rats and probably related to the increased digestive secretions. The physiological effects of spices and their role in health benefits have been reviewed (Platel and Srinivasan 2004; Srinivasan, 2005).

1.3. Role of Harmones

Leptin and ghrelin are the two harmones that have been recognized to have a major influence on energy balance. Leptin is a mediator of long term regulation of energy balance suppressing food intake. While ghrelin is a fast acting harmone, seemingly playing a role in meal initiation. Understanding the mechanisms by which various harmones and neurotransmitters have influence on energy balance has been a subject of intensive research. Ghrelin, 28-amino acid octanotated peptide is predominantly produced in the mucosa membrane of upper gastrointestinal tract and it stimulates the production of neuropeptide Y. Lepin, 16 k Da peptide, a harmone secreted by adiposyte as a product of obese gene has an implication in the regulation of food intake, energy expenditure and body fat storage. Circulating leptin concentrations are well correlated with body fat storage in humans and animals (Maffei et al., 1995; Considine et al., 1996; Havel et al., 1996). The meal time has an impact on leptin levels (Schoeller et al., 1997; Raben et al., 2003). Plasma leptin concentration decreases after fasting and increases after feeding. Several factors such as type of food, meals time, food intake, physiologic conditions, diseased conditions influence the leptin levels which will be reflected through the brain receptors mechanism. Generally, the role of leptin in the brain is at the hypothalamus for energy expenditure and food intake, but yet another role is in the hippocampus for improvement of memory and learning.

In animal models, Soliman (2001) has found that in adult rats, several factors such as gender, body weight, blood glucose level and serum insulin concentration are involved in the regulation of circulating leptin level. Serum leptin levels were higher in females than males in control group and were statistically significant. While, in diabetic mellitus induced group, it was not clear. However, positive correlation was found between leptin levels and insulin harmone levels. But, inverse relationship was observed between leptin and blood glucose levels. Exner et al., (2000) have reported that leptin suppressers cause semi-starvation induced hyperactivity in rats. Farr et al., (2006) in animal models seen that leptin plays a role in memory. In diseased conditions lower leptin levels contributed to memory impairment.

In healthy human studies, Keim et al., (1998) have observed that leptin levels decrease was coincided with increase in hunger. Arosio et al., (2007) have studied the effect of modified sham feeding on ghrelin in healthy human subjects and they have observed that ghrelin levels was related to orosensorial stimulation. Harmone levels are also influenced by diseased conditions and several studies brings out clearly the changes in leptin levels. Meyer et al., (1997) have studied the role of kidney in leptin metabolism. The results revealed that kidneys account for a substantial proportion of overall systematic leptin removal from the circulation. Aguilera et al., (2004) in their study on ghrelin level and appetite found that the ghrelin plasma levels increase in dialysis patients. Karakas et al., (2005) have seen that circulating leptin levels are associated with chronic obstructive pulmonary disease.

In diabetic women subjects, Konukoglu et al., (2004) have seen the relationship between leptin and zinc levels and their effect on oxidative stress and insulin. The results revealed that obese diabetic subjects had significantly higher plasma leptin and insulin levels with lower zinc levels compared to non-obese diabetic and non-diabetic controls. Zinc may be the mediator for the leptin effects and may be through free radical induced mechanism. Shirai et al., (2004) have reported the mechanism of regulation of leptin production in adipocytes. The data supported the mechanism that molonyl CoA levels act as a signal of the availability of fuels in adipocytes and act as a trigger of leptin production. The role of leptin in body weight control and its relevance on obesity has been reviewed (Friedman and Halaas, 1998). The role of leptin and ghrelin harmones on food intake and body weight in humans and their mechanism of action has been reviewed by Klok et al.,(2007). Anorexigenic leptin harmone increased while orexigenic ghrelin harmone decreased showing the differential action of these two appetite regulation harmones. It has been seen that alcohol has an appetizing effect (Westertrep planteg and Verwegen, 1999; Poppit et al, 1996; Raben et al, 2003), but Classendorff et al., (2005) have reported that alcohol has an acute inhibitory influence on ghrelin secretion. If the alcohol is below 5%, it falls under food class and generally these levels are found in fermented foods. Probably at higher levels it exerts an inhibhitary effect on meal consumption thereby, reduced ghrelin secretion. Though many reports are available, the detail discussion do not fall under the scope of this chapter.

1.4. Effect of High Altitude

Climatic extremes can exert profound effect on human physiology. Referring particularly to high altitudes, though acclamatisation of personnel to the environment is suggested, followed, the longer periods of stay leads to acute mountain sickness, pulmonary oedema cerebral oedema and high altitude retinopathy. Stress at high altitudes is induced by hypoxia, cold, solar radiations, etc. The physical activity at high altitude such as mountaineering, trekking, exercises as well as stay at high altitudes leads to anorexia followed by weight loss. The reduced appetite, exhaustion, intestinal complaints and increased basal metabolism with hormonal changes may be the reasons for weight loss at high altitude. Though malabsorption of nutrients occurs, it is of lesser practical significance. Oxidative stress mediated through free radicals may be important factor and protective cellular antioxidants defence mechanism can overcome the oxidative damage (Simon-Schnass, 1992). The reduced appetite or lack of appetite reduces the food intake leading to inadequacy in energy requirements. This is the point where the nutritional needs in terms of high calories, vitamins, minerals have a special, specific place for the personnel deployed at high altitudes. Generally, more than 4000 KCals with the supplementation of vitamin A and vitamin E which have antioxidant effect and high carbohydrate diet are recommended. Consolazio et al., (1969) and Askew (1996) have reported the beneficial effects upon symptoms, mood and performance from the carbohydrate rich diet. However, the energy and protein intakes at high altitude decrease over the period by 30-40% which may lead to negative nitrogen balance even with the best food available. Therefore, though proper steps are taken, firstly for food availability, secondly to nutritional requirements, priority should be to address the related problems of lack of appetite so that food intake in turn energy intake can be improved upon.

Exposure to high altitude leads to altitude illness which is a combination of symptoms of headache, nausea, vomiting and over the period of stay, it leads to lack of appetite and decreased food intake. Westerterp-Plantenga (1999) have found in their high altitude simulation study that the reduced energy intake at 5000-6000 feet above sea level was due to the reduced appetite. Orosensory stimulation plays a role in overcoming this problem. However, alteration in orosensory response of an individual leading to weight loss on exposure to high altitudes has been reported. (Rao and Prabhakar, 1992; Sharma et al., 1977). The threshold values for different tastes have found to be altered (Grandjean, 1955; Maga and Lorenz, 1972). Singh et al., (1996) have reported in their study on rat models that the decrease in food intake at high altitudes will be through the shift in taste preference. Also suggested the provision of palatable carbohydrate diet which may reduce the problem of hypophagia and weight loss. It has been found that the thresholds increased for glucose and sodium chloride while reduced for bitter and sour tastes (Singh et al., 1997). The exposure to high altitudes brought about the changes in hedonics responses with increased palatability for sweetness. Thus, the orosensory stimulation foods may be the better choice and pungent spices have a greater influence to improve the food intake at high altitudes.

In a study on high altitude low landers, Shukla et al., (2005) have found that appetite regulatory harmones significantly changes over a period of stay at high altitude. Leptin levels increased while ghrelin level decreased at an altitude of 4300m. On induction to altitude of 3600m, leptin levels increased by 8.6%, but, when moved to 4300m, increased by 54.9%. While, ghrelin levels decreased by 34.9% at 3600 m and 42.6% at 4300 m. There was a concomitant decrease in body weight by 2 kgs in 9 days. Ricci etal (2000) have reported 14, 17 and 22% decrease in plasma leptin levels of women volunteers at 30, 60 and 90 minutes respectively when exposed to cold. Suri et al., (2002) study on suppressed appetite at high altitudes, reported that zinc supplementation reduces the plasma leptin levels at high altitudes which will be the causative factor for appetite.

In Antarctica, at low temperatures, high wind velocity, low humidity, very active life was observed with weight gain initially (Vats et al., 2005). Serum plasma leptin levels decreased from 5.66 ± 0.59 to 4.4 ± 0.37 ng/ml. after 48 hrs of stay at Antarctica which shows the increase in appetite. But, after one month stay leptin levels increased to 7.49 ± 1.18 and a significant increase in neuropeptide Y. Thus, positive energy balance in the Antarctica expedition may be due to the changes in leptin and neuropeptide Y levels and the changes in these appetite regulatory peptides may be the adaptive mechanism against cold stress. The differential roles and mechanisms of food, stimulants, harmones as well as exposure to high altitudes emphasizes the fact that appetite regulation is an important, desirable phenomenon for better physiological action in turn the health.

2. APPETISERS

Appetiser is a component or a food item which exerts stimulating action thereby creates the urge to consume food. Basically, the stimulating components can act as appetisers. Spices are the most active components which acts as a stimulant and increase the salivary flow and gastric juice secretion thereby improves digestion and relieves anorexia. Many of the herbs called as blood cleansers or purifiers are used traditionally. Bogbean leaves, chicory leaves, dandelion leaves and fenugreek seeds are often bitter but increases the secretion of digestive juices, stimulates stomach and restore the appetite. Thus the decoction of these leaves before meals is practiced (Sarah Garland, 1979). Spices are used in meals to create a state of wellness. Cooking of foods with spices is the oldest form of aromatherapy, since aroma can stimulate gastric secretions that create appetite. Ayurveda emphasis the prevention of disease through a holistic approach through the persuasion of mental, physical and emotional harmony. Ayurveda categorizes foods into six basic tastes called rasas and all these rasas should be a part of every meal and these tastes must be balanced in a meal as per the person's constitution which is specific to the person. Different spices and spice based foods contribute to the taste, for example, fennel contributes to sweet, tamarind to sour, fenugreek to bitter, mustard to spicy, asofetida to astringent and ginger as pungent. Similar to Ayurvedic practices in Indian cooking of foods, Chinese cooking also have similar school of thought of balancing the five basic tastes in a meal to achieve health and well being. Today, the traditional concepts with 100 bioactive ingredients is showing its face as functional foods. In a realistic sense, appetisers also fall into the group of functional foods, where spices inturn its active ingredient influence appetising effect bringing the physiological changes. The active principles responsible for stimulating action is summarized in Table 1. On the other hand, some drugs are used as appetite stimulants most commonly for treating the anorexia in the patients of cancer (Desport et al, 2003), Acquired Immuno Deficiency Syndrome (Bayer, 2001), renal disease (Axelsson et al, 2007). Appetite stimulants such as megestrol, marinol, cyproheptadine, thalidoimide, oxandrolone and carticosteriods are being used in patients with AIDS, anorexia cachexia syndrome and advanced cancer (Persons and Nichols, 2007). However, the present chapter covers the food components based appetisers which acts as stimulants and improves the food intake. These natural appetisers will have wider application for normal persons as well as for personnel deployed at high altitudes.

Since ancient times, the spices as ginger, pepper, jeera, chillies, ajowan are known for their flavour, pungent taste and beneficial effects. The general approach is to use spices as stimulants in soups, but the low levels of less than 1% used imparts flavour and helps to release more saliva thereby aids digestion. Commercially, soups are available in the form of mixes and can be reconstituted in boiling water prior to consumption. Considering the food habits, psychological based acceptance and consumer demands, several types of soups are being marketed. The product profile is presented in Table 2. Tomato, carrot, onion, chilli and other vegetable soup mixes refers to vegetarian soups while chicken based soups fall into non-vegetarian category. Recently, noodles based soups have also gained the marketing. The other ingredients in the soup mix impart texture and body and many a time an adverse feeling of fullnesss is felt which results in less food intake later. For example, from Table 3, it can be observed starch is the major ingredient which gets gelatinsed during reconstitution and impart thickening but contributes to the fullness feeling. It can also be observed that though major emphasis is on vegetarian and non vegetarian soup mixes, but the difference in ingredients reveal is mainly with reference to flavour enhancer, acidity regulator and the relative quantities. The ingredient composition brings out the fact that spices occupies a position at the lower end indicating the low level of spices. Higher levels of spices may intensify stimulation thereby manage appetite loss. Yoshioka et al (1999) have studied the effect of red pepper based appetiser on energy intake and their result revealed that carbohydrate and energy intakes at lunch and snack meals decreased and was related to the increase in sympathetic nervous system activity. According to Cecil et al (1999), high carbohydrate and high fat soups consumption leads to appetite suppression and reduced meal intake. The clinical trials conducted on young men with 5 types of soups with different components say corn starch, maltodextrin, whole grain and amylase showed the reduced food intake and premeal appetite decreased by all treatments (Anderson et al, 2010).

Table 2. Profile of commercially available soup mixes

Hot and Sour Vegetable Soup
Home style Rich tomato Soup
Home style Mixed Vegetable Soup
Sweet Corn Vegetable Soup
Thick Tomato Soup
Creamy Mushroom Soup
Lemon Coriander Soup
Sweet corn Chicken Soup
Manchow Soup
Mixed Vegetable Soup
Thai Noodles Soup
Masala Noodles Soup
Chilli Soup
Spinach and Carrot Soup*
Mixed Vegetable Soup*
Baby corn Spring Onion Soup*
Tomato Soup*
Sweet corn Chicken Soup
Hot and Sour Chicken Soup
Creamy Chicken Soup

* Soup concentrates.

Appetisers have been developed with spices ginger, pepper, cumin, ajowan, chillies as one of the ingredients at a level of 10-15%. These spices at higher levels could manage appetite loss, motion sickness and prevent vomiting. The heat generation to some extent protects the body heat in cold region. But the other problem due to hotness could be addressed by using dietary fibre, cooling constituents such as raisins, dates, lemon, pseudolemon etc. In the appetisers based on pepper in the form of convenience mixes which can be reconstitutable in hot water, the active ingredient pepper was at 1.5 to 2.8% with pipperine levels of 0.08 to 0.155% (Wadikar et al, 2008). These appetisers on reconstitution in water were rated good with the score of more than 3 on 5 point hedonic scale. However, the base level field rating of acceptability were lower as compared to laboratory and at altitude the acceptance ratings was higher (Premavalli et al, 2009). Pepper based ready-to-eat appetisers in the form of pepper munch and lemon munch developed with 3.5-4.5% pepper, as a stimulating ingredient have been liked very much with a sensory score of 3.4 to 3.7 on 5 point hedonic scale.

Table 3. Ingredient profile of commercial soup mixes

No.	Soup Mixes	Ingredients
	Vegetarian	
1	Sweet corn Vegetable Soup	Corn flour, Dehydrated Vegetables, sugar, salt, Fat powder, Edible vegetable fat, hydrolyzed vegetable protein, green chilli powder, garlic powder, yeast extract powder, soy sauce powder, flavor enhancer- 627 and 631, spices and condiments, traces of wheat and nuts
2	Thick Tomato Soup; Home style Rich tomato Soup	Refined wheat flour, Corn flour, tomato powder, sugar, salt, Fat powder, Edible vegetable fat, onion powder, beet root juice powder, garlic powder, yeast extract powder, dehydrated coriander leaves, Acidity regulator-330, Flavor enhancer- 627 and 631/635, spices and condiments, traces of soy and nuts
3	Hot and Sour Vegetable Soup; Home style Hot and Sour Vegetable Soup	Corn starch, maltodextrin, sugar, iodized salt, soy sauce powder, onion, tomato powder, color 150d, edible vegetable oil, carrot flakes, green bell pepper, wheat flour, noodle bits, garlic powder, cabbage bits, mixed spices, acidifying agents-330, coriander leaves, flavour enhancer-627, traces of almond and milk
4	Home style Mixed vegetable soup; Mixed Vegetable Soup	Wheat flour, corn starch, sugar, salt, edible vegetable oil, milk solids, cabbage, carrot, peas, onion powder, garlic powder, acidifying agent-330, Flavor enhancer- 635/627/631, mixed spices, traces of soy and nuts
5	Babycorn spring onion soup concentrate	Babycorn, spring onion, ginger, garlic, sugar, salt, chilli powder, citric acid, corn flour, spices
	Non Vegetarian	
6	Sweet corn chicken soup	Corn flour, Dehydrated Vegetables, salt, dehydrated chicken shreds, edible vegetable fat, dried glucose syrup, hydrolyzed vegetable protein, green chilli powder, garlic powder, yeast extract powder, soy sauce powder, flavor enhancer- 627 and 631, spices and condiments, traces of wheat, milk and nuts
7	Classic Hot and Sour Chicken Soup	Corn starch, refined wheat flour, sugar, salt, soy sauce powder, dehydrated Vegetables, dried glucose syrup, dried chicken, hydrolyzed vegetable protein, green chilli powder, garlic powder, yeast extract powder, flavor enhancer- 627 and 631, acidity regulator [296 and 451(i)], spices and condiments, softening agent (500-ii)

Ginger, a pungent and stimulant spice used widely in Indian culinary since time immemorial. Early Chinese and Japanese research found that fresh ginger decoction produced a stimulant action on gastric secretion (Chang and Butt, 1987). German scientists have reported that chewing 9g of crystallized ginger had a profound effect on saliva production (Blumberger and Glatzel, 1964). Ginger is also used for treatment of asthma, breathing problems, diarrhea, nausea, motion sickness and appetite loss (Sifton 1999, Steward et al, 1991). Ready-to-eat appetisers in the form of ginger munch and fruit munch with 6-8% of ginger levels had excellent acceptance with a rating of 7.5 to 8 score on 9 point hedonic scale (Wadikar et al, 2010). Ginger based ready to drink beverage produced by aseptic process and ready to reconstitute mix with an active ingredient at 7% level were excellent products with an established shelf life of 6 months. Cumin seeds posses the active principle as cuminaldehyde and influences the bile action. Ready-to-eat cumin munch with 25% of appetiser level as a combination of ginger and cumin had very good acceptability by the consumers. Ajowan being antiflatulent and stimulant, acts as digestive and improves appetite. Ready-to-eat appetiser ajowan munch with the appetiser level of 10% has been found to be liked very much by the panelists. Thus the development of appetisers is a challenging task with varied processing and spices provide variety and the level of active ingredients above 6% had better potential. Ready-to-eat munches had shelf life of 9-12 months while ready-to-reconstitute mixes and ready-to-drink beverage had a shelf life of 6 months.

In general, the acceptance rating was higher at high altitudes than the base level subjects and ginger based products were preferred to pepper based products. The food intake was found to be higher with ginger based product, probably due to the appetiser level. The application of two statistical models of Latin square method, for relative preferences of ready-to-eat munches has shown that all the munches were accepted very well and order of preference were ginger munch, lemon munch, cumin munch, fruit munch and pepper munch and evaluation method (Bailey, 1996) was the most promising. Such type of appetising products are not found so far in literature. However, Bawadi et al (2009) studied on the development of meal planning exchange list for Middle east traditional foods in Jordon. In their study, forty types of appetisers and forty types of deserts were included with 5 different reciepes for each. The dishes preparation, their proximate composition and their comparison with Food Analysis software concluded a valid exchange system for traditional desserts and appetisers for used by dieticians and health care providers. But the level of appetising components to be used and their effect has not been attempted so far.

3. ROLE OF APPETISERS

Appetisers on administration to the animal or human system is expected to reflect the appetising effect in terms of increased food intake as well as changed hormonal levels. The hormones ghrelin and leptin play a significant role in appetite regulation. The role of leptin and ghrelin on food intake and body weight and their mechanism of action have been reviewed by Klok et al (2007). But the reverse study on the role of natural appetisers on the hormonal changes which reflects study on the role of natural appetisers is still open for research. The study on administration of ready-to-drink appetisers based on ginger, ajowan and karpuravalli in male wister rats under fasting condition showed a decrease in serum leptin levels. The fasting leptin levels ranged from 0.75 to 2.5ng/ml, but decreased by 3.4 to 10.8% after consumption of appetisers. Food consumption and weight gain was found to be higher in rats fed with the appetizer as compared to control group and the changes were significant ($p < 0.5$). In human study, the evaluation of the effect of ginger based appetiser administration on serum plasma leptin levels has been investigated and it was a laboratory study (Wadikar and Premavalli, 2010). The results revealed that the plasma leptin level in fasting subjects ranged from 4.6 to 8.13ng/ml and the average fasting plasma leptin level was 6.02 ± 5.57. The plasma leptin level after consumption of appetiser decreased in all the groups irrespective of the type of appetiser. It has been observed that the reduction of plasma leptin was lowest in jeera munch (6.4%) followed by fruit munch (10.7%), ginger munch (11.4%) and appetiser drink (14.9%). This reduction was statistically significant ($P<0.05$) in case of fruit munch, ginger munch and appetiser drink. In the present study, it has been observed that leptin levels were higher in female than male volunteers, which may be probably due to higher fat tissue mass. These mean plasma leptin level for males was 4.86 ± 3.54 as against normal range of 2.4 ± 1.1ng/ml, while for females it was 10.50 ± 6.84 as against 6.6 ± 3 ng/ml, which reflects to be higher than the normal range. Edward and Abdishakur (2000) also reported higher plasma leptin levels in females as compared to males. Singh et al (2001) has also found plasma leptin levels of 8.35 ± 0.35ng/ml in normal lean non-athletic females while another study (Vats et al, 2005) with 22 male subjects study reported 5.66 ± 0.59ng/ml plasma leptin levels in base region. The post prandial leptin level after consumption of appetisers decreased irrespective of the gender and age of the subjects. The reduction in leptin was lesser in the lower age group (6.07%) as compared with the higher age group (11.40%). The plasma leptin levels increase with the increase in altitude (Shukla at al, 2005). In the present investigation, the munching of appetisers led to the decreased leptin levels thereby increased the appetite. The study concluded that the fasting plasma leptin levels were dependent on the age and sex of the individuals. All the four evaluated appetisers resulted in the reduction of post prandial plasma leptin levels indicating the appetising effect. In this chapter, a new direction and dimension is shown for appetite regulation and this approach of food based natural appetisers inturn their effect on harmonal control proves to be more promising than the direct harmonal control through drugs for regulation of appetite.

REFERENCES

Aguilera, A., Cirugeda, A., Amair, R., Sansone, G., Alegre, L., Codoceo, R., Auxiliadora Bajo, M., Gloria del Peso, Diez, JJ., Jose A. Sanchez-Tomero and Selgas, R.(2004). Ghrelin Plasma Levels and Appetite in Peritoneal Dialysis Patients. *Advance in Peritoneal Dialysis,* 20, 194-199.

Anderson G. H. (1995). Sugars, sweetness and food intake. *American Journal of Clinical Nutrition*, 62(1):195S-202S.

Anderson G. H., Cho C.E., Akhavan T., Mollard R.C., Luhovyy B.L., Finochhiaro E.T. (2010). Relation between estimates of corn starch digestibility by the Englyst in vitro method and glycemic response, subjective appetite and short term food intake in young men. *American Journal of clinical Nutrition*, 91(4):932-939.

Arosio, M., Ronchi, C L., Beck-Peccoz, P., Gebbia, C., Giavoli,C., Cappiello, V., Conte, D., and Peracchi M. (2007). Effect of Modified Sham Feeding on Ghrelin Levels in Healthy

Human Subjects. *The Journal of Clinical Endocrinology and Metabolism*, 89(10):5101-5104.

Askew, E.W. (1996) Nutrition and performance in hot, cold and high altitude environments, In 'Nutrition in Exercise and Sport'. 3rd edn. I Wolinsky (Ed), CRC Press, Boca Raton, FL: 597-619.

Augusti KT. (1996) Therapeutic values of onion (Allium cepa) and garlic (Allium sativum). *Indian J. Exp. Biol.*, 34: 634-40.

Axelsson J, Carrero JJ, Lindholm B, Heimburger O and Stenvinkel P (2007). Malnutrition in patients with end-stage renal disease- Anorexia, cachexia and catabolism. *Current Nutrition and Food Science*, 3:37-46.

Bailey R. A. (1996). *Orthogonal partition for design experiments, designs, codes and cryptography*, 8, 45-77.

Bawadi H.A., Al-Shwaiyat N.M., Tayyem R.F., Mekary R., Tuuri G. (2009) Developing a food exchange list for Middle Eastern appetizers and desserts commonly consumed in Jordan. *Nutrition and Dietetics*, 66 (1):20-26.

Bayer RE (2001).Therapeutic Cannabis (Marijuana) as an antiemetic and appetite stimulant in persons with acquired immunodeficiency syndrome (AIDS). In 'Cannabis Therapeutics in HIV/AIDS' (ed. Ethan Russo), The Haworth Integrating Healing Press, an imprint of The Haworth Press, Inc., pp.5-16.

Beard J (2008) Mineral micronutrient status and Food intake studies with Animal models. Eds. Ruth B.S., Harris and Richard D Mattes, CRC Press, London. p323-332.

Beasley, J.M., Ange, B.A., Anderson, C.A.M., Miller III, E.R., Erlinger, T.P., Holbrook, J.T., Sacks, F.M. and Appel, L.J. (2009). Associations between macronutrient intake and self-reported appetite and fasting levels of appetite hormones: results from the optimal macronutrient intake trial to prevent heart disease. *Am. Epidemiol.* 169, 893-900.

Bhat GB and Chandrashekhar N (1987). Effect of black pepper and piperine on bile secretion and composition in rats. *Die Nahrung*, 31(9):913-916.

Bhavanishankar T N. and Sreenivasamurthy V. (1985) Inhibitory effect of curcumin on intestinal gas formation by Clostridiuim perfringens. *Nutr. Rep. Int.*, 32, 1285-92.

Blumberger, W. and Glatzel, H. (1964). The Physiology of Spices and Condiments: The Action of Ginger on the Amount and Condition of the Saliva. Nutritio et Dieta (*Euro. Rev. Nutri. Dietetics*), 64:181-192.

Blundell, J.E. and Naslund, E. (1999). Glucagon like peptide -1, satiety and appetite control. *Brit. J. Nutri.* 81:259-260.

Blundell, J.E., and Halford, J.C.G. (1998). Appetite: Physiological and Neurological aspects. In: Salder M. (Ed) Encyclopedia of Human Nutrition: Academic Press London, 121-126.

Bosscher D (2006) Limit food intake by inducing satiety. *Agro food Industry high tech.* 17(5) VI-VII.

Bryant, H.R. and Green, B.G. (1997) Perceived irritation during ingestion of capsaicin or piperine: comparison of trigeminal and non trigeminal areas. *Chemical Senses* 22: 257-266.

Calissendorff, J., Danielsson,O., Brismar, K. and Rojdmark,S. (2005). Inhibitory effect of alcohol on ghrelin secretion in normal man. *European Journal of Endocrinology*, 152, 743-747.

Camire ME and Blackmore M (2007). *Breakfast foods and satiety.* 61(2):24-25.

Cassady BA, Hollis JH, Fulford AD, Considine RV and Mattes RD (2009). Mastication of almonds: effects of lipid bio-accessibility, appetite and hormone response. *American Journal of Clinical Nutrition*, 89(3):794-800.

Cecil, J.E., Francis, J. Read NW. (1999). Comparison of the effects of a high-fat and high-carbohydrate soup delivered orally and intra-gastrically on gastric emptying, appetite, and eating behavior. *Physiology and Behavior*, 67(2), 299-306.

Chang, H. M. and But, P.P.H. (Ed)(1987). Pharmacology and Applications of Chinese Materia Medica. *World Scientific* vol.2, Singapore.

Chelladurai ASS. (1991). Spices in Homeopathy medicines. *Indian Spices*, 28: 5-6.

Chopra RN, Chopra IC, Handa KL, Kapur LD. (1958). Chopra's indigenous drugs of India, 2nd ed., Calcutta : Dhur and Sons.

Considine RV, Sinha MK, Heiman ML, Kriauciunas A, Stephens TW, Nyce MR, Ohannesian JP, Marco CC, Mckee LJ, Bauer TL et al (1996) Serum immunoreactive-leptin concentrations in normal weight and obese humans *N. Engl. J. Medicne*, 334:292-295

Consolazio C. F., Matoush L.O., Johnson H.L., Krzywicki J.H., Daws T.A. and Issac G.J. (1969) Effects of high carbohydrate diets on performance and clinical symptomatology after rapid ascent to high altitude. *Fed. Pro.* 28:937.

Cunningham K (1998). Sugar and diet: what is the latest scientific knowledge? *Leatherhead Food RA Food Industry Journal*, 1(1):25-32.

Cunningham KM, Daly J, Horowitz M and Read NW (1991a). Gastrointestinal adaptation to diets of differing fat composition in human volunteers. *Gut*, 32:483- 486.

Cunningham KM, Horowitz M and Read NW (1991b). The effect of short term dietary supplementation with glucose on gastric emptying in humans. *British Journal of Nutrition,* 65:15-19.

Delin CR and Lee TH (1992). Wine and ethanol: issues in nutrition, *Australian and New Zealand Wine Industry Journal,* 7(1):34, 36-38,49,42-43,45.

Desport JC, Gory-Delabaere G, Blanc-Vincent MP, Bachmann B, Beal J, Benamouzig R, Colomb V, Kere D, Melchior JC, Nitenberg G, Raynard B, Schneider S and Senesse P (2003). Standards, options and recommendations for the use of appetite stimulants in oncology (2000). *British Journal of Cancer*, 89(s1):S98-S100.

Dorthy T and Carolyn G (2008) Minerals and food intake, a human perspective. Eds. Ruth B.S., Harris and Richard D Mattes, CRC Press, London. p.337-346.

Edward A. and Abdishakur, A.(2000). A comparison of plasma leptin levels in obese and lean individuals in the United Arab Emirates. *Nutrition Research*, 20(2):157.

Exner, C., Hebebrand, J., Remschmidt,H, Wewetzer, C., Ziegler, A, Herpertz, S., Schweigher, U., Blum,W.F., Preibisch, G., Heldmaier, G. and Klingenspor, M. (2000). Leptin suppresses semi-starvation induced hyperactivity in rats: implications for anorexia nervosa. *Molecular Psychiatry*, 5, 476-481.

Farr, S. A., Banks, W. A., Morley, J. E. (2006). Effects of leptin on memory processing. *Peptides, 27,* 1420-1425.

Friedman J.M. and Halaas J. L. (1998). Leptin and the regulation of body weight in mammals. *Nature*, 395: 765-770.

Glatzel, H. (1968) Physiological aspects of flavour compounds. *Indian Spices* 5:13-21.

Grandjean E, Maga JA and Lorenz K (1955). The effect of altitude on various nervous functions. London, England: *Proceedings of the Royal Society of London*, Ser, B. 143:12-3.

Gustafson DR, McMohan DJ, Morrey J and Nan R (2001) Appetite is not influenced by a unique milk peptide: caesinomacropeptide (CMP). *Appetite*, 36(2)157-163.

Hall WL, Millward DL, Long SJ and Morgan LM (2003). Casien and whey exert different effects on plasma amino acid profiles, gastrointestinal hormone secretion and appetite. *British Journal of Nutrition*, 89(2):239-248.

Havel PJ, Kasim KS, Mueller W, Johnson PR, Gingerich RL, Stern JS (1996). Relationship of plasma leptin to plasma insulin and adiposity in normal weight and overweight women. *Journal of Clin Endocrinal Metabolism*, 81, 4406-4413.

Hearty, A.P., McCarthy, S.N., Kearney, J.M. and Gibney, M.J. (2007). Relationship between attitudes towards healthy eating and dietary behavior, lifestyle and demographic factors in a representative sample of Irish adults. *Appetite*, 48, 1-11.

Heasman, M. and Mellentin, J. (1998). Single ingredients, global markets. *International-Food-Ingredients*, 1, 16-18.

Hirasa K and Takemasa M (Eds.) (1998). Spice Science and Technology. Marcel Dekker, Inc. New York.

Hlebowicz J (2009) Postprandial blood glucose response in relation to gastric emptying and satiety in healthy subjects. *Appetite*, 53(2):249-252.

Karakas, S., Karadag, F., Karul, A.B., Gurgey, O., Gurel, S., Guney, E. and Cildag, O. (2005). Circulating leptin and body composition in chronic obstructive pulmonary disease, *International Journal of Clinical Practice*, 59(10):1167-1170.

Kawada T, Sakabe S, Watanabe T, Yamamoto M and Iwai K (1998). Some pungent principles of spices cause the adrenal medulla to secret catecholamine in anesthesized rats. *Proc. Soc. Exp. Biol. Med.*; 188: 229-233.

Keim, N.L., Stern, J.S. and Havel, P. J. (1998). Relation between circulating leptin concentrations and appetite during a prolonged, moderate energy deficit in women[1-3]. *American Society for Clinical Nutrition*, 78, 794.

Klok MD, Jakobsdottir S and Drent ML (2007). The role of leptin and ghrelin in the regulation of food intake and body weight in humans: a review. *Obesity reviews*, 8(1):21-34.

Konukoglu, D., Turhan, S.M., Ercan, M. and Serin, O. (2004). Relationship between plasma leptin and zinc levels and the effect of insulin and oxidative stress on leptin levels in obese diabetic patients. *Journal of Nutritional Biochemistry*, 15: 757-760.

Krishnamurthy A. (1969). The Wealth of India: A dictionary of materials and Industrial products, *Raw materials*- Vol. VIII, CSIR, New Delhi.

le Roux, C.W. and Bloom, S.R. (2005). Peptide YY, appetite and food intake. *The Nutrition Society*, 64, 213-216.

Little TJ, Horowitz M and Feinle-Bisset C (2007). Modulation by high fat diets of gastrointestinal function and hormones associated with the regulation of energy intake: implications for patho-physiology of obesity. *American Journal of Clinical Nutrition*, 86(3):531-541.

Maffei M, Halaas j, Ravussin E, Pratley RE, Lee GH, Zhang Y, Fei H, Kim H, Lallone R, Ranganathan S, Kern PA and Friedman JM. (1995) Leptin levels in human and rodent: measurement of plasma leptin and ob RNA in obese and weight reduced subjects. *Nat. Med.* 1:1155-1161.

Maga J.A. and Lorenz K. (1972). Effects of altitude on taste thresholds. *Percept Mot Skills*. 34:667-670.

Marciani L, Faulks R, Wickham MSJ, Bush D, Pick B, Wright J, Cox EF, Fillery-Travis A, Gowland PA and Spiller RC (2009). Effect of intra-gastric acid stability of fat emulsions on gastric emptying, plasma lipid profile and post prandial satiety. *British Journal of Nutrition,* 101(6):919-928.

Meyer, C., Robson, D., Rackovsky, N., Nadkarni, V., and Gerich, J. (1997). Role of the kidney in human metabolism. *American Journal of Physiology*, 273 (Endocrinol Metab. 36):E903-E907.

Nadkarni KM, Nadkarni AK. (1976). Indian Materia Medica. Mumbai: Popular Prakashan Pvt. Ltd.

O'Neill, J. (2008). The lifelong benefits of inulin and oligofructose, *Ceral Food World*, 53(2):65-68.

Park, M.I., Camilleri, M., O'Connor, H., Oenning, LV., Burton, D., Stephens,D. and Zinsmeister,A.R. (2007). Effect of different macronutrients in excess on gastric sensory and motor functions and appetite in normal-weight, overweight, and obese humans. *American Society for Nutrition*, 85, 411-418.

Persons RK and Nichols W (2007). Should we use appetite stimulants for malnourished elderly patients? The Journal of Family Practice, 56(9):761-762

Platel K and Srinivasan K. (2000) Influence of dietary spices and their active principles on pancreatic digestive enzymes in albino rats. *Nahrung;* 44: 42-46.

Platel K. and Srinivasan K. (2001). Studies on the influence of dietary spices on food transit time in experimental rats. *Nutr. Res.;* 21: 1309-1314.

Platel, K. and Srinivasan, K. (2004) Digestive stimulant action of spices: A myth or reality? *Indian Journal of Medical Research*. 119:167-179.

Poppitt SD, Eckhardt JW, McGonagle J, Murgatroyd PR, Prentice AM (1996). Short term effects of alcohol consumption on appetite and energy intake. *Physiology and Behavior*, 60(4):1063-1070.

Poppitt SD, McCormack D, Buffenstein R. (1998). Short-term effects of macronutrient preloads on appetite and energy intake in lean women. *Physiol. Behav.* 64(3):279-85.

Prajapati ND, Purohit SS, Sharma AK, TArun kumar (2003). A Handbook of Medicinal Plants: a complete source book, 1st edn. Agrobios (India), Jodhpur.

Premavalli, K. S (2005). 'Ginger as a spice and Flavorant' Chapter 16; In 'Ginger: the genus Zingiber': eds. Ravindran PN and Nirmal Babu, Medicinal and Aromatic Plants – *Industrial Profiles*, CRC Press, USA.

Premavalli, K. S (2007). 'Turmeric: as a spice and Flavorant' Chapter 13; In 'Turmeric: the genus Curcuma'. eds. Ravindran PN, Nirmal Babu and K. Sivaraman Medicinal and Aromatic Plants – Industrial Profiles, CRC Press, USA.

Premavalli, K.S., Wadikar, D.D. and Nanjappa, C. (2009) Comparison of the acceptability ratings of appetizers under laboratory, base level and high altitude field conditions. *Appetite* 53(1): 127-130

Prentice AM and Poppitt SD (1996) Importance of energy density and macronutrients in the regulation of energy intake. *International Journal of Obesity*, 20(Suppl. 2):S18-S23

Raben, A., Agerholm-Larsen, L., Flint, A., Holst, J.J. and Astrup, A. (2003). Meals with similar energy densities but rich in protein, fat, carbohydrate, or alcohol have different effects on energy expenditure and substrate metabolism but not on appetite and energy intake[1-3]. *American Society for Clinical Nutrition*, 77, 91-100.

Ramachandran K, Ambasta SP. (1986). The useful plans of India, New Delhi: Council of Scientific and Industrial Research.

Rao B.S. and Prabhakar E. (1992). Effects of body weight loss and taste on VMH-LH electrical activity of rats. *Physiology and Behavior*, 52:1187-1192.

Ratliff J, Mutungi G, Puglisi MJ, Volek JS and Luz-Fernandez M (2009) Carbohydrate restriction with or without additional dietary cholesterol provided by eggs reduces insulin resistance and plasma leptin without modifying appetite hormones in adult men. *Nutrition Research*, 29(4):262-268.

Rema J, Krishnamoorthy B. (1992) Economic uses of tree spices. *Indian Spices,*; 29 : 2-4.

Ricci MR, Fried SK and Mittleman KD (2000). Acute cold exposure decrease plasma leptin in women. *Metabolism*, 49: 421-423.

Roberfroid MB (2007). Inulin type fructans: functional food ingredients. *Journal of Nutrition*, 137(11):2493S-2502S.

Sarah Garland (1979). The herb and spice book, eds, Felicity Laurd and Nonie Niesewand, Frances Lincoln Publishers Ltd. P-270.

Shastri BN (1962). The Wealth of India: A dictionary of materials and Industrial products, *Raw materials-* Vol. VI, CSIR, New Delhi

Schneider M.A., Deluca V Jr, Grah ST. (1956). The effect of spice ingestion upon stomach. *American J. Gastroenterology*, 26 : 722-32.

Schoeller DA, Cella LK, Sinha MK, Caro JF, (1997). Entrainment of the diurnal rhythm of plasma leptin to meal timings. *Journal of clinicalInvest*, 100:1882-1887

Sharma KN, Jacob HL, Gopal V, Duasharma S, (1977). Nutritional state / taste interactions in food intake: behavioural and physiological evidence for gastric / taste modulation. In: kare MR, Maller O, eds. The chemical senses and nutrition, New York, NY: Academic press Inc: 167-168.

Shirai, Y., Yaku,S. and Suzuki,M. (2004). Metabolic regulation of leptin production in adipocytes : a role of fatty acid synthesis intermediates. *The Journal of Nutritional Biochemistry*, 14, 651-656.

Shukla, V., Singh, S.N., Vats, P., Singh, V.K., Singh, S.B., and Banerjee, P.K. (2005). Ghrelin and leptin levels of sojourners and acclimatized lowlanders at high altitude. *Nutritional Neuroscience*, 8(3):161-165.

Sifton, D.W. (1999). The PDR family guide to natural medicines and healing therapies. pp237-238. Three Rivers Press, New York, USA.

Simon-Schnass I. M. (1992). Nutrition at high altitude, *The Journal of Nutrition*, 122:778-781

Singh, S.B., Sharma, A., Sharma, K.N., and Selvamurthy, W. (1996) Effect of high-altitude hypoxia on feeding responses and hedonic matrix in rats, *Journal of Applied Physiology*, 80(4):1133-1137

Singh, S.B., Sharma, A., Yadav, D.K., Verma, S.S., Srivastava, D.N., Sharma, K.N., and Selvamurthy, W. (1997) High altitude effects on human taste Intensity and Hedonics. *Aviation Space Environmental Medicine*, 68(12):1123-1128.

Singh, S.N., Vats, P., Susi, S., Kumaria, M.M.L., Radheyshyam, Banerjee, P.K., and Sridharan, K. (2001). Leptin levels in normal and overweight Indians. *Indian Journal of Pharmacology*, 33:61

Soliman, N. A. (2001). Effect of experimentally induced diabetes mellitus on serum leptin level and the role of insulin replacement therapy. *The Egyptian Journal of Hospital Medicine*, 3, 190-208.

Srinivasan, K. (2005). Spices as influencers of body metabolism: an overview of three decades of research. *Food Research International*, 38, 77-86.

Stewart, J.J., Wood, M.J., Wood, C.D. and Mims, M.E. (1991). Effects of ginger on motion sickness susceptibility and gastric function. *Pharmacology* 42:111-120.

Stubbs J, Stephen W and Nik MM (2008) Macronutrients feeding behavior and weight control in humans. Eds. Ruth B.S., Harris and Richard D Mattes, CRC Press, London. p.295-316.

Stubbs RJ, van Wyk MC, Johnstone AM, Harbron CG. (1996). Breakfasts high in protein, fat or carbohydrate: effect on within-day appetite and energy balance. *Eur. J. Clin. Nutr.* 50(7):409-17.

Suri S., Salhan A, Singh SN, and Selvamurthy W. (2002). Changes in plasma leptin and zinc status of the women mountaineers at altitude. Defence Science Journal, 52 (2):173-179.

Thampi PSS. (1991). Spices of the Blue Mountains. *Indian Spices*, 28: 2-5.

Vats, P., Singh, S.N., Singh, V.K., Radheyshyam, Upadhyay, T.N., Singh, S.B., and Banerjee, P.K. (2005). Appetite regulatory peptides in Indian Antarctic expeditioners. *Nutritional Neuroscience*, 8(4):233-238.

Wadikar D. D. and Premavall, K.S. (2010). Effect of appetiser administration on plasma leptin level in human volunteers. *Int. J. Food Sci. Nutri.*, doi: 10.3109/09637486.2010.511606

Wadikar D.D., Nanjappa, C. Premavalli, K.S., and Bawa, A. S. (2010). Development of ginger based ready-to-eat appetizers by Response surface methodology. *Appetite*, 55:76-83

Wadikar DD, Majumdar TK, Nanjappa C, Premavalli KS and Bawa AS (2008). Development of pepper based shelf stable appetizers by Response surface methodology (RSM). LWT *Food Sci and Technology*, 41:1400-11

Warrier P. K. (1989). Spices in Ayurveda. *Indian Spices*, 26:11-5.

Westerterp-Plantenga, M.S. (1999). Effect of extreme environments on food intake in human subjects. *Proceedings of the Nutrition Society*; 58:791-798.

Westerterp-Plantenga,M.S. and Verwegen C.R.T. (1999). The appetizing effect of an aperitif in overweight and normal-weight humans. *American Society for Clinical Nutrition*, 69, 205-212.

Yoshioka M, St-Pierre S, Drapeau V, Dionne I, Doucet E, Suzuki M and Tremblay A (1999) Effects of red pepper on appetite and energy intake. *British Journal of Nutrition*, 82:115-123.

Chapter 4

ASSOCIATION BETWEEN SOUP INTAKE AND OBESITY-RELATED PARAMETERS

Motonaka Kuroda,[*,1] *Masanori Ohta,*[2]
Hitomi Hayabuchi[3] *and Masaharu Ikeda*[2]

[1]Institute of Food Sciences and Technologies, Ajinomoto Co., Inc.,
Kawasaki, 210-8681, Japan
[2]Institute of Industrial and Ecological Sciences, University of Occupational
and Environmental Health, Kitakyushu, 807-8555, Japan
[3]Faculty of Human Environmental Science, Fukuoka Women's University,
Fukuoka, 813-8529, Japan

ABSTRACT

In this review, we discuss epidemiological studies examining the correlation between soup intake and obesity-related parameters. Several epidemiological studies conducted in Western countries have shown a negative correlation between soup intake and obesity-related parameters, such as body mass index (BMI), serum cholesterol, and serum triacylglycerol, suggesting that soup intake reduces the risk of obesity in Western countries. After adjusting for confounding factors, multiple linear regression in a cross-sectional study of 103 Japanese men aged 24–75 years showed that the frequency of soup intake was significantly and inversely associated with BMI, waist circumference, and waist-to-hip ratio. On the other hand, no significant associations were found with other metabolic risk factors. These findings suggest a negative correlation between soup intake and obesity-related physical parameters in Japanese men. In addition, after adjusting for confounding factors in a cross-sectional study of 504 Japanese adults aged 20–76 years (103 men and 401 women), multiple regression analysis revealed that the frequency of soup intake was significantly and inversely associated with plasma leptin concentration. These results indicate that soup intake is negatively correlated with obesity-related parameters such as BMI, waist circumference, waist-to-hip ratio, and plasma leptin concentration, suggesting that soup intake may reduce the risk of obesity in Japanese adults.

---

[*] Corresponding author: Motonaka Kuroda. 1-1 Suzuki-cho, Kaswasaki-ku, Kawasaki city, Kanagawa, 210-8681, Japan. TEL: +81-44-223-4158 FAX: +81-44-246-6196. E-mail address: motonaka_kuroda@ajinomoto.com.

1. INTRODUCTION

Obesity is a condition known to increase the risk of cardiovascular disease, diabetes mellitus, stroke, and other chronic diseases (Garrow, 1998; Giding, 1995; Bray, 1996; Kannel and Wilson, 1995; Rimm et al, 1995; Huang et al., 1998; Golay and Felber, 1994). It is a particularly serious problem in Western countries. The prevalence of obesity in Japan, although lower than in Western countries, is increasing, especially in men (Ministry of Health, Labour and Welfare, 2002). The etiology of obesity is multifactorial, but positive energy balance over time is reported to be the primary cause (Ravussin et al., 1988; Bouchard et al., 1990; Grundy, 1998).

Soup is a food which consists mainly of soup stock containing meat, fish, and/or vegetables. Its consumption is common worldwide, and the examples are potage in France, minestrone in Italy, Tom yam goong in Thailand, and *miso* (fermented soybean paste) soup in Japan.

Since it is known that soup is one of low-energy density food, it is expected that soup is effective to improvement of obesity. Many studies have been performed on the association between soup consumption and obesity-related parameters (e.g., BMI, serum triacylglycerol, serum total cholesterol, and serum low density lipoprotein cholesterol (LDL). In this review, we will summarize epidemiological studies on the correlation between soup intake and obesity-related parameters.

2. ASSOCIATION BETWEEN SOUP INTAKE AND OBESITY-RELATED PARAMETERS IN WESTERN COUNTRIES

Several epidemiological studies performed in Western countries have investigated the correlation between soup intake and obesity-related parameters, such as BMI. Bertrais et al. conducted a cross-sectional study of 5037 French adults (Bertrais et al., 2001). The study included 2188 men aged 45-60 years and 2849 women aged 35-60 years who reported twelve 24-h dietary records during a 2-year period. The participants were divided into three group: those who ate soup on 0-2 days out of 6 days were classified as occasional or non-consumers; those who consumed soup 3-4 days out of 6 were defined as regular consumers; and those who consumed soup 5-6 days out of 6 were defined as heavy consumers. In male participants (n=2188), the average amount of soup consumed by occasional or non-consumers (n=1076), regular consumers (n=925), and heavy consumers (n=187) was 13.5 g/day, 70.2 g/day, and 142.6 g/day, respectively. In female participants (n=2849), the respective amount of soup intake by non-consumers (n=1355), regular consumers (n=1304), and heavy consumers (n=190) was 15.5 g/day, 70.7 g/day, and 150.6 g/day. In addition, they conducted a factor analysis to investigate the association between soup intake and obesity-related parameters. The results indicated a higher frequency of BMI > 27 kg/m^2 in occasional and non-soup consumers, with a higher frequency of BMI < 23 kg/m^2 in heavy soup consumers, suggesting that soup intake decreased the risk of obesity in French adults.

In addition, soup intake was inversely associated with BMI in French adults and serum cholesterol concentration in French men. Giacosa and Filiberti conducted a cross-sectional study of 698 Italian adults (Giacosa and Filiberti, 1997). The results indicated that a high prevalence of obesity (13%) was observed among participants who did not eat soup, while obesity among soup eaters was lower (4%). The authors also indicated that soup eaters had a lower incidence of hypercholesterolemia, hypertriglyceridemia, and hypertension. These results and the results obtained by Bertrais et al. suggest a negative correlation between soup intake and the prevalence of obesity in adults in European countries.

Bessa et al. conducted a case-control study in 1675 Portuguese children to investigate the correlation between intake of various fluids and risk of obesity (Bessa et al., 2008). The participants were 833 boys aged 5 to 10 years and 842 girls aged 5 to 10 years. Dietary intake was assessed using a food frequency questionnaire (FFQ) that included information on milk, vegetable soup, cola, ice tea and other sugar-sweetened beverages. The amount of soup consumption in obese girls (318.4± 179.4 g/day) was significantly lower than that in non-obese girls (357.1±197.2 g/day) ($p=0.010$), while there was no significant difference in boys (351.9±202.4 g/day for obese boys; 378.0±201.7 g/day for non-obese boys, $p=0.226$). These results indicate a significant increase in the probability of obesity among girls (odds ratio [OR] = 0.68, CI 95%, 0.48-0.96, $p=0.030$) with low soup consumption (equal or lower than the median) compared to those with high consumption (higher than the median) after adjusting for confounders.

These previous studies suggest that the intake of soup reduces the risk of obesity. In fact, soup intake is considered beneficial in weight reduction programs. An intervention study in 1050 overweight Americans by Jordan et al. demonstrated a significant correlation between the frequency of soup consumption over a period of 10 weeks (Jordan et al., 1981) and weight loss. Participants included 898 females and 159 male subjects. The median age was 37 years. Participants were sorted into four groups matched for age, gender, and percent overweight. Subjects in all four groups were provided with a basic weight control program consisting of a 10-week correspondence course in behavior modification. Each week all participants received a food diary by mail and a description of some behavioral techniques to be used in the coming week. The first intervention group was instructed to eat soup "whenever appropriate but at least four times a week" for the duration of the program; the second intervention group was instructed to eat soup "at least four times a week for lunch" for the duration of the program. The two other groups were controls. Data were analyzed for 472 subjects who continued the program. We obtained the frequency of specific food usage, the number of kcal ingested, and the time and duration of meals from the food diaries. To investigate the correlation between soup intake and weight loss during the program, we conducted a linear regression analysis on the average soup meal per week and the weight loss in 10 weeks. The correlation between the number of soup meals and weight was significant (regression coefficient = 1.2, $p < 0.01$). These results indicate that soup intake can be an efficient aid in weight loss programs.

Foreyt et al. also reported that soup consumption has beneficial effects on weight loss (Foreyt et al., 1986). The authors conducted a 12-week intervention study with 52 weeks of follow-up on 122 US adults aged 21 to 55 years (91 females and 31 males). The subjects were randomly stratified by gender into one of three groups: (a) traditional behavioral weight loss (traditional group), (b) soup with behavioral weight loss (soup group), and (c) non-treatment group (control group). As shown in Table 1, the soup group lost an average of 7.8 kg (woman, 6.3 kg; men, 10.9 kg) and the traditional group lost an average of 8.6 kg (women, 7.1 kg; men, 12.5 kg) at 12 weeks. At 52 weeks, weight loss in the soup group averaged 6.8 kg (women; 5.4 kg; men, 10.0 kg) and those in the traditional group, 6.2 kg (women, 4.2 kg; men, 11.1 kg). These results show that members of the soup group regained an average of 1.0

kg, while members of the traditional group regained an average of 2.4 kg, suggesting that soup intake can help people lose weight and maintain the weight loss.

Table 1. Average weights (kg) at initial, 12-, and 52-week periods[a]

time	soup				traditional				controls		
Women											
initial	90,4	±	15,1		87,7	±	14,9		92,0	±	19,1
12 weeks	84,1	±	14,6	*	80,6	±	14,3	*	93,2	±	19,7
52 weeks	85,0	±	16,0	#	83,5	±	16,3	#	—		
Men											
initial	109,6	±	13,6		106,8	±	9,0		107,5	±	9,7
12 weeks	98,7	±	13,8	*	94,3	±	8,5	*	107,0	±	10,3
52 weeks	99,6	±	19,0		95,7	±	10,4	#	—		

[a]Values expressed as mean ± standard deviation. *$p<0.05$ (1 to 12 week). #$p<0.05$ (1 to 52 week).

Table 2. Food and beverage groups

Food groups	Beverage groups
Confections	Milk
Rice	Coffee and black tea
Breads	Soft drinks
Noodles	Alcoholic beverages
Potatoes	
Fruits	
Meat and meat products	
Fish, including shrimp, squid, and octopus	
Processed and marine products	
Eggs	
Tofu (soybean curd)	
Natto (fermented soybean)	
Cheeses	
Yogurt	
Butter and margarine	
Dressings and mayonnaise	
Vegetables including green-yellow and pickled vegetables	
Seaweeds	
Mushrooms	
Salted products	
Soy sauce and other sauces	
Miso (soybean paste)	
Sugars	
Oils	

These epidemiological and intervention studies conducted in Western countries indicate that soup intake is inversely correlated with obesity-related parameters, such as BMI, body weight, and serum cholesterol, suggesting that soup intake is an efficient means to decrease the risk of obesity.

3. ASSOCIATIONS BETWEEN SOUP INTAKE AND OBESITY-RELATED METABOLIC RISK FACTORS IN JAPANESE MEN

3.1. Introduction

Soup consumption is higher in Asia than it is in Western countries, but there are scant data on the correlation between the frequency of soup intake and the development of obesity-related metabolic risk factors in Japanese men. Reports from Western countries suggest that intake of soup not only promotes weight loss (Jordan et al., 1981; Foreyt et al., 1986) but also reduces the risk of obesity and improves biomarkers of related comorbidities (e.g., high BMI, waist circumference, and waist-to-hip ratio). To examine the association between soup intake and obesity-related metabolic risk factors, we conducted a cross-sectional study in Japanese men (Kuroda et al., 2011).

3.2. Materials and Methods

The Kitakyushu Municipal Health Promotion Committee recruited volunteers to take part in a 12-week lifestyle change program. The objective of the program was to encourage enduring lifestyle changes to prevent lifestyle-related diseases. The program offered us opportunities for detailed analyses of lifestyle factors and their relationship to disease. Because other studies have shown that soup intake is negatively correlated with BMI and promotes weight loss (Jordan et al., 1981; Foreyt et al., 1986), we investigated whether soup intake was negatively associated with obesity-related risk factors (e.g., BMI, waist circumference, waist-to-hip ratio, and cholesterol, triacylglycerol, and glucose levels). The Ethics Committee at the University of Occupational and Environmental Health approved the study protocol, and all participants provided written informed consent.

The program, which ran from 1999 to 2005, involved 236 Japanese men. Those who were taking anti-inflammatory agents or drugs to lower lipids or treat hypertension were excluded, leaving 103 participants between the ages of 24-75 years. The researchers recorded baseline data on metabolic and lifestyle risk factors, soup intake, and dietary patterns.

Data on dietary intake and lifestyle patterns during the preceding month were collected and analyzed using WELL-200 software (version 1, 1999, Fukuda Denshi Co., Tokyo, Japan), a program that includes two semi-quantitative questionnaires. A 74-question FFQ (Takahashi et al., 2001) was used to determine the usual amount and frequency of food and nutrient intakes from 28 food and four beverage groups. Lifestyle factors were measured with a 58-question survey. The food and beverage groups are shown in Table 3. Portion sizes were standardized, e.g., 80 g of meat. Soups included in the questionnaire included miso (fermented soybean paste), sumashi (made with soy sauce), consommé, potage, stew, and

Chinese-style as well as other soups. The mean salt intake from soup (1.2 g per ounce) was based on the Tokushima prefecture nutrition survey (Tokushima prefecture, 1998). Nutrient intake was calculated using the weighted average amount consumed from each food group and a weighted mean food composition table (Takahashi et al., 2001). The nutrient content of each food was based on the 4th edition of the food composition table (1996).

Table 3. Characteristics and nutrient intake in a cohort of Japanese adult males aged 24–75 years old (n=103)[a]

	Median	25th percentile	75th percentile
Age (y)	52,0	44,0	64,5
Height (cm)	165,9	162,1	170,1
Weight (kg)	68,2	63,6	73,4
Body mass index (kg/m^2)	24,4	23,2	26,3
Waist circumference (cm)	87,5	83,8	93,6
Hip circumference (cm)	93,9	90,6	97,0
Waist / hip ratio	0,94	0,91	0,98
Systolic blood pressure (mmHg)	138,0	126,3	149,8
Diastolic blood pressure (mmHg)	84,5	78,3	92,0
Total cholesterol (mg/dL)	200,0	181,5	221,5
HDL-cholesterol (mg/dL)	56,0	47,0	64,0
LDL-cholesterol (mg/dL)	144,0	126,0	172,0
Triacylglycerol (mg/dL)	112,0	75,0	166,0
Glucose (mg/dL)	102,0	98,0	108,5
Glycated hemoglobin (%)	5,0	4,7	5,4
Nutrient intake			
Energy intake (kcal/day)	2061,7	1773,8	2466,3
Carbohydrates (g/day)	265,5	224,3	324,8
Fat (g/day)	54,5	45,0	64,6
Protein (g/day)	70,6	58,2	78,6
Total dietary fiber (g/day)	18,2	13,3	23,4
Alcohol energy (kcal/day)	100,0	0,0	247,5
NaCl (g/day)	12,3	10,7	14,0
Soup intake (times/week)	7,0	2,5	14,0
Energy expenditute (kcal/day)	2038,2	1817,8	2237,9
Current smokers, n (%)	45 (43.7)		

[a]Values expressed as median and inter-quartile range (i.e., 25th and 75th percentiles), except for current smokers (n, %).
HDL: high-density lipoprotein; LDL: low-density lipoprotein.

The questionnaire on physical activity covered the frequency and duration of high- and moderate-intensity and sedentary activities. For example, high-intensity activities included jogging, lifting heavy weights, and moderate-effort bicycling; moderate-intensity activities included carrying light loads and easy biking; sedentary activities included watching television, working on the computer, and reading. Participants also answered questions on work environment, commuting time, hours of sleep, medical history, and any current subjective symptoms. The validation study compared estimates of energy expenditure from the questionnaire and activity records. The correlation between the two sources was 0.65

(Ainsworth et al., 1993). We evaluated physical activity and calculated energy expenditure as previously described (Laporte et al., 1983; Siconolfi et al., 1985; Albanes et al., 1990; Washburn et al., 1991; Ainsworth et al., 1993). Energy expenditure was based on basal metabolism (BM) and reported physical activity. The formula used to calculate BM was

$$BM = BMstandard \times BSA \times 24$$

where BMstandard is the standard value of BM (kcal/m^2/hr), BSA is the body surface area, and 24 is the number of hours/day. BSA was calculated as

$$BSA = BW0.444 \times BH0.663$$

where BW is body weight and BH is body height.

The formula for estimated energy expenditure (EEE) was derived from Rafamantanantsoa et al. (2002):

$$EEE = 1.111 \times BM \times (1 + physical\ activity\ index)$$

For this equation, physical activity was classified into four groups, and assigned the following values: light (1 hour of walking, mostly seated working) = 0.35; moderate (walking for approximately 2 hours, seated while working, and working while standing) = 0.50; relatively heavy (many hours of walking and 1 hour of intense physical work) = 0.75; and heavy (2 hours of intense training or mostly heavy physical work) = 1.00.

We measured body height and waist and hip circumferences to the nearest 0.1 cm with participants standing without shoes. Body weight was measured in light indoor clothes and without shoes to the nearest 0.1 kg. We used a body composition analyzer (BF-220, Tanita, Tokyo, Japan) to determine body fat and weight. BMI was calculated as the body weight in kilograms divided by the square of body height in meters (kg/m^2). After approximately 5 min of rest, we measured systolic and diastolic blood pressures with a mercury sphygmomanometer. Blood pressure was taken at least twice and the mean value was used for analyses.

Participants were asked to fast for more than 12 hours before blood collection. Fasting blood samples were collected in evacuated tubes without additives and centrifuged at 3000 ×g for 10 min at room temperature to separate the serum. Blood samples were also collected in EDTA-coated blood tubes and centrifuged at 3000 ×g for 15 min to obtain plasma. The serum and plasma samples were stored at −25°C until analysis.

All data were analyzed using STATVIEW (version 5, 1998, SAS Institute, Inc., Cary, NC, USA). Variables that were not normally distributed (e.g., BMI) were expressed as medians with 25th and 75th percentiles. We performed Spearman's rank correlation analysis on the frequency of soup intake, which was not normally distributed. Multiple linear regression analysis was used to examine the associations between soup intake and metabolic risk factors. Given the wide age range of participants, we also performed age-stratified analyses.

After adjusting for age, current smoking (no or yes [one or more cigarettes per day]), energy intake (kcal/d), energy from alcohol consumption (kcal/d), and energy expenditure (kcal/d), we used partial regression coefficients (σ) to analyze BMI, waist circumference, and waist-to-hip ratio. We also calculated the σ for soup intake to analyze associations with blood pressure, total cholesterol, LDL, high density lipoprotein cholesterol (HDL), triacylglycerol, glucose, and glycated hemoglobin. Adjustments were made for age, current smoking (no/yes), energy intake, energy from alcohol consumption, energy expenditure, and BMI. All results were considered significant at $P < 0.05$.

3.3. Results and Discussion

The baseline characteristics of the participants (n = 103) and age-stratified groups are shown in Table 3. The median frequency of soup intake was 7.0 times per week. The median waist circumference was 87.5 cm and median waist-to-hip ratio was 0.94 cm. The median BMI was 24.4 kg and was higher than the mean BMI (23.5 kg/m^2) for Japanese adult males (Ministry of Health, Labour, and Welfare, 2002). The median total cholesterol level of 200.0 mg/dL was similar to the average value (199.6 mg/dL) for Japanese adult males. In addition, the median systolic (138.0 mmHg) and diastolic (84.5 mmHg) blood pressures were higher than the average systolic (133.9 mmHg) and diastolic (82.0 mmHg) blood pressures for Japanese adult males. Among all participants, the ratios of energy intake from fat (23.7%), carbohydrates (52.7%), and protein (70.1 g) were within the ranges recommend in Japanese dietary guidelines (i.e., 20–25% for fat, > 50% for carbohydrates, and > 70 g/day for protein).

Table 4 shows the associations between the frequency of soup intake and metabolic risk factors. Spearman's rank correlation analysis suggested a negative association between soup intake and waist-to-hip ratio. No correlations with other variables were observed. Multiple regression analysis showed a significant inverse association between the frequency of soup intake and BMI (p = –0.106, P = 0.040), waist circumference (p = –0.340, P = 0.024), and waist-to-hip ratio (p = –0.003, P = 0.0010) after adjusting for age, current smoking, energy intake, energy from alcohol intake, and energy expenditure. Frequency of soup intake was not significantly associated with other metabolic risk factors (e.g., triacylglycerol, glucose, glycated hemoglobin, total cholesterol, HDL-C, or LDL-C).

Previous studies in Western countries report an inverse association between soup intake and BMI (Bertrais et al., 2001; Giacosa and Filberti, 1997; Bessa et al., 2008), suggesting that soup intake reduces the risk of obesity. The results in this study also indicate a negative association between soup intake and obesity-related biomarkers in Japanese men. Results revealed a mean frequency of soup intake of 8.2 times/week, or average consumption of approximately 1222 g/week based on a usual soup volume (mainly miso soup) of approximately 150 g (Murakami et al., 2007). This value exceeds that (344.4 g/week) reported in a study in France (Bertrais et al. 2001).

The age-stratified analysis (Table 4) showed an inverse correlation between the frequency of soup intake and BMI, waist circumference, and waist-to-hip ratio in younger and older participants. Several prior studies have suggested an inverse relationship between soup intake and BMI. However, this report is believed to be the first to show a negative correlation between soup intake and waist circumference and waist-to-hip ratio.

Table 4. Results of Sperman's rank correlation analysis and multiple regression analyses for the association between frequency of soup intake and various metabolic risk factors in a cohort of Japanese adult males aged 24–75 years old[a]

	Spearman's rank correlation Correlation Coefficient	P-value	Multiple regression analysis Partial regression coefficient	P-value
BMI (kg/m^2)[b]	−0.093	0,347	−0.106	0,040
Waist circumference (cm)[b]	−0.135	0,172	−0.34	0,024
Waist / hip ratio[b]	−0.236	0,017	−0.003	0,0010
Systolic blood pressure (mmHg)[c]	−0.014	0,890	0.021	0,944
Diastolic blood pressure (mmHg)[c]	−0.007	0,946	−0.021	0,916
Total cholesterol (mg/dL)[c]	0,114	0,298	0,390	0,528
HDL-cholesterol (mg/dL)[c]	0,079	0,427	0,202	0,460
LDL-cholesterol (mg/dL)[c]	0,083	0,400	0,188	0,763
Triacylglycerol (mg/dL)[c]	0,114	0,248	3,028	0,185
Glucose (mg/dL)[c]	−0.056	0,574	0,077	0,870
Glycated hemoglobin (%)[c]	0,014	0,887	0,0004	0,976

[a]The oartial regression coefficient and P-values are for independent variables in the multiple regression analysis.
[b]Adjusted for age, energy intake, alcohol intake, current smoking (yes/no), and estimated energy expenditure in multiple regression analyses.
[c]Adjusted for age, energy intake, alcohol intake, current smoking (yes/no), estimated energy expenditure, and BMI in multiple regression analyses.
HDL: high-density lipoprotein; LDL: low-density lipoprotein.

Whether soup intake has a direct or indirect influence on obesity remains unclear. More detailed studies are needed to identify the causes of the negative correlation between the frequency of soup intake and obesity-related parameters, but several factors seem to be plausible.

Prior studies suggest that soup consumption reduces energy intake by increasing satiety (Rolls et al., 1990; Himaya and Louis-Sylvestre, 1998; Mattes, 2005; Flood and Rolls, 2007). Thus, caloric displacement might account for improvements in obesity-related parameters. Since the main soup consumed in this study was miso soup, another possibility relates to the role of food components in soups contained in miso (fermented soybean paste). Kondohnand and Torii (Kondoh and Torii, 2008) found that intake of monosodium glutamate suppressed weight gain and fat deposition in male Spague-Dawley rats, and that intake of isoflavone improved obesity-related parameters in rodents (Kim et al., 2006; Davis et al., 2007). Jenkins et al. (Jenkins et al., 2002; McVeigh et al., 2006; Taku et al, 2007) found similar results in humans. These studies suggest that the association between soup intake and obesity-related parameters is related to the components contained in miso, such as monosodium glutamate and isoflavone.

Several studies conducted in European countries have demonstrated an inverse association between soup consumption and serum cholesterol levels (Bertrais et al., 2001; Giacosa and Filiberti, 1997), triacylglycerol (Giacosa and Filiberti, 1997), and blood pressure (Giacosa and Filiberti, 1997). However, there were no significant relationships between soup consumption and such obesity-related risk factors as blood pressure, triacylglycerol, glucose, glycated hemoglobin, and serum cholesterol. These inconsistencies might be due to genetic influences, differences in habitual dietary patterns, or the ages of study participants. Soup consumption can be associated with higher salt intake, but this study found no correlation between the frequency of soup intake and blood pressure. However, the Spearman's rank correlation analysis indicated a positive correlation between soup consumption and salt intake (correlation coefficient = 4.47, $P < 0.0001$). Further epidemiological studies and clinical interventions are needed to clarify the relationship between soup intake and blood pressure.

Our study (Kuroda et al., 2010) was the first to show associations between soup intake and obesity-related parameters in Japanese adult males, but outcomes must be considered in light of certain limitations of the study. Participants might have had preexisting metabolic risk factors that motivated them to take part in the lifestyle modification program. The study's cross-sectional design also precludes assessment of a causal association between soup intake and obesity-related parameters.

4. ASSOCIATIONS BETWEEN SOUP INTAKE AND PLASMA LEPTIN LEVELS IN JAPANESE ADULTS

4.1. Introduction

As indicated in chapter 2, epidemiological studies conducted in Western countries show a negative correlation between intake of soups and obesity-related biomarkers, such as serum cholesterol (Bertrais et al., 2001). They also show an inverse association with obesity-related physical biomarkers, such as BMI, waist circumference, and waist-to-hip ratio in Japanese adult males (Kuroda et al., 2010a). However, few data exist on the effect of soup intake on hormones, such as leptin, in Japanese adults.

Leptin, a peptide hormone released from white adipose tissue, acts in the hypothalamus to reduce appetite and food intake, and increase energy expenditure (Mora, and Pessin, 2002; Margetic et al., 2002; Seufert, 2004). Higher leptin levels in obese people indicate the presence of leptin resistance (Ahima, and Filer, 2000; El-Haschimi, and Lehnert, 2003). Studies have also shown a strong positive correlation between serum leptin levels and BMI in middle-aged Finnish males (Haffner et al., 1999), Swedish adults (Soderberg et al, 1999), African American adults (Racette et al., 1997), U.S. adults (Considine et al., 1996 ; Ganji et al., 2009; Beasley et al., 2009), Japanese-American adults (McNeely et al., 1999), middle-aged Japanese, males and females (Mabuchi et al., 2005), overweight Japanese men (Miyatake et al., 2004), obese Japanese children and adolescents (Ikezaki et al., 2002), and Chinese adolescents (Zhang et al., 2009).

Nonetheless, the same degree of adiposity produces wide variations in leptin levels (Considine et al., 1996), indicating that genetic and environmental factors play a role in leptin expression. The positive correlation between leptin levels and subsequent weight gain (Chu et al., 2001) suggest that leptin is a primary marker of obesity.

The correlation between the intake of food or nutrients and blood leptin levels has been explored in many epidemiological studies. Several Western reports failed to find significant associations between nutrient intake and blood leptin concentrations (Miller et al., 2001; Yannakoulia et al., 2003), but data show a significant positive association between leptin and the intake of total fat and polyunsaturated fatty acids in middle-aged American men with a BMI < 25 kg/m^2 (Chu et al., 2001). A positive association has also been reported between fat intake and serum leptin levels in postmenopausal breast cancer survivors (Wayne et al.,

2008). Conversely, a Western study by Wayne et al. (Wayne et al., 2008) found no significant correlation between dietary fiber intake and blood leptin concentrations, and Murakami et al. (Murakami et al., 2007) demonstrated an inverse association between dietary fiber intake and leptin levels in young Japanese women.

The types of food consumed also affect leptin levels. Western studies have reported an inverse association between leptin levels and consumption of whole grains (Jensen et al., 2006), vegetables (Ambroszkiewicz et al., 2004), and fish (Winnicki et al., 2002). They also demonstrate a significant positive correlation between the intake of meat and serum leptin concentrations (Aeberli et al., 2006). Similarly, an inverse association has been found between intakes of vegetables and pulses and leptin concentrations in young Japanese women (Murakami et al., 2007a). Data on the association between soup intake and leptin levels in Japanese adults are scarce. A cross-sectional study on the correlation between soup intake and plasma leptin concentration was conducted in this population to address this gap.

4.2. Methods

The Kitakyushu Municipal Health Promotion Committee conducted a 12-week lifestyle modification program focused on the prevention of lifestyle-related diseases. Subjects included adult residents of Kitakyushu City in Fukuoka, Japan. A total of 1040 subjects participated in the program between 1999 and 2005 (n = 1040). Baseline data on leptin, soup intake, and dietary habits collected from 504 individuals (103 males aged 24-75 years and 401 females aged 20-76 years) were used for the analysis. The study protocol was approved by the Ethics Committee of the University of Occupational and Environmental Health, and all subjects provided written informed consent.

We assessed dietary patterns and lifestyle during the preceding month using WELL-200 software (Fukuda Denshi Co., Tokyo, Japan) as described in the previous chapter. Participants fasted for more than 12 hours prior to blood collection. Fasting blood samples were collected in EDTA blood tubes and centrifuged at 3000 ×g for 15 min to obtain plasma. Plasma samples were stored at $-25°C$ until analysis. Leptin concentrations were analyzed using a commercial radioimmunoassay kit (Linco Research, St. Charles, MO, USA). Body height was measured to the nearest 0.1 cm with the subjects standing without shoes. Subjects wore light indoor clothing for body weight measurements to the nearest 0.1 kg. BMI was calculated as body weight in kilograms divided by the square of body height in meters (kg/m^2).

Data were analyzed with the STATVIEW version 5 statistical package (SAS Institute, Inc., Cary, NC, USA). All values were expressed as means ± standard deviations. Calculations were performed on the baseline data of subjects by tertile of plasma leptin concentration. We used one-way analysis of variance (ANOVA) with Bonferroni's post hoc test to measure differences in each tertile. Multiple regression analysis was used to examine the association of macronutrient intakes with plasma leptin concentrations. The partial regression coefficients for soup intake were calculated after adjusting for the following variables: gender and age (Model 1); current smoking, alcohol consumption, and energy expenditure in addition to factors in Model 1 (Model 2); fat intake in addition to factors in Model 2 (Model 3); energy intake in addition to factors in Model 3 (Model 4); and BMI in addition to variables in Model 4 (Model 5).

Table 5. Background data of the participants with tertile of plasma leptin concentration[a]

	Total			T1 (Low group)			T2 (Middle group)			T3 (High group)		
Men (n=103)												
n	103			35			34			34		
Age	52,6	±	12,5	53,7	±	11,1	51,2	±	13,7	52,9	±	12,9
Height (cm)	166,5	±	6,5	166,2	±	5,7	167,4	±	5,8	165,9	±	7,8
Weight (kg)	69,3	±	9,1	62,9	±	5,4[A]	70,3	±	7,6[B]	74,9	±	9,7[C]
Body mass index (kg/m^2)	25,0	±	2,9	22,8	±	1,5[A]	25,1	±	2,2[B]	27,2	±	3,0[C]
Plasma leptin concentration (ng/ml)	4,61	±	2,60	2,27	±	0.52[A]	4,11	±	0.6[B]	7,53	±	2.33[C]
Nutrient intake												
Energy intake (kcal/day)	2156,6	±	543,4	2112,1	±	599,6	2189,4	±	520,1	2169,6	±	518,1
Carbohydrates (g/day)	284,4	±	84,5	266,4	±	85,8	293,1	±	83,9	294,3	±	83,0
Fat (g/day)	57,0	±	18,1	54,6	±	13,4	61,9	±	24,0	54,5	±	17,1
Protein (g/day)	70,1	±	16,7	70,9	±	15,9	70,0	±	18,6	69,5	±	15,8
Total dietary fiber (g/day)	18,5	±	6,6	19,5	±	6,2	18,3	±	7,1	17,6	±	6,4
Alcohol energy (kcal/day)	202,0	±	297,5	255,1	±	417,4	154,9	±	191,1	194,4	±	229,1
Soup intake (times/week)	8,15	±	5,25	8,83	±	4,96	8,62	±	6,27	6,97	±	4,28
Energy expenditute (kcal/day)	2032,2	±	263,4	2133,7	±	183.1[A]	2022,3	±	295.4[AB]	1937,5	±	268.8[B]
Current smokers (ratio: %)	45 (43.7)			15 (42.9)			15 (44.1)			15 (44.1)		
Women (n=401)												
n	401			134			134			133		
Age	53,9	±	11,3	53,1	±	11,4	53,9	±	12,4	54,8	±	9,9
Height (cm)	154,2	±	5,5	154,5	±	5,4	153,9	±	4,9	154,0	±	6,2
Weight (kg)	55,7	±	9,0	50,0	±	5.3[A]	55,1	±	6.3[B]	62,0	±	10.2[C]
Body mass index (kg/m^2)	23,4	±	3,4	20,9	±	2.0[A]	23,2	±	2.4[B]	26,1	±	3.6[C]
Plasma leptin concentration (ng/ml)	8,57	±	4,21	4,53	±	1.20[A]	7,96	±	0.87[B]	13,22	±	3.58[C]
Nutrient intake												
Energy intake (kcal/day)	1906,5	±	432,1	1838,7	±	391,4	1939,6	±	451,3	1938,4	±	448,2
Carbohydrates (g/day)	263,5	±	65,6	255,4	±	60,0	267,2	±	66,3	267,8	±	70,0
Fat (g/day)	58,0	±	17,3	55,8	±	17,5	57,8	±	16,5	60,5	±	17,8
Protein (g/day)	69,6	±	14,9	67,7	±	14,5	70,6	±	15,5	70,4	±	14,9
Total dietary fiber (g/day)	21,8	±	7,5	22,2	±	7,3	21,9	±	7,7	21,2	±	7,5
Alcohol energy (kcal/day)	45,6	±	112,0	42,2	±	85,2	58,6	±	161,9	35,2	±	63,4
Soup intake (times/week)	7,45	±	5,13	7,77	±	5.18[AB]	8,09	±	5.38[A]	6,42	±	4.66[B]
Energy expenditute (kcal/day)	1706,4	±	204,2	1748,9	±	185.4[A]	1727,9	±	208.2[A]	1642,0	±	203.8[B]
Current smokers (ratio: %)	19 (4.7)			10 (7.5)			5 (3.7)			4 (3.0)		

[a]Values expressed as mean ± s.d. except for current smokers.
[b]Values with different superscript indicate significantly different ($p<0.05$) as a result of ANOVA with Bonferoni's post-hoc test.

4.3. Results and Discussion

Table 5 shows baseline data of participants by tertile of plasma leptin concentration. The average frequency of soup consumption for all subjects was 7.59 times per week. The mean plasma leptin concentration was 7.76 ng/mL. For men, it was 4.61 ng/mL; for women, 8.57 ng/mL. Average daily energy intake for all subjects was 1957.6 kcal. Mean daily intake of protein and fat was 69.7 g and 57.8 g, respectively. Mean daily intake of carbohydrates and dietary fiber was 267.8 g and 21.1 g, respectively. Body weight and BMI differed significantly between males and females. Higher plasma leptin levels were associated with higher body weight and BMI. Soup intake in the T2 subgroup of women was significantly higher than that in T3 subgroup. In the T1 subgroup of men, energy expenditure was significantly higher than it was in the T3 subgroup. In the T1 and T2 subgroups of women, energy expenditure was significantly higher than it was in the T3 subgroup.

Table 6 shows the independent associations between the frequency of soup intake and plasma leptin concentrations. After adjusting for gender and age, there was a significant inverse association between the frequency of soup intake and plasma leptin concentrations (Model 1; p = –0.076, P = 0.026). Significant inverse associations between soup intake and plasma leptin levels were also seen in Model 2 (p = –0.083, P = 0.013), Model 3 (p = –0.083, P = 0.013), Model 4 (p = –0.089, P = 0.009) and Model 5 (p = –0.054, P = 0.041).

Table 6. Multiple regression analysis on association between soup intake and plasma leptin concentration[a]

	Partial regression coefficient	Adjusted R^2	P-value
Model 1[b]	-0,076	0,144	0,026
Model 2[c]	-0,083	0,195	0,013
Model 3[d]	-0,083	0,203	0,013
Model 4[e]	-0,089	0,202	0,009
Model 5[f]	-0,054	0,536	0,041

[a]Partial regression coefficient and P-values are for independent variables in the multiple regression analysis.
[b]Model 1 adjusted for gender and age.
[c]Model 2 adjusted for variables in Model 1 and current smoking (yes/no), alcohol intake, and energy expenditure.
[d]Model 3 adjusted for variables in Model 2 and fat intake.
[e]Model 4 adjusted for variables in Model 3 and energy intake.
[f]Model 5 adjusted for variables in Model 4 and BMI.

Prior studies in Western countries have shown inverse associations between soup intake and BMI and fat intake (Bertrais et al., 2001; Giagosa and Filiberti, 1997), suggesting that soup intake reduces the risk of obesity. Soup consumption in Japan is estimated to be greater than it is in Western countries. The usual volume of Japanese soup (mainly miso soup) consumed is approximately 150 g, with an intake of approximately 1100 g per week. This amount is much greater than the 344 g/week of soup intake reported in a study in France (Bertrais et al., 2001). Findings in this study also suggest that soup intake may play a role in reducing obesity in Japan.

Results indicate an inverse association between the frequency of soup intake and plasma leptin concentrations after adjusting for fat intake (Model 3), energy intake (Model 4), and BMI (Model 5). These findings suggest an independent relation between soup consumption and plasma leptin concentrations. It remains unclear whether soup intake has a direct or indirect influence on plasma leptin levels.

Earlier studies suggest that soup consumption helps decrease energy intake by evoking feelings of satiety (Rolls et al., 1990; Himaya and Louis-Sylvestre, 1998; Mattes, 2005; Flood and Rolls, 2007). The lower leptin levels in this study might be due to satiety induced reductions in energy intake. However, the significant negative correlation between soup intake and plasma leptin concentrations, even after adjusting for energy intake (Table 6, Model 4), is likely influenced by other factors as well.

Another possibility relates to the role of food components in soups contained in miso (fermented soybean paste), since the main soup consumed in this study was miso soup. Kodoh and Torii (Kondoh and Torii, 2008) reported that intake of monosodium glutamate suppressed weight gain, fat deposition, and plasma leptin levels in male Spague-Dawley rats. In addition, previous studies found that the intake of isoflavone improved obesity-related parameters in rodents (Kim et al., 2006; Davis et al., 2007) and in humans (Jenkins et al., 2002; McVeigh et al., 2006; Taku et al, 2007). These studies suggest that the association between the soup intake and obesity-related parameters is related to the components contained in miso, such as monosodium glutamate and isoflavone. However, more detailed studies are needed to identify the cause of the effect. This is the first report to show an association between soup intake and plasma leptin levels in Japanese adults. However, its cross-sectional design precludes the ability to assign causation, and future studies should be designed to avoid this limitation.

5. GENERAL DISCUSSION

It remains unclear whether soup intake influences obesity-related parameters directly or indirectly. Since previous studies have indicated that soup consumption contributes to a decrease in energy intake by evoking feelings of satiety (Rolls et al., 1990; Himaya and Louis-Sylvestre, 1998; Mattes, 2005; Flood and Rolls, 2007), one possibility is that obesity-related parameters improved because energy intake decreased as a result of the satiety-inducing effects of soup. Himaya and Louis-Sylvestre (Himaya and Louis-Sylvestre, 1998) compared the influence of three solid/liquid preloads to no-preload on hunger rating and energy intake of lunch in 12 lean men (average BMI = 21.9 kg/m^2) and 10 overweight men (average BMI = 27.9 kg/m^2) aged 18-24 years). The preloads (vegetables and water, strained vegetable soup, chunky soup) were of the same composition (energy = 95 kcal) and volume but differed in the distribution of nutrients between the liquid and the solid. As shown in Figure 1, hunger ratings were reduced by the preloads, and there was a significantly greater suppression of hunger after the chunky soup than after the vegetables and water ($p < 0.01$). As shown in Figure 2, chunky soup significantly reduced the energy intake of lunch compared to the no-preload condition in both the lean and overweight groups ($p < 0.05$), and significantly reduced the energy intake of lunch compared to vegetable and water in the overweight group ($p<0.05$). These results indicate that the preload with chunky soup can reduce energy intake, suggesting that it has a satiating effect.

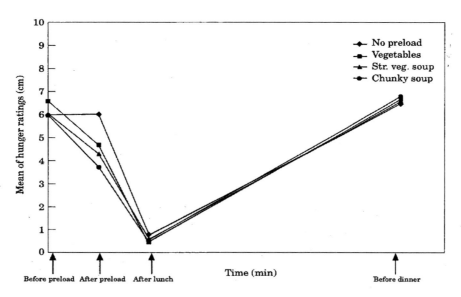

Figure 1. Hunger rating as a function of time and nature of preload. Str. veg. soup, strained vegetable soup.

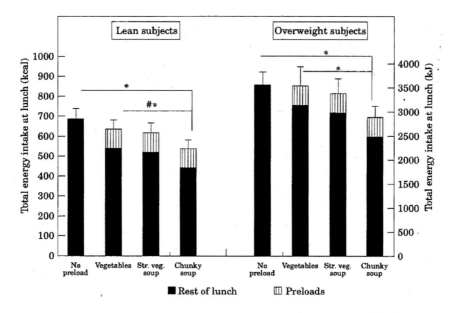

Figure 2. Energy intakes at lunch as a function of nature of preload. The data for lean subjects and overweight subjects are shown separately. #*Just failed to reach significance; *$p<0.05$. Str. veg. soup, strained vegetable soup.

In addition, Flood and Rolls (Flood and Rolls, 2007) investigated the effect of different forms of soup preloads on meal energy intake, including broth and vegetables served separately, chunky vegetable soup, chunky pureed vegetable soup, or pureed vegetable soup.

The subjects were 30 normal weight men and 30 normal weight women. As shown in Figure 3, soup consumption significantly reduced total meal energy intake (preload + test meal) compared to having no soup (p<0.0001). The type of soup had no significant effect on total meal energy intake. These results indicate that soup preload can reduce the energy intake, suggesting that it has a satiating effect.

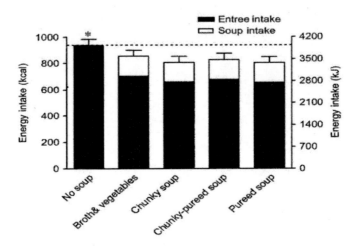

Figure 3. Mean (±SEM) energy intake at lunch (soup and entrée intake) for women and men combined (n=60). Subjects consumed significantly less total energy at lunch when soup was eaten as a first course, compared to when no soup was eaten *(p<0.0001).

Epidemiological studies have also shown that soup intake is inversely correlated with energy intake. Bertrais et al. (Bertrais et al., 2001) found an inverse correlation between soup intake and total energy intake in women (p < 0.02), and an inverse correlation with fat intake in both men (p = 0.05) and women (p = 0.0001). Interestingly, there was a positive correlation between soup intake and carbohydrate intake in both men (p = 0.001) and women (p = 0.03). These results indicate that soup intake decreases energy and fat intake by its satiating effect.

The cause of the satiating effect of soup is unclear. However, several reasons can be considered. One possibility is the low energy density of soup. In a cross-sectional study of 1136 female Japanese women aged 18-22 years, Murakami et al. (Murakami et al., 2007a) reported an inverse association between dietary energy density and BMI (p = 0.004) and waist circumference (p < 0.0001). Therefore, it is possible that the satiating effect of soup is due to its low energy density.

In addition, data show a significant increase in plasma cholecystokinin levels after soup intake, suggesting that some of the satiating effect of soup is mediated by elevated endogenous cholecystokinin (Nolan et al., 2003). However, in this study, the plasma cholecystokinin level increased when the participants consumed approximately 800 mL of soup. Therefore, the contribution of cholecystokinin to the satiating effect should be carefully considered. Although several hypotheses can be proposed for the mechanism of the association between soup intake and obesity-related parameters, further studies are needed to confirm the mechanism.

CONCLUSION

Epidemiological studies carried out in Western countries indicate an inverse correlation between soup intake and obesity-related parameters such as BMI, serum cholesterol, and serum triacylglycerol. In addition, studies performed in Japan also indicate that soup intake is inversely associated with obesity-related parameters, such as BMI, waist circumference, waist-to-hip ratio, and plasma leptin. These results indicate that soup intake reduces the risk of obesity.

REFERENCES

Aeberli I, Molinari L, Spinas G, Lehmann R, I'Allemand D, Zimmermann M. (2006). Dietary intakes of fat and antioxidant vitamins are predictors of subclinical inflammation in overweight Swiss children. *Am. J. Clin. Nutr.*, 84, 748-755.

Ainsworth BE, Leon AS, Richardson M T, Jacobs DR, Paffenbarger, RS Jr. (1993). Accuracy of the college alumnus physical activity questionnaire. *J. Clin. Epidemiol.*, 46, 1403-1411.

Albanes D, Conway JM, Taylor PR, Moe PW, Judd J. (1990). Validation and comparison of eight physical activity questionnaires. *Epidemiology*, 1, 65-71.

Ambroszkiewicz J, Laskowska-Klita T, Klemarczyk W. (2004). Low serum leptin concentration in vegetarian prepubertal children. *Roczniki Akademii Medycznej w Bialymstoku* 49, 103-105.

Ashima RS, Filer JS. (2000). Leptin. *Annu. Rev. Physiol.*, 62, 413-437.

Beasley JM, Ange BA, Anderson CA., Miller ER, Holbrook JT, Appel LJ. (2009). Characteristics associated with fasting appetite hormones (obestatin, ghrelin, and leptin). *Obesity*, 17, 349-354.

Bertrais S, Galan P, Renault N, Zarebska M, Preziosi P, Hercberg S. (2001). Consumption of soup and nutritional intake in French adults. *J. Hum. Nutr. Dietet.*, 14, 121-128.

Bessa M, Valente H, Cordeiro T, Padrao P, Moreira A, Lopes C, Moreira P. (2008). Fluid intake and overweight risk in children. *Acta Med. Port.* [in Portuguese] 21, 161-170.

Bouchard C, Tremblay A, Despres JP, Nsadeau A, Lupien PJ, Theriault G, Dussault J, Moorjani S, Pinaults S, Fournier G. (1990). The response to long-term overfeeding in identical twins. *New Engl. J. Med.* 322, 1477-1482.

Bray GA. (1996). Health hazards of obesity. *Endocrinol. Metab. Clin. Nutr. Am.* 25, 907-919.

Chu NF, Stampfer MJ, Spiegelman D, Rifai N, Hotamisligil GS, Rimm EB. (2001). Dietary and lifestyle factors in relation to plasma leptin concentrations among normal weight and overweight men. *Int. J. Obes.*, 25, 106-114.

Chu NF, Spiegelman D, Yu J, Rifai N, Hotamisligil GS, Rimm EB. (2001). Plasma leptin concentrations and four-year weight gain among US men. *Int. J. Obes. Relat. Metab. Disord.*, 25, 346-353.

Considine RV, Sinha MK, Heiman ML, Kriauciunas A., Stephens TW, and Nyce MR. (1996). Serum immunoreactive-leptin concentrations in normal-weight and obese humans. *New Eng. J. Med.*, 334, 292-295.

Davis J, Higginbotham A, O'Connor T, Moustaid-Moussa N, Tebbe A, Kim YC, Cho KW, Shay N, Adler S, Peterson R, Banz W. (2007). Soy proteen and isoflavones influence adiposity and development of metabolic syndrome in obese male ZDF rats. *Ann. Nutr. Metab.*, 51, 42-52.

El-Haschimi K, Lehnert H. (2003). Leptin resistance- or why leptin fails to work in obesity. *Exp. Clin. Endocrinol. Diabetes*, 111, 2-7.

Flood JE, Rolls BJ. (2007). Soup preloads in a variety of forms reduce meal energy intake. *Appetite* 49, 626-634.

Foreyt JP, Reeves RS, Darnell LS, Wohlleb JC, Gotto AM. (1986). Soup consumption as a behavioral weight loss strategy. *J. Amer. Diet .Assoc.* 86, 524-526.

Ganji V, Kafai MR, McCarthy E. (2009). Serum leptin concentrations are not related to dietary patterns but are related to sex, age, body mass index, serum triglycerol, serum insulin, and plasmaglucose in the US population. *Nutr. Metab.* 6, 3-12.

Garrow JS. (1988). Health implications of obesity. In: *Obes Related Diseases*. Churchill Livingstone: London; pp1-16.

Giacosa A, Filiberti R. (1997). Rilevamento dei comportamenti alimentari sul terrotorio. *Med. Doctor* 8, 40-45.

Giding SS. (1995). A perspective on obesity. *Am. J. Med. Sci.* 310(Suppl1), S68-71.

Golay A, Felber JP. (1994). Evolution from obesity to diabetes. *Diabetes Metab.* 20, 3-14.

Grundy SM. (1998). Multifactorial causation of obesity: implications for prevention. *Am. J. Clin. Nutr.* 67(Suppl1), 563S-572S.

Haffner SM, Mykkanen L, Rainwater DL, Karhapaa P, Laakso M. (1999). Is leptin concentration associated with the insulin resistance syndrome in nondiabetic men? *Obes. Res.*, 7, 164-169.

Health Promotion and Nutrition Division, Health Service Bureau, Ministry of Health and Welfare. (1996). Recommended Dietary Allowances for the Japanese, 5th revision, Dai-ichi shuppan, Tokyo.

Himaya A, Louis-Sylvestre J. (1998). The effect of soup on satiation. *Appetite*, 30, 199-210.

Huang Z, Willett WC, Manson JE, Rosner B, Stampfer MJ, Speizer FE, Colditz GA. (1998). Body weight, weight change, and risk for hypertension in women. *Ann. Intern. Med.* 128, 81-88.

Ikezaki A, Hosoda H., Ito K, Iwama S, Miura N, Matsuoka H. et al. (2002). Fasting plasma ghrelin levels are negatively correlated with insulin resistance and PAI-1, but not with leptin, in obese children and adolescents. *Diabetes*, 51, 3408-3411.

Iso H, Date C, Noda H, Yoshimura T, Tamakoshi A. (2005). Frequency of food intake and estimated nutrient intake among men and women: The JACC study. *J. Epidemiol.* 15(Suppl1), S24-S42.

Jenkins DJ, Kendall CW, Jackson CJ, Connelly PW, Parker T, Faulkner D, Vidgen E, Cunnane SC, Leiter LA, Josse RG. (2002). Effects of high- and low- isoflavone soyfoods on blood lipids, oxidized LDL, homocysteine, and blood pressure in hyperlipidemic men and women. *Am. J. Clin. Nutr.*, 76, 365-372.

Jensen MK, Koh-Banerjee P, Franz M, Sampson L, Gronbaek M, Rimm EB. (2006). Whole grain, bran, and germ in relation to homocysteine and markers of glycemic control, lipids, and inflammation. *Amer. J. Clin. Nutr.*, 83, 275-283.

Jordan HA, Levitz LS, Utgoff KL, Lee HL. (1981). Role of food characteristics in behavioral change and weight loss. *J. Amer. Dietet. Assoc*, 79, 24-29.

Kagawa Nutrition University Publishing, (1994) Food composition table (4th edition), edited by Kagawa Nutrition University Publishing.

Kannel WB, Wilson PW. (1995). An update on coronary risk factors. *Med. Clin. Nutr. Am.* 79, 951-971.

Kim HK, Nelson-Dooley C, La-Fera MA, Yang JY, Zhang W, Duan J, Hartzell DL, Hamrick MW, Baile CA. (2006). Genistein decreases food intake, body weight, and fat pad weight and causes adipose tissue apotosis in ovariectomized female mice. *J. Nutr.* 136, 409-414.

Kondoh T, Torii K. (2008). MSG intake suppresses weight gain, fat deposition, and plasma leptin levels in male Spague-Dawley rats. *Physiol. Behav.* 95, 135-144.

Kuroda M, Ohta M, Okufuji T, Takigami C, Eguchi M, Hayabuchi H, Ikeda M. (2011). Frequency of soup intake is inversely associated with body mass index, waist circumference and waist-to-hip ratio, but not with other metabolic risk factors in Japanese men. *J. Amer. Dietet. Assoc.* in press.

Kuroda M, Ohta M, Okufuji T, Takigami C, Eguchi M, Hayabuchi H, Ikeda M. (2010). Frequency of soup intake and amount of dietary fiber intake are inversely associated with plasma leptin concentrations in Japanese adults. *Appetite.* 54, 538-543

LaPorte RE, Black-Sandler R, Cauley JA, Link M, Bayles C, Marks B. (1983). The assessment of physical activity in older woman: analysis of the interrelationship and reliability of activity monitoring, activity surveys, and caloric intake. *J. Gerentol.*, 38, 394-197.

Mabuchi, T., Yatsuya, H., Tamakoshi, K., Otsuka, R., Nagasawa, N., Zhang, H. et al. (2005). Association between serum leptin concentration and white blood cell count in middle-aged Japanese men and women. *Diabetes Metab. Res. Rev.*, 21, 441-447.

Margetic S, Gazzola C, Pegg GG., Hill RA. (2002). Leptin: a review of its peripheral actions and interactions. *Int. J. Obes. Relat. Metab. Disord.*, 26, 1407-1433.

Mattes R. (2005). Soup and satiety. *Physiol. Behav.*, 83, 739-747.

McNeely MJ, Boyko EJ, Weigle DS, Shofer JB, Chessler SD, Leonnetti DL et al. (1999). Association between baseline plasma leptin levels and subsequent development of diabetes in Japanese Americans. *Diabetes Care*, 22, 65-70.

McVeigh BL, Dillingham BL, Lampe JW, Duncan AM. (2006). Effect of soy protein varying in isoflavone content on serum lipids in healthy young men. *Am. J. Clin. Nutr.*, 83, 244-251.

Miller GD, Frost R, Olive J. (2001). Relation of plasma leptin concentrations to sex, body fat, dietary intake, and peak oxygen uptake in young adult men and women. *Nutrition*, 17, 105-11.

Ministry of Health, Labour, and Welfare. (2004). The National Nutrition Survey in Japan, 2002 [in Japanese]. Tokyo, Japan: Ministry of Health and Welfare.

Miyatake N, Takahashi K, Wada J, Nishikawa H, Morishita A, Suzuki H et al. (2004). Changes in serum leptin concentration in overweight Japanese men after exercise. *Diabetes Obes. Metab.*, 6, 332-337.

Mora S, Pessin JE. (2002). An adipocentric view of signaling and intracellular trafficking. *Diabetes Metab. Res. Rev.*, 18, 345-356.

Murakami K, Sasaki S, Takahashi Y, Uenishi K, Yamasaki M, Hayabuchi H et al. (2007a). Nutrient and food intake in relation to serum leptin concentration among young Japanese women. *Nutrition*, 23, 461-468.

Murakami K, Sasaki S, Takahashi Y, Uenishi K, Yamasaki M, Hayabuchi H, Goda T, Oka J, Baba K, Ohki K, Kohri T, Muramatsu K, Furuki M. (2007b). Hardness (difficulty of chewing) of the habitual diet in relation to body mass index and waist circumference in free-living Japanese women aged 18-22 y. *Am. J. Clin. Nutr.* 86, 206-213.

Nolan LJ, Guss JL, Liddle RA, Pi-Sunyer FX, Kissileff HR. (2003). Elevated plasma cholecystokinin and appetite ratings after consumption of a liquid meal in humans. *Nutrition.* 19, 553-557.

Okazaki T, Himeno E, Nanri H, Ikeda M. (2001). Effects of a community-based lifestyle-modification program on a cardiovascular risk factors in middle-aged women. *Hypertens. Res.*, 24, 647-653.

Racette SB, Kohrt WM, Landt M, Holloszy JO. (1997). Response of serum leptin concentrations to 7 d of energy restriction in centrally obese African Americans with impaired or diabetic glucose tolerance. *Amer. J. Clin. Nutr.*, 66, 33-37.

Rafamantanantsoa HH, Ebine N, Yoshioka M, Higuchi H, Yoshitake Y, Tanaka H, Satoh S, Jones PJH. (2002). Validation of three alternative methods to measure total energy expenditure against the doubly labeled water method for older Japanese men. *J. Nutr. Sci. Vitaminol.* 48, 517-523.

Ravussin E, Lillioja S, Knowler WC, Christin L, Freymond D, Abbott WG, Boyce V, Howard BV, Bogardus C. (1988). Reduced rate of energy expenditure as a risk factor for body-weight gain. *New Engl. J. Med.* 318, 467-472.

Rimm EB, Stampfer MJ, Giovannucci E, Ascherio A, Spiegelman D, Colditz GA, Willett WC. (1995). Body size and fat distribution as predictors of coronary heart disease among middle-aged and other US men. *Am. J. Epidemiol.* 141, 1117-1127.

Rolls BJ, Fedoroff IC, Guthrie JF, Laster LJ. (1990). Foods with different satiating effects in humans. *Appetite*, 15, 115-126.

Seufert J. (2004). Leptin effects on pancreatic beta-cell gene expression and function. *Diabetes*, 53, Suppl 1, S152-158.

Siconolfi SF, Lasater TM, Snow RC, Carleton RA. (1985). Self-reported physical activity compared with maximal oxygen uptake. *Am. J. Epidemiol.*, 122, 101-105.

Soderberg S, Ahren B, Stegmayr B, Johnson O, Wiklund PG, Weinehall L et al. (1999). Leptin is a risk marker for first-ever hemorrhagic stroke in popular-based cohort. *Stroke*, 30, 328-337.

Takahashi K, Yoshimura Y, Kaimoto T, Kunii D, Komatsu T, Yamamoto S. (2001). Validation of a food frequency questionnaire based on food group for estimating individual nutrient intake. *Jpn. J. Nutr. Dietet.*, 59, 221-232.

Taku K, Uenishi K, Sato Y, Taki Y, Endoh K, Watanabe S. (2007). Soy isoflavones lower serum total and LDL cholesterol: a meta-analysis of 11 randomized controlled trials. *Am. J. Clin. Nutr.*, 85, 1148-1156.

Tokushima Prefecture, The results of the prefecture nutrition survey in Tokushima, 1997 [in Japanese]. (1998). Tokushima, Japan: Tokushima prefecture.

Washburn RA., Smith KW, Goldfield SR, McKinlay JB. (1991). Reliability and physiological correlates of the Harvard Alumni Activity Survey in a general population. *J. Clin. Epidemiol.*, 44, 1319-1326.

Wayne SJ, Neuhouser ML, Ulrich CM, Koprowski C, Baumgartner KB, Baumgartner RN, et al. (2008). Dietary fiber is associated with serum sex hormones and insulin-related peptides in postmenopausal breast cancer survivors. *Breast Cancer Res. Treat*, 112, 149-158.

Winnicki M, Somers VK, Accurso V, Phillips BG, Puato M, Palatini P. (2002). Fish-rich diet, leptin, and body mass. *Circulation*, 106, 289-291.

Yannakoulia M, Yiannakouris N, Bluher S, Matalas AL, Klimis-Zacas D, Mantzoros CS. (2003). Body fat mass and macronutrient intake in relation to circulating soluble leptin receptor, free leptin index, adiponectin, and resistin concentrations in healthy humans. *J. Clin. Endocrinol. Metab.*, 88, 1730-1736.

Zhang S, Liu X, Brickman WJ, Christoffel KK, Zimmerman D, Tsai H-J et al. (2009). Association of plasma leptin concentrations with adiposity measurements in rural Chinese adolescents. *J. Clin. Ecdocrin. Metab.*, doi:10.1210/jc.2009-1060.

In: Appetite: Regulation, Role in Disease and Control
Editor: Steven R. Mitchell, pp. 97-112
ISBN 978-1-61209-842-5
© 2011 Nova Science Publishers, Inc.

Chapter 5

SEROTONIN NEUROTRANSMISSION IN ANOREXIA NERVOSA

*Darakhshan Jabeen Haleem**

Department of Biochemistry, Neurochemistry and Biochemical Neuropharmacology Research Unit, University of Karachi, Karachi 75270, Pakistan

ABSTRACT

5-Hydroxytryptamine (5-HT; serotonin) system is the major neurotransmitter system of interest in research on anorexia nervosa (AN). The AN patients show extreme dieting weight loss, hyperactivity, depression, obsession and loss of impulse control. Pharmacological studies show that manipulations that tend to increase brain serotonin functions are anorexiogenic. The hypothesis of suppression of appetite through excessive release of 5-HT to receptors is not supported by data on subjects with clinical symptoms of AN as cerebrospinal fluid (CSF) levels of 5-hydroxyindoleacetic acid (5-HIAA), a major metabolite of 5-HT, are reduced in AN patients and returned to normal in recovered patients. Loss of appetite in AN may simply follow self imposed dieting and diet restriction (DR). The hypothalamus is believed to be the site of the brain transducing satiety signals of serotonin. Studies on animal models show that acute starvation although increases brain serotonin metabolism but excessive DR over a period of few weeks decreased 5-HT metabolism and synthesis in the brain and hypothalamus and elicited hyperactivity. Based upon these finding animal models of DR-induced AN and activity based AN have been developed. This article highlights some of the important investigations on serotonin neurotransmission in animal models of AN. It focuses particularly on the role of serotonin in the regulation of appetite, activity and mood to understand ways in which DR-induced changes of brain serotonin may account for behavioral changes observed in AN patients with a hope that information contained herein would stimulate relevant research on AN for more rational and successful prevention/treatment of this tragic often fatal disease.

---

* Address for correspondence: Prof Dr Darakhshan Jabeen Haleem. Department of Biochemistry, University of Karachi. Karachi 75270. Pakistan. e-mail:darakhshan_haleem@yahoo.com. djhaleem@uok.edu.pk.

1. ANOREXIA NERVOSA

Anorexia nervosa (AN) is a frequent disorder among adolescent girls and young women. According to the DSM-IV, diagnostic criteria, the disease is described by weight loss or failure to attain expected weight gain during periods of growth, intense fear of gaining weight or becoming fat, body image disturbance and amenorrhea. Arising during the period of growth and maturation, AN leads to interruptions of somatic and psychological development and to serious medical complications and high mortality (Bemporad, 1997, Haleem, 1996, Halmi et al, 2005, Kaye, 2008). The disease usually starts quite harmlessly and may begin as a simple attempt to lose weight in order to look more beautiful and attractive (Ploog and Pirke, 1987). Failure to see the turning point when fasting becomes unreasonable may lead to malnutrition and AN (Haleem, 1996).

Individuals with AN severely restrict food intake, particularly fats and carbohydrates, but rarely stop eating completely; rather they restrict their caloric intake to a few hundred calories a day. They tend to be vegetarians, have monotonous choices in food intake, select unusual combinations of foods and flavors, and have ritualized eating behaviors (Lilenfeld et al, 1998; Strober et al, 2000). They also have elevated rates of lifetime diagnoses of anxiety and depressive disorders, and obsessive-compulsive disorder (Kaye et al, 2004; Godart et al, 2002). They have an obsessive and rigid personality style and have difficulty shifting sets. Although they do well on goal directed behavior, they have difficulties incorporating feedback and modifying their behavior and often feel that they should be able to do things perfectly without making mistakes (Strupp et al, 1986; Kingston et al, 1996).

Computed tomography and magnetic resonance imaging studies show that underweight patients with anorexia nervosa have enlarged sulci and ventricles, cortical atrophy and decreased grey and white matter volumes (Kerem and Katzman, 2003). Changes in brain metabolism as measured by magnetic resonance spectroscopy seem to be related to poor cognitive function (Ohrmann et al, 2004)

The eating disorder mainly affects young women and is often theorized to be caused by cultural pressures for thinness (Becker et al, 2003). It is described as symptomatic triad of anorexia, emaciation and amenorrhea (Kohl et al, 2004). Besides these three symptoms hyperactivity is often also associated with AN (Kron et al, 1978, Casper and Lyubomirsky, 1997; Walsh and Devlin, 1998).

Hyperactivity, defined by an excess of physical activity, can take different forms, most striking is the restlessness which can induce social, professional and family consequences (Kohl et al, 2004). It is often considered as a strategy to lose weight, but studies on animal models have shown that it could be explained by more complicated mechanisms (Haleem, 2009). Many studies show that hyperactivity follows DR and weight loss suggesting that it is a consequence of DR. Although patients with anorexia nervosa are not all hyperactive but a trend for a significantly higher frequency of compulsive exercising is reported in patients with anorexia nervosa than those with bulimia nervosa.

Studies carried out to estimate the prevalence of high level exercise in the eating disorders indicate that a large majority of patients with anorexia nervosa were exercising excessively during an acute phase of the disorder. The prevalence being highest in AN, lowest in eating disorders not otherwise specified, and intermediate in bulimia nervosa (Dalle et al, 2008). Hyperactive patients are more dissatisfied by their body image, they use less means of purging (laxatives, vomiting; the symptoms of bulimia nervosa) but start starving earlier than patients without hyperactivity suggesting a link between hyperactivity and severity of AN. Factors such as social and cultural requirements, sports environment, family influences have been shown to promote the emergence and maintenance of hyperactivity (Brewerton et al, 1995). On the other hand, the experience of intense guilt when exercise is missed was greater in patients with the purging form of anorexia nervosa than those with the restricting form of anorexia nervosa (Mond and Calogero, 2009). Excessive exercise is therefore thought to be an important issue in the development as well as treatment of AN (Bratland-Sanda, 2010).

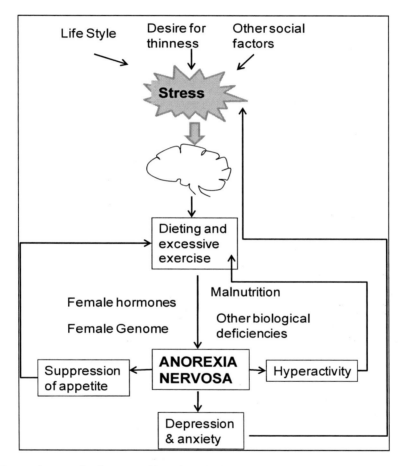

Figure 1. Factors that may lead to AN: Life style and other social pressures produce a desire of starvation and excessive exercise, resultant biological deficiencies make particularly female sex vulnerable to AN. Behavioral changes in AN patients can further exaggerate the severity of the disease.

On the basis of some clinical and neurochemical changes, hyperactivity in AN is sometimes explained in terms of a kind of obsessive compulsive disorder (Kaye, 2008). Other studies explain excessive exercise in anorexia nervosa as an addiction (Ehrlich et al, 2009). All together these studies suggest that excessive exercise and starvation as a simple attempt to lose weight may produce biological deficiencies that particularly make female sex vulnerable to AN (Figure 1). The behavioral changes in AN patients such as refusal to eat, hyperactivity and depression can further exaggerate the severity of the disease leading to a fatal condition.

2. SEROTONIN SYNAPSE

The 5-hydroxytryptamine (5-HT; serotonin) system involved in the regulation of appetite and mood is the major neurotransmitter system of interest in research on AN. Cell bodies of serotonin containing neurons are concentrated in the midbrain raphe. The dorsal and median raphe nuclei located dorsally in the brain stem contain a very high density of serotonergic cell bodies. Their axons innervate almost every area of the central nervous system (CNS) including the hypothalamus, the site of the brain transducing satiety signal of serotonin (Curzon, 1990; Haleem, 1996; Leibowitz, 1986; Sugrue, 1987). Hippocampus (Haleem et al, 2007a) and striatum (Haleem 2006; Haleem et al, 2007b) the regions of the brain involved in adaptation to stress and motor control respectively are also innervated by serotonergic neurons.

Tryptophan, the precursor of 5-HT is an essential amino acid; for which the initial source is dietary protein (Figure 2). The uptake of tryptophan by brain is brought about by a stereospecific, saturable, facilitated transport mechanism shared by all large neutral amino acids (LNAAs) (Oldendorf, 1973; Yudilevich et al, 1972). All together, eight LNAAs namely tryptophan, tyrosine, phenylalanine, threonine, valine, leucine, isoleucine and methionine share common transport carrier. Increase in the concentration of any of these amino acids, therefore, decreases the transport of others.

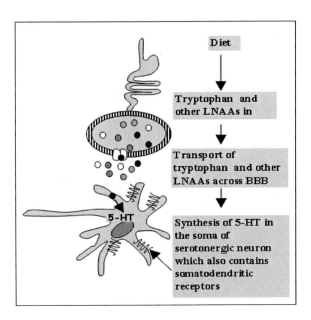

Figure 2. Transport of dietary tryptophan to the brain: The essential amino acid absorbed from gastrointestinal tract circulates largely (90%) in bound form with plasma albumin. It crosses blood brain barrier via a stereo specific, saturable, facilitated transport mechanism shared by all large neutral amino acids (LNAAs). Localization of somatodendritic 5-HT-1A receptors that control synthesis and release of the neurotransmitter via a feedback mechanism is also shown.

The first step of serotonin biosynthesis (Figure3) involves hydroxylation of tryptophan to form 5-hydroxytryptophan (5-HTP) in presence of enzyme tryptophan hydroxylase (TH) which is highly localized within 5-HT producing neurons. 5-HTP is converted to 5-HT by a non specific enzyme L-aromatic amino acid decarboxylase which is ubiquitously distributed. Activity of the decarboxylase is much greater than that of TH and normally very little 5-HTP is found in the mammalian brain. The predominant metabolite of 5-HT in the brain is 5-hydroxyindole acetic acid (5-HIAA).

We now know that serotonin plays a number of very important roles in normal brain function, which include modulation of mood states, hunger, sex, sleep, memory, emotion, anxiety, endocrine effects, and many others. Regarding the behavioral changes that occur in AN, a role of serotonin in the regulation of appetite, control of motor activity and elicitation of depression/ anxiety becomes important. Serotonin receptors are widely expressed throughout the brain and in various nuclei of the hypothalamus, hippocampus and striatum responsible for the modulation of appetite, mood and motor activity (Nicholas and Nicholas, 2008). Localization of different receptor subtypes is shown in Figure 3.

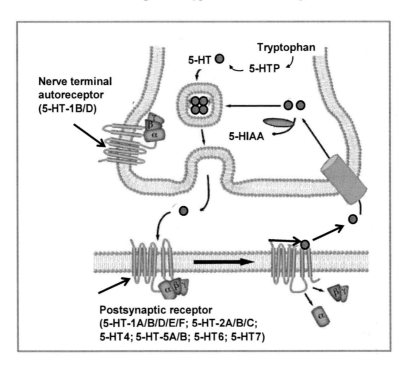

Figure 3. Serotonin Synapse: The neurotransmitter synthesized from the essential amino acid tryptophan is stored in the synaptic vesicles. After release and reuptake it may either be degraded to 5-HIAA or restored in the vesicles. Localization of postsynaptic receptors and nerve terminal autoreceptors is also shown.

With the exception of the 5-HT-3 receptor, a ligand-gated ion channel, all other serotonin receptors are G protein-coupled receptors that activate an intracellular second messenger cascade to produce an excitatory or inhibitory response. The 5-HT-1A receptor is a G-protein-coupled receptor widely distributed in regions that receive serotonergic input from the raphe nuclei: the frontal cortex, septum, amygdale, hippocampus, striatum and hypothalamus (Nicholas and Nicholas 2008). It also serves as somatodendritic (Verge et al, 1985) autoreceptor (Figure 2) of raphe nuclei reducing the firing rate of serotonergic neurons (Haleem et al, 1990; Haleem, 1990).

3. SEROTONIN IN ANIMAL MODELS OF AN

Development of appropriate animal model of AN has been difficult as the etiology of this eating disorder likely involves a complex interaction between genetic, environmental, social and cultural factors. Separation stress, activity and diet restriction (DR) are often used to develop animal model of AN (Seigfried et al, 2003). Restricted Food access in combination with voluntary excess to running wheels is reported to result in hyperactivity, hypophagia and severe body weight loss

In some early investigations on the effects of starvation on brain serotonin it was shown that brain serotonin metabolism is increased following acute 24 h starvation (Curzon et al, 1972) because starvation-induced lipolysis increases plasma levels of free fatty acids. These free fatty acids displace tryptophan, the precursor of 5-HT, from its binding sites with plasma albumin to make free tryptophan available more for transport to the brain. Increase in brain tryptophan concentration increases 5-HT synthesis because tryptophan hydroxylase, the rate limiting enzyme of 5-HT biosynthesis, is only half saturated with its substrate (Fernstrom and Wurtman, 1971).

Unlike acute starvation, DR for only one week decreased 5-HT content and synthesis in the hypothalamus of rat brain (Haleem and Haider, 1996). The decreases of tryptophan and 5-HIAA were not significant. Tryptophan is an essential amino acid its source is only dietary. It may be expected that limited availability of tryptophan to the brain during DR decreases brain 5-HT synthesis. Although DR of one week (short term) duration did not significantly decrease plasma and brain levels of tryptophan in male rats but DR of longer duration (5 weeks) decreased both plasma and brain levels of tryptophan and the decreases were greater in female than male rats (Haider and Haleem, 2000).

Data on the effects of DR on brain serotonin (Haleem and Haider, 1996; Haider and Haleem, 2000) was supported by clinical data on subjects with symptoms of AN, as AN patients exhibited low basal levels of 5-HIAA, a major metabolite of 5-HT, in the cerebrospinal fluid (CSF), which returned to normal after weight recovery (Kaye et al, 1988; 2001). Although availability of tryptophan, the precursor of 5-HT and an essential amino acid, increased in anorexia associated with different diseases (Rossi-Fanelli and Cangiano, 1999; Haider et al, 2004) but AN patients exhibited low levels of plasma tryptophan which increased after weight recovery (Attia et al, 2005). Moreover, acute tryptophan depletion reduced anxiety levels in AN patients (Kaye et al, 2003) suggesting that a decrease in the availability of precursor amino acid tryptophan has a significant role in the precipitation of anorexia nervosa.

The synthesis and release of 5-HT is under the control of an effective feedback mechanism (Figure 2) involving stimulation of somatodendritic autoreceptors (Verge et al, 1985). The stimulation provides an inhibition of nerve impulse flow within the serotonergic neurons (Blier et al, 1987). Administration of 8-hydroxy-2-di (n-propylamino) tetralin (8-OH-DPAT), a selective 5-HT-1A agonist, therefore decreases the synthesis, turnover and release of 5-HT in brain regions where these neurons project (Hjorth et al, 1988; Hutson et al, 1989) including the hypothalamus, hippocampus and caudate (Haleem, 1999) An increase in the effectiveness of these somatodendritic receptors may also decrease the availability of 5-HT in terminal regions .

An increase in the effectiveness of feedback regulation on 5-HT synthesis has been shown to be involved in stress-induced behavioral depression (Samad et al, 2007). Conversely, a decrease in the effectiveness of these receptors increasing the availability of 5-HT in terminal regions is involved in adaptation to stress (Haleem, 1999). Moreover, SSRIs that are known to produce their therapeutic effect by decreasing the effectiveness of feedback control over 5-HT (Artigas, 1993) appear to prevent relapse of weight restoration in AN patients (Kaye et al, 2001). We therefore investigated the responsiveness of somatodendritic 5-HT-1A receptors following long term DR and reported (Haleem, 2009) that an exaggerated feedback control over 5-HT synthesis and release is responsible for the decrease in the synthesis and availability of 5-HT in the raphe and terminal regions respectively in rat model of DR-induced AN. It is also possible that smaller availability of the essential amino acid tryptophan during long term DR increases the responsiveness of somatodendritic 5-HT-1A receptors as an adaptive mechanism to conserve 5-HT from being excessively released in conditions of precursor deficiency.

4. SEROTONIN AND THE SUPPRESSION OF APPETITE IN AN

It was observed in some early neurochemical investigations that brain tryptophan levels are increased following ingestion of carbohydrate rich diet because diet-induced insulin secretion decreases circulating levels of LNAAs (Fernstrom and Wurtman, 1972; Haleem, 1994; Wurtman and Wurtman, 1996) which compete with tryptophan for transport to the brain (Figure 2). Data from human studies also showed that tryptophan/LNAAs ratio in circulation increases following a carbohydrate breakfast (Piji et al, 1993). The increase in brain tryptophan is followed by an increase in 5-HT synthesis because TH, the rate limiting enzyme of 5-HT biosynthesis (Figure 3) exists only half saturated with its substrate (Haleem et al, 1993). Microdialysis showed that in the hypothalamus of rat brain an increase in 5-HT release occurred during eating as well as during pre ingestive event (Schwartz et al, 1990). Because pharmacological manipulations that tend to increase 5-HT functions are anorexiogenic (Blundell et al, 1995), these studies suggested that brain 5-HT is increased following the ingestion of meal to generate a satiety signal for the termination of meal (Haleem, 1996).

The 5-HT-1B and 5-HT-2C receptors located postsynaptically (Figure 3) are the main candidate receptors mediating the inhibitory influence of 5-HT on food intake (Kennett et al, 1988; Clifton et al, 2000, Vickers et al, 2003). D-fenfluramine, a useful anorexiogenic agent (Rowland and Carlton, 1986) stimulates 5-HT release and inhibits its reuptake (Gibson et al, 1993). Hypophagic effects of d-fenfluramine are also thought to be mediated via excessive release of 5-HT at 5-HT-1B and 5-HT-2C receptors (Simansky and Nickolas, 2002; Tecott, 2007).

A decrease in 5-HT content in the hypothalamus following DR in a rat model of AN although relevant with clinical studies does not explain suppression of appetite observed in AN patients because an increase in 5-HT neurotransmission would be expected to elicit satiety signal (Haleem, 1996). It was therefore argued that DR-induced decreases of brain serotonin may induce a compensatory upregulation of hypophagic serotonin receptors (Figure 4) which leads to the suppression of appetite (Haleem, 2009)

Clinical data are relevant that disturbance of serotonin receptor responsiveness may contribute to the pathophysiology of AN. For example, results from positron emission tomography (PET) studies showed that AN patients have reduced 5-HT-2A receptor binding in the mesial temporal lobe and some other cortical regions, which persists after weight recovery (Frank et al, 2002; Bailor et al, 2007) suggesting that the alterations may be traits that are independent of the state of the illness (Kaye et al, 2005). Association studies revealed polymorphism in the promoter of the 5-HT2A and 5-HT2C receptor that was associated with AN (Gorwood et al, 2002, Hu et al, 2003, Rosmond et al, 2002, Westberg et al, 2002), although this could not be confirmed by others (Campbell et al, 1998; Nacmias et al, 1999).

5. SEROTONIN AND HYPERACTIVITY IN AN

The dopamine system has traditionally been considered crucial to the control of motor activity (Haleem, 2006). The serotonergic system is known to inhibit dopamine neurotransmission at the level of origin of dopamine system in the midbrain as well as in the terminal region. A potential role of 5-HT-2C receptors in the attenuation of motor activity was suggested because 5-HT-2C receptors are found in high density in the ventral tegmental area, the origin of dopaminergic neurons (Pierucci et al, 2004). Moreover, drugs with agonist activity towards 5-HT-2C receptors elicited hypolocomotion and akinesia (Haleem, 1993) and markedly decreased cocaine induced hyperactivity in experimental animals (Fletcher et al, 2004).

Dopamine release in the caudate and other terminal regions was decreased by drugs with preferential agonist activity towards 5-HT-2C receptors (Millan et al, 1998). Conversely, drugs with preferential antagonist activity towards 5-HT-2C receptors increased dialysate levels of dopamine in the striatum (Alex et al, 2005). 5-HT-1A agonists that decreased 5-HT availability in the caudate also released dopamine neurotransmission from the inhibitory influence of 5-HT and attenuated/ reversed Parkinsonian like effects of dopamine D2 antagonists (Haleem et al, 2007b).

An increase in the responsiveness of somatodendritic 5-HT-1A receptor has been seen in rat model of DR-induced AN (Haleem, 2009). It is therefore possible that DR-induced exaggerated feedback control over the synthesis and release of 5-HT resulting in a decrease of 5-HT in the caudate releases dopamine neurotransmission from the inhibitory influence of serotonin to elicit hyperactivity (Figure 4).

6. SEROTONIN AND DEPRESSION/ANXIETY IN AN

AN patients often show anxiety/depression, obsession and loss of impulse control (Kaye et al, 2004). The brain serotonin acting via the hippocampus is strongly implicated in the neuronal regulation of mood and anxiety state (Dranovsky and Hen, 2006) and adaptation to stress (Haleem and Parveen, 1994, Haleem, 2011).

Young male rats supplied daily with 50% chow for 5 weeks exhibited a decrease in 5-HIAA concentration and 5-HIAA/5-HT ratio in the hippocampus which was associated with anxiety and depression like behavior in an elevated plus maze and forced swim test respectively (Jahng et al, 2007). Exposure to an uncontrollable stressor increases the responsiveness of somatodendritic 5-HT-1A receptors to decrease the availability of 5-HT in terminal regions including the hippocampus (Haleem and Parveen, 1994; Haleem et al, 2007a). Rats fed on a DR schedule of 2h/day for 5 days also exhibited an increase in the responsiveness of somatodendritic 5-HT-1A receptor (Haleem, 2009). Conversely, adaptation to stress was associated with a decrease in the sensitivity of somatodendritic 5-HT-1A receptors (Haleem, 1999). It is therefore tempting to suggest that DR-induced increase in the sensitivity of somatodendritic 5-HT-1A receptors resulting in a decrease of 5-HT in the hippocampus may have a causal role in the elicitation of depression/ anxiety.

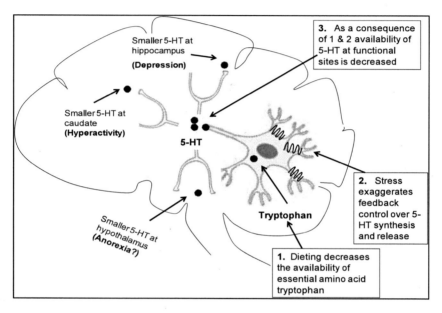

Figure 4. Serotonin in the modulation of behavior in AN: A decrease in the availability of essential amino acid tryptophan may induce exaggerated feedback control over the synthesis and release of 5-HT. Resultant decrease in the availability of 5-HT in the caudate and hippocampus may have a role in the hyperactivity and depression respectively in AN.

7. SEROTONIN AND VULNERABILITY OF FEMALE GENDER TO AN

The AN most commonly develops during adolescence or young adulthood in proximity to puberty (Klein and Walsh, 2003). It is a time of profound biological, psychological and socio cultural change that demands a considerable degree of flexibility to successfully manage transition to adulthood (Connan, 2003).The biological changes may significantly enhance the risk of onset of AN particularly in women is supported by twin studies which found essentially no genetic influence on overall levels of eating attitude and other behaviors in 11 year old twins, but significant genetic effects (>50%) in 17 year old twins (Klump et al, 2000). The changes associated with adolescence differ in males and females and may therefore contribute to the sexual dimorphism of AN.

If a decrease in of serotonin neurotransmission due to exaggerated feedback control over 5-HT synthesis and release is involved in the elicitation of AN, the sex differences of somatodendritic 5-HT-1A receptors that regulate serotonin neurotransmission become important. Sexual dimorphism in the serotonin was first reported in early 1960's (Kato, 1960). An increasing amount of later work supported the view that central serotonin metabolism synthesis and functional responses are greater in female than male rats (Haleem, 2011).

Sex differences also occur in the regulation of serotonin neurotransmission via 5-HT-1A receptors. Expression of serotonin-1A receptor messenger RNA was greater in males in the hypothalamus and amygdala, and less in males in the hippocampus (Zhang et al, 1999). The concentrations of 5-HT and 5-HIAA were greater in female than male rats but the sensitivity of 5-HT-1A receptors that control the availability of 5-HT in the terminal regions is greater in female sex (Haleem, 1990). It would suggest that a greater sensitivity of somatodendritic 5-HT-1A receptor can make female sex more vulnerable to stress and other psychological disorders including AN.

CONCLUSION

Self imposed starvation and excessive exercise may lead to AN. Besides anorexia, emaciation and amenorrhea, AN patients also exhibit hyperactivity and a decrease in serotonin content in the CSF. Studies on animal models show that long and short term DR to decrease body weight 20-25% below normal decreases brain serotonin metabolism and elicits hyperactivity. The decreases of brain 5-HT are not always explainable in terms of limited availability of its precursor tryptophan which is an essential amino acid. An increase in the responsiveness of feedback control over 5-HT synthesis and release mediated via somatodendritic 5-HT-1A receptors also has an important role in DR-induced decreases of 5-HT. it is however possible that exaggerated feedback control over 5-HT synthesis and release occurs as an adaptation to limited availability of tryptophan. Data accumulated in the present article suggest that DR-induced decreases of serotonin neurotransmission may lead to hyperactivity and mood changes as observed in AN. How can DR or decreases of brain serotonin suppress appetite is not clear. It is suggested that tryptophan supplementation as it can decrease the responsiveness of somatodendritic 5-HT-1A receptors may be of use in the treatment of AN. Investigations on the role of serotonin in AN may help to identify novel therapeutic agents for more rational and successful prevention/treatment of this tragic often fatal disease.

ACKNOWLEDGMENT

The author would like to thank Higher Education Commission Pakistan and Karachi University for providing grant.

REFERENCES

Alex K. D., Yavanian G. J., McFarlane H., Pluto C., and Pehec E. (2005) Modulation of Dopamine Release by Striatal 5-HT2C Receptors. *Synapse* 55, 242–251.

Artigas F. (1993) 5-HT and antidepressants: New views from microdialysis studies. *Trends Pharmacol. Sci.* 14, 262-263.

Attia E. , Wolk S., Cooper T., Glasofer D. and Walsh B. T. (2005) Plasma tryptophan during weight restoration in patients with Anorexia nervosa. *Biol. Psychiat.* 57, 674-78.

Bailer U. F., Frank G. K., Henry S. E., Price J. C., Meltzer C. C., Mathis C. A., Wagner A., Thornton L., Hoge J., Ziolko S. K., Becker C. R., McConaha C. W. and Kaye W. H. (2007) Exaggerated 5-HT-1A but normal 5-HT2A receptor activity in individuals III with anorexia nervosa. *Biol. Psychiat.* 61, 1090-1099.

Becker A. E., Burwell R. A., Navara K.. and Gilman S. E. (2003) Binge-eating and binge-eating disorder in a small-scale indigenous society: The view from Fiji. *International Journal of Eating Disorders*, 34, 423-431.

Bemporad J. R. (1997) Cultural and historical aspects of eating disorders. *Theor. Med.* 18, 401–420.

Blier P., de Montigny C. and Chaput Y. (1987) Modification of the serotonin system by antidepressant treatment: implications for therapeutic responses in major depression *J. Clin. Psychopharmacol. Suppl.* (6), 24S-35S.

Blundell J. E., Lawton C. L. and Halford C. (1995) Serotonin, eating behavior, and fat intake. *Obes. Res. 3(Suppl 4)*, 471S–476S.

Bratland-Sanda S., Sundgot-Borgen J., Rø Ø, Rosenvinge J. H., Hoffart A. and Martinsen E. W. (2010) Physical activity and exercise dependence during inpatient treatment of longstanding eating disorders: an exploratory study of excessive and non-excessive exercisers. *Int. J. Eat. Disord.* 43(3), 266-273.

Brewerton T. D., Stellefson E. J., Hibbs N., Hodges E. L.and Cochrane C. E. (1995) Comparison of eating disorder patients with and without compulsive exercising. *Int. J. Eat. Disord.* 17(4), 413-416.

Campbell, D. A,, Sundaramurthy, D., Markham, A. F., Pieri, L. F. (1998) Lack of association between 5-HT2A gene promoter polymorphism and susceptibility to anorexia nervosa. *Lancet*, 351, 499

Casper R. C. and Lyubomirsky S. (1997) Individual psychopathology relative to reports of unwanted sexual experiences as predictor of a bulimic eating pattern. *Int. J. Eat. Disord.* 21, 229–36.

Clifton P. G., Lee M. D. and Dourish, C. T. (2000) Similarities in the action of Ro 60-0175, a 5-HT2C receptor agonist and d-fenfluramine on feeding patterns in the rat. *Psychopharmacology* (Berlin) 152, 256-267.

Connan F., Campbell I., Katzman M., Lightman S. and Treasure J. (2003) A neurodevelopmental model for anorexia nervosa. *Physiol. Behav.* 79(1), 13–24.

Curzon G. (1990) Serotonin and appetite *Ann. NY. Acad. Sci.* 600, 521-530.

Curzon G., Joseph M. H. and Knott P. J. (1972) Effects of immobilization and food deprivation on rat brain tryptophan metabolism. *J. Neurochem.* 19, 1967-1974.

Dalle G. R., Calugi S. and Marchesini G. (2008) Compulsive exercise to control shape or weight in eating disorders: prevalence, associated features, and treatment outcome. *Compr. Psychiatry.* 49(4), 346-352.

Dranovsky A. and Hen R. (2006) Hippocampal Neurogenesis: Regulation by Stress and Antidepressants *Biological Psychiatry* 59 (12), 1136-1143.

Ehrlich S.; Salbach-Andrae H., Eckart S., Merle J. V., Burghardt R., Pfeiffer E., Leonora F. L., Uebelhack R., Lehmkuhl U. and Hellweg R. (2009) Serum brain-derived neurotrophic factor and peripheral indicators of the serotonin system in underweight and weight-recovered adolescent girls and women with anorexia nervosa. *J. Psychiatry Neurosci.* 34(4), 323-329.

Fletcher P. J., Chintoh A. F., Sinyard J. and Higgins GA (2004) Injection of the 5-HT2C receptor agonist Ro60-0175 into the ventral tegmental area reduces cocaine-induced locomotor activity and cocaine self-administration. *Neuropsychopharmacology.* 29(2), 308-18.

Frank G. K., Kaye W. H., Meltzer C. C., Price J. C., Greer P., McConaha C. and Skovira K (2002) Reduced 5-HT2A receptor binding after recovery from anorexia nervosa. *Biol. Psychiatry* 52, 896–906

Fernstrom J. D. and Wurtman R. J. (1971) Brain serotonin content: increase following ingestion of carbohydrate diet. *Science* 174(13), 1023–1025.

Fernstrom J. D. and Wurtman R. J. (1972) Brain serotonin content: physiological regulation by plasma neutral amino acids. *Scienc* 178(59), 414–416.

Gibson E. L., Kennedy A. J. and Curzon G. (1993) D-fenfluramine and D-norfenfluramine-induced hypophagia: Differential mechanism and involvement of postsynaptic 5-HT receptors. *Eur. J. Pharmacol.* 242, 83-89.

Godart N. T., Flament M. F., (2002) Perdereau F, Jeammet P. Comorbidity between eating disorders and anxiety disorders: a review. *Int. J. Eat. Disord.*, 32(3), 253–270.

Gorwood P., Ades J., Bellodi L., Cellini E., Collier D. A., Bella D., Di Bernardo M., Estivill X, Fernandez-Aranda F. and Gratacos, M. (2002) The 5-HT(2A) -1438G/A polymorphism in anorexia nervosa: a combined analysis of 316 trios from six European centers. *Mol. Psychiat.*, 7, 90-94.

Haider S. and Haleem D. J. (2000) Decreases of brain serotonin following a food restriction schedule of 4 weeks in male and female rats. *Med. Sci. Monit.* 6, 1061-1067.

Haider S., Saleem S., Shameem S., Ahmed S. P., Perveen T. and Haleem D. J. (2004) Is anorexia in thioacetamide-induced cirrhosis related to an altered brain serotonin concentration? *Pol. J. Pharmacol.* 56, 73-78.

Haleem D. J. (1993) Function specific supersensitivity of m-chlorophenyl piperazine-induced serotonergic neurotransmission in female compared to male rats. *Life Sciences* 52(25), PL279-PL284.

Haleem D. J. (1994) Decreases of plasma tryptophan concentrations following restricted feeding do not decrease serotonin and its metabolite in rat brain. *Die Nahrung*, 38(6), 606-611.

Haleem D. J. (1996) Serotonin Appetite and Anorexia Nervosa. *J. Coll. Phys. Sur. Pak.*, 6,167-172.

Haleem D. J. (1999b) Attenuation of 8-OH-DPAT-induced decreases in 5-HT synthesis in brain regions of rats adapted to a repeated stress schedule. *Stress* 3, 123-129.

Haleem D. J. (2006) Serotonergic modulation of dopamine neurotransmission: a mechanism for enhancing therapeutics in schizophrenia. *J. Coll. Physicians Surg. Pak.* 16, 556-562.

Haleem D. J. (2009) Exaggerated feedback control decreases brain serotonin concentration and elicits hyperactivity in a rat model of diet-restriction-induced anorexia nervosa. *Appetite* 52(1), 44-50.

Haleem D. J. (2011) Raphe-Hippocampal Serotonin Neurotransmission In The Sex Related Differences Of Adaptation To Stress: Focus on Serotonin-1A Receptor. *Current Neuropharmacology*, 9 (in press).

Haleem D. J. and Haider S. (1996) Food restriction decreases serotonin and its synthesis rate in the hypothalamus. *NeuroReport* 7, 1153-1156.

Haleem D. J., Kennett G. A. and Curzon G. (1990) Hippocampal 5-HT synhesis is greater in females than in males and is more decreased by 5-HT-1A agonist 8-OH-DPAT. *J. Neural. Transm.* 79, 93-101

Haleem D. J., Parveen T (1994) Brain regional serotonin synthesis following adaptation to repeated restraint. *Neuroreport* 5(14), 1785-8.

Haleem DJ, Samad N, Perveen T, Haider S and Haleem MA. (2007a) Role of serotonin-1A receptors in restraint-induced behavioral deficits and adaptation to stress in rats. *Int. J. Neuroscience* 117, 243-57.

Haleem D. J., Samad N. and Haleem M. A. (2007b) Reversal of haloperidol-induced tardive vacuous chewing movements and supersensitive somatodendritic serotonergic response by buspirone in rats. *Pharmacol., Biochem. and Behav.* 87(1), 115-121.

Halmi K., Agras W.S., Crow S., Mitchell J., Wilson G., Bryson S. and Kraemer H. C. (2005) Predictors of treatment acceptance and completion in anorexia nervosa. *Arch. Gen. Psychiatry,* 62, 776–781.

Hu X., Giotakis O., Li T., Karwautz A.., Treasure J. and Collier D. A. (2003) Association of the 5-HT2c gene with susceptibility and minimum body mass index in anorexia nervosa. *NeuroReport*, 14, 781-783.

Jahng J. W., Kim J. G., Kim H. J., Kim B. T., Kang W. D. and Lee J. H. (2007) Chronic food restriction in young rats results in depression and anxiety like behaviors with decreased expression of serotonin reuptake transporter. *Brain Res* 1150, 100-107.

Kato R. (1960) Serotonin content of rat brain in relation to sex and age. J Neurochem 5, 202P.

Kaye W. (2008) Neurobiology of Anorexia and Bulimia Nervosa Purdue Ingestive Behavior Research Center Symposium Influences on Eating and Body Weight over the Lifespan: Children and Adolescents. *Physiol. Behav.* 94(1), 121–135.

Kaye W. H., Barbarich N. C., Putnam K., Gendall K. A., Fernstrom J., Fernstrom M., McConaha C. W. and Kishore A. (2003) Anxiolytic effects of acute tryptophan depletion in anorexia nervosa. *Int. J. Eat Disord.* 33(3), 257–267.

Kaye W., Bulik C., Thornton L., Barbarich N., Masters K., Fichter M., Halmi K,. Kaplan A., Strober M., Woodside D. B., Bergen A., Crow S., Mitchell J., Rotondo A., Mauri M., Cassano G., Keel P. K., Plotnicov K., Pollice C., Klump K., Lilenfeld L. R., Devlin B., Quadflieg R. and Berrettini W. H. (2004) Co morbidity of anxiety disorders with anorexia and bulimia nervosa. *Am. J. Psychiatry* 161, 2215–2221.

Kaye W. H., Frank G. K., Bailer U. F., Henry S. E., Meltzer C. C., Price J. C, Mathis C. A. and Wagner A. (2005) Serotonin alterations in anorexia and bulimia nervosa: new insights from imaging studies. *Physiol. Behav.* 85, 73-81.

Kaye W. H., Gwirtsman H. E., George D. T., Jimerson D. C. and Ebert M. H. (1988) CSF 5-HIAA concentrations in anorexia nervosa: reduced values in underweight subjects normalize after weight gain. *Biol. Psychiat.* 23, 102-105.

Kaye W. H., Nagata T., Weltzin T. E., Hsu L. K., Sokol M. S., McConaha C., Plotnicov K. H., Weise J. and Deep D. (2001) Double blind placebo controlled administration of fluoxetine in restricting and restricting purging type anorexia nervosa. *Biol. Psychiat.* 49, 644-652.

Kennett G. A. and Curzon G. (1988) Evidence that hypophagia induced by m-CPP and TFMPP requires 5-HT2C and 5-HT-1B receptors: hypophagia induced by RU 24969 only requires 5-HT-1B receptors. *Psychopharmacology Berl.* 96, 93-100.

Kerem N. C., Katzman D. K. (2003) Brain structure and function in adolescents with anorexia nervosa. *Adolesc. Med.* 14, 109-118.

Kingston K., Szmukler G., Andrewes D., Tress B. and Desmond P. (1996) Neuropsychological and structural brain changes in anorexia nervosa before and after refeeding. *Psychol. Med.* 26(1), 15–28.

Klein D. and Walsh B. (2003) Eating disorders. *Int. Rev. Psychiatry* 15, 205–216.

Klump K. L., McGue M. and Iacono W. G. (2000) Age differences in genetic and environmental influences on eating attitudes and behaviors in preadolescent and adolescent female twins. *Journal of Abnormal Psychology* 109(2), 239–251.

Kohl M., Foulon C. and Guelfi J. D. (2004) Hyperactivity and anorexia nervosa: behavioural and biological perspective. *Encepahle.* 30(5), 492-499.

Kron L., Katz J. L. Gorzynski G. and Weiner H. (1978) Hyperactivity in anorexia nervosa: A fundamental clinical feature. Comprehen Psychiatry 19(5), 433-440

Leibowitz S. F. (1986) Brain monoamines and peptides: role in the control of eating behavior. *Fed. Proc.* 45, 1396-1403.

Lilenfeld L. R., Kaye W. H., Greeno C. G., Merikangas K. R., Plotnicov K., Pollice C., Rao R., Strober M., Bulik C. M. and Nagy L. A. (1998) Controlled family study of anorexia nervosa and bulimia nervosa: psychiatric disorders in first-degree relatives and effects of proband comorbidity. *Arch. Gen. Psychiatry* 55(7), 603–610.

Millan M. J., Dekeyne A. and Gobert A. (1998) Serotonin (5-HT)2C receptors tonically inhibit dopamine (DA) and noradrenaline (NA), but not 5-HT, release in the frontal cortex in vivo. *Neuropharmacology* 37 (7) 953-955.

Mond J. M. and Calogero R. M. (2009) Excessive exercise in eating disorder patients and in healthy women. Aust N Z J Psychiatry. 43(3), 227-234This article is not included in your organization's subscription. However, you may be able to access this article under your organization's agreement with Elsevier.

Nacmias B.; Ricca V.; Tedde A.; Mezzani B.; Rotella C. M and Sorbi S. (1999) 5-HT2A receptor gene polymorphisms in anorexia nervosa and bulimia nervosa. *Neuroscience letters* 277(2), 134-136.

Nichols D. E. and Nichols C. D. (2008) Serotonin Receptors Chem. Rev. 108, 1614–1641

Ohrmann P., Kersting A., Suslow T, Lalee-Mentzel, J; Donges Uta-S., Fiebich Martin., Arolt V., Heindel W. and Pfleiderer B. (2004) Proton magnetic resonance spectroscopy in anorexia nervosa: correlations with cognition. *NeuroReport* 15, 549-553.

Oldendorf W. H. (1973) Carrier-mediated blood-brain barrier transport of short-chain monocarboxylic organic acids. *Am. J. Physiol.* 224(6), 1450-1453

Pierucci M., Di Matteo V. and Esposito E. (2004) Stimulation of serotonin2C receptors blocks the hyperactivation of midbrain dopamine neurons induced by nicotine administration. *J. Pharmacol. Exp. Ther.* 309(1),109-118.

Piji H., Koppeschaar H. P., Kohen A. F., Lestra J. A., Schoemaker H. C. and Frolich, M. (1993) Evidence of brain serotonin mediated control of carbohydrate consumption in normal weight and obese humans. *Int. J. Obes. Relat. Metabol. Disord.* 17, 513-520.

Ploog D. W. and Pirke K. M. (1987) Psychobiology of anorexia nervosa. *Psychol. Med.* 17, 843-859.

Rosmond R., Bouchard C. and Björntorp P. (2002) 5-HT2A Receptor Gene Promoter Polymorphism in Relation to Abdominal Obesity and Cortisol. *Obesity Research* 10, 585–589.

Rossi-Fanelli F. and Cangiano C. (1991) Increased availability of tryptophan in brain as common pathogenic mechanism for anorexia associated with different diseases. *Nutrition* 7, 364-367.

Rowland N. E. and Carlton, J. (1986) Neurobiology of an anorectic drug: fenfluramine. *Prog. Neurobiol.,* 27, 13-62.

Samad N., Batool F. and Haleem D. J. (2007) Neurochemical and behavioral effecs of 8-OH-DPAT following exposure to restraint stress in rats. *Pharmacol. Reports* 59: 173-80.

Schwartz D. H., Hernandez L. and Hoebel B. G. (1990) Tryptophan increases extracellular serotonin in the lateral hypothalamus of food deprived rats. *Brain Res. Bull.* 25, 803-807.

Siegfried Z., Berry E. M., Hao S. and Avraham Y. (2003) Animal models in the investigation of anorexia. *Physiol. Behav.* 79, 39-45.

Simansky K. J. and Nicklous, D. M. (2002) Parabrachial infusion of D-fenfluramine reduces food intake. Blockade by the 5-HT(1B) antagonist SB-216641. *Pharmacol. Biochem. Behav.* 71, 681-690.

Strober M., Freeman R., Lampert C., Diamond J. and Kaye W. (2000) Controlled family study of anorexia nervosa and bulimia nervosa: evidence of shared liability and transmission of partial syndromes. *Am. J. Psychiatry* 157(3), 393–401.

Strupp B. J., Weingartner H., Kaye W. and Gwirtsman H. (1986) Cognitive processing in anorexia nervosa, a disturbance in automatic information processing. *Neuropsychobiology*, 15(2), 89–94.

Sugrue M. F. (1987) Neuropharmacology of drugs affecting food intake. *Pharmacol. Ther.* 32, 145-182.

Tecott L. H. (2007) Serotonin and the orchestration of energy balance Cell Metab 6,352-361

Verge D., Daval G., Patey A., Gozlan H., Mestikawy S. and Hamon M. (1985) Presynaptic 5-HT autoreceptors on serotonergic cell bodies and/or dendrites but not terminals are of the 5-HT-1A subtype. *Eur. J. Pharmacol.* 113, 463-464.

Vickers S. P., Easton N., Webster I.J., Wyatt A., Bickerdike M. J., Dourish C. T. and Kennett G. A. (2003) Oral administration of the 5-HT-2C receptor agonist m-CPP reduces body weight gain in rats over 28 days as a result of maintained hypophagia. *Psychopharmacology* (Berlin) 167: 274-280.

Yudilevich D. L., De Rose N. and Sepulveda, F. V. 91972) Facilitated transport of amino acids in a single capillary circulation, 1972, *Brain Res.*, 44, 569-578.

Walsh B. T. and Devlin M. J. (1998) Eating disorders: progress and problems *Science,* 280(5368), 1387-1390.

Westberg L., Bah J., Rastam M., Gillberg C., Wenz E., Melke J., Hellstrand M., Eriksson E. (2002) Association between a polymorphism of the 5-HT2C receptor and weight loss in teenage girls. *Neuropsychopharmacology*, 26, 789-793.

Wurtman R. J. and Wurtman J. J. (1996) Brain serotonin, carbohydrate craving, obesity and depression. *Adv. Exp. Med. Biol.* 398, 35–41.

Zhang L., Ma W., Barker J. L. and Rubinow, D. R. (1999) Sex differences in expression of serotonin receptors (subtypes 1A and 2A) in rat brain: a possible role of testosterone. *Neuroscience.* 94, 251-259.

Chapter 6

OLDER AND AGING CONSUMERS DIET AND ITS INFLUENCE ON HEALTH: THE SPANISH CASE

Teresa García and Ildefonso Grande
Universidad Pública de Navarra, Pamplona, Spain

ABSTRACT

The purpose of this research is to identify and to valuate how healthy is the diet of some different groups of older and aging consumers living in Spain and to provide some actions, if any, to correct misbehaviors in food intake. Some variables affecting the diet as age, income, location and education are revisited. A large sample of older consumers' food expenditures is statistically treated using secondary data collected by the Spanish National Institute of Statistics by means of multivariate analysis techniques. Different levels of healthy diet are found regarding the consumers demographics.

Keywords. Diet, Aging consumers, Health, Multivariate analysis

1. INTRODUCTION

European consumers have undergone a major lifestyle transformation over the last decades reflected in increased concern for health issues, a healthy lifestyle, conservation of the environment, responsible consumption, etc. and the elderly consumer segment is no exception to these changes.

These changes in the socio-economic environment have created a growing segment of older consumers with higher incomes that has attracted the interest of marketers. There is a large body of research pointing to the importance of the elderly consumer segment across Europe as a target for the various components of the industrial sector. This obviously applies to the entire agrifood industry, including producers, manufacturers, distributors, caterers, and all those engaged in agriculture for nutritional purposes.

Although throughout history the concern of humankind has been to obtain the necessary nutrients to ensure the proper bodily functioning, today's nutritional demands are shaped in a different manner. That is, a diet that, in addition to enabling us to carry out our activities, also includes foods to enhance our health and reduce the risk of contracting certain ailments, called functional foods. The aforementioned objectives feature prominently among the demands of the elderly consumer segment.

Accoding Verbeke (2004) these functional foods match these demands which have been launched on the back of the current direct link between diet and health. Frewer et al. (2003), Verbeke (2004) and Urala and Lähteenmäki (2005) point out there is a significant probability to accept functional products as age raises because consumers trust they are healthier.

The population ageing process affecting several European countries, including Spain, is leading to continually improving in living conditions: better health and, what is supposedly more important from the management perspective, improvements in economic status. (Bódalo, 2003; Ong et al., 2008; Jauhiainen, 2008). Spain's socio-economic development over the last decades of the 20th century matched that of other societies and has meant a considerable increase in overall income levels. This in turn has created a "well-being society" with newly emerging needs that prove a challenge not only to retailers but also to the administration.

As time passes people begin to show signs of wear and tear both physical and mental, between which there may be a mutual cause and effect relationship. The earliest research into the possible impact of people's physical condition on their food purchase habits dates back to the early 1960s. The financial position of the elderly, along with the physical and mental limitations resulting from the inevitable ageing process, are all conditioning factors of their food consumption (Burger et al.; 2003, Lundkvist et al., 2010).

Despite the importance of income as a consumption determinant, it would be an exaggeration to use it to explain all the variation in the eating habits of the elderly. Research has therefore gone into identifying further factors and exploring their impact. Quandt et al. (1998) and Bódalo (2003) report age, gender, social class, rural or urban habitat, access to support networks, etc... as factors to be taken into consideration. Findings in a similar vein were obtained by Poortinga (2007).

According to Gil (2004), the elderly as we have known them until now are doomed to disappear and be replaced by new generations of better educated, more productive and more able elderly citizens. This author suggests that such a cultural revolution among the elderly would take several generations and require them to have a level of education that were not significantly lower in quantitative terms than that of the succeeding younger generations.

High educational level means more qualified job and higher income. Customers belonging this group should be more concern with food intake (Grande, 2002). This will happen as soon as the overpopulated baby boomer generation reaches old-age (Harris and Blisard, 2002). In Spain, this generation is made up of those born between the 1959 Stabilisation Plan and the 1978 Constitution.

Donkin et al. (1998) and Mckay et al. (2006) concluded that living on one's own, gender, and level of education all influence food consumption. In their view, this is due, on the one hand, to the fact that men living alone do not take the trouble to cook and, on the other that single women take more care of their appearance.

Suggest that some of these consumers are living on limited means and that their consumption habits are marked by a series of socio-demographic and geographics factors, making them immune to the marketing efforts of agrifood firms. It is observed that older and elderly people spend in hogher proportion in basic food (Bódalo, 2003 and Grande, 2002), specially in fresh products. The expenditure in more elaborated products is lower than the observed in other groups of consumers.

Age

Time and the aging process affect the purchase basket composition. Quantity and quality are affected by health status. Age and consumer preferences have been researched decades ago. Some outstanding researchers are Gillett (1970), Zeithaml and Gilly (1987), Schewe (1988), Bone, (1991), Moschis (1992, 1994) y Wolfe (1997). They conclude that the age affects the lifestyle and the consumer behavior, but emphasize that researchers should take into consideration not only the chronological age, but self-perceived age and health status. More recently Pieniak et al. (2010), point out that the older the consumer the more concerned with the diet and the food intake.

Spanish evidence suggests that food expenses diminish as the consumers age increase, probably because very old consumer's income is lower than the recently retired income. Financial risk and lower calories need are additional explanations.

Grande (1993) states that despite retirement age is the most repeated argument to consider a person as a third age integral, chronological age is only one side. Biological age conditions the health status, social age has an effect on the roles and habits, and self perceived age conditions the lifestyles. However, only the chronological age is the objective parameter determined by the birth date. Others are subjective and they should be measured for each person. In Spain there is not available information for measuring subjective age perceptions. Ad hoc research should be conducted for this purpose.

Age perception is also related with the number of persons which the consumer lives with. The impact of living alone or in a couple has effects on the quality of one's diet, etc. (Wyne, 1999; Larsson and Silverstein, 2004). Furthermore, the needs of those living on high pensions cannot be compared with those living on the basic pension, especially women living on the basic widow's pension.

Gender

Regarding the gender Moss et al. (2007) and Hare et al. (2001), point out that gender appears to mark a real difference in food expenditure. Rousset et al. (2006) stressed the differences found between in the consumption habits of elderly men and women especially in relation to food. According to a study conducted by these authors in France, this effect is due to the fact that women tend to care more about their health and appearance, etc.

Grande (2002) concluded that there are some similarities with the French results and he suggests that consumer behaviour dealing with the gender has a cultural basis. Women over 65 years old were born and raised within scarcity times, and they were educated in some typical roles attached to women, as housewives, to take care of their husbands and children, and so on. Currently observed behaviour in older women is greatly conditioned by obsolete values and lifestyles.

Geographical Areas

There many differences across Spanish geographical areas regarding the income, the consumer preferences and their lifestyles. Spain is a melting pot of cultures. This country gathers regions with different cultural and historical backgrounds. Northern areas are more developed than those located in the south of Spain. Northern areas are typically industrial and the services industry is very relevant. In southern areas agriculture is the main activity. It is expected to meet differences in food expenditures based on geographical locations.

The level of life in capital towns is higher than the observed in small towns or rural areas. Older consumers living there had a better qualified jobs, they earned higher incomes and the retirement pensions are higher that obtained by farmers or fishermen.

As noted by Marcellini et al. (2007), the definition of rural and urban areas varies across Europe from one country to another. These authors suggest that the term rural should be used to describe the kind of setting in which agriculture is the main source of household income. Such settings impose certain consumption patterns, involving the consumption of home-grown produce, affecting the whole household, the elderly included (Wilson et al., 2004).

The size of the place of residence also has an impact on food availability, because one's food supply usually depends on where one live. Many rural areas are still under endowed in terms of retail services (Donkin el al., 1999; Marcellini et al., 2007; Coveney and O'Dwyer, 2009). Capital towns provide more opportunities for purchasing services and goods than smaller or rural areas. Some goods or services are not available in lesser developed areas. It could be expected that *per capitae* food expenses increase as the size of the populations raise.

According to Entrena (1999), the long-term trend in relative terms is for declining food expenditure. It can therefore be assumed to depend on other factors besides income. McKie (1999) believes that diet, and thereby food expenditure is the result of physical and economic conditions and other personal restrictions affecting ease of outlet access, deriving from health and income status, availability of transport, and the ability to cook for oneself or to shop alone. In addition, the election of foods by all these factors, have a great influence in the health of the older people (Hare et al., 1999).

2. OBJETIVES AND METHODOLOGY

Based on a review of the literature and findings for different countries, the purpose of the present study is to determine whether the underlying factors of food expenditure among elderly consumers in Spain are the same as those reported for other countries. Our objective is to detect factors, if any, affecting the expenditures in food and to valuate in what extent the diet is healthy or not. According the literature review a number of hypotheses can be stated.

- Ho = Income is a relevant variable that affects the older and elderly consumers food expenditures. The higher the incomes, the higher the expenditures in healthy food, as fish, skimmed milk or olive oil.

- H1= Diets are not healthy in the same way across locations. These are relevant to explain the observed differences in food expenditures.
- H2 = The size of the municipality affects the food expenditure. The larger is the population, the larger is the expenditure, and conversely.
- H3= Age explain differences in food expenditures. The older the consumer is, the lower is the food expenditure.

Observed evidences in other countries highlight that women spend more money in food and their diet is healthier. The hypothesis of the gender influence on expenditures cannot be tested in the Spanish case. Age and gender interact. The life expectancy is higher for women and, consequently, there more widows than widowers. The pensions of the widows are lower than the widowers´, and lower income means lower expenditures. Moreover, most of the widows never joined the labour force, there were traditional housewives and their pensions are lower than received by men.

For testing these hypotheses we have analyzed a random sample of older and elderly consumers. Data source is the National Survey of Household Budget in 2008. This panel is a stratified sample of households and collects information of the expenditures in several hundreds of products and services. These data are collected over the course of the year. They are corrected to eliminate the influence of inflation and differences in price levels due to the household location within the country. The final output is an extremely reliable database for analyses. Data are collected from a sample composed by 1237 households. All households are composed by people aged 65 and over. The household size is one or two persons, no matter the civil status, none under 65.

The considered food expenditures measure the budget in the following categories: rice, bread, pasta, some ox, cow, veal, pork, lamb, poultry, fish, seafood, fat milk, skimmed milk, yogurt, cheese, eggs, butter, margarine, olive oil, citrus fruits, bananas, apples, pears, beans, potatoes, sugar, marmalade, chocolate, ice cream, coffee, tea, cocoa, spring water, soft drinks, juices, alcoholic beverages, wine, and beer.

The statistical method for the empirical test has been principal component analysis using the expenditures as continuous variables. The supplementary nominal variables have been gender of the head of the family, education municipality size and location. Age and income are the supplementary continuous variables. The following charts display the clusters found.

Older consumers are broken down into three clusters. The first one holds 786 households, the 63.54% of the sample. The relevant characteristic for this cluster is their lower education level. There are 1094 households in the sample in which the head of the family has primary education. They are the 88.43 % of the sample. In this cluster, the 64.99 % of the households have primary education, 711 in total. Proportion of this sort of households in the group is 90.46 %, 771 divided by 786. The proportions are different enough to let us to conclude that the lowest education level is a relevant characteristic in this group. The characterizing continuous variables are age and income. The mean of the age is over the average value of the sample, and income is lower than the observed in the sample.

The consumer profile of cluster 1 characterizes a group belonging to lower social class, less educated and older than the average. The expenditures in food reveal that overall they spend less money in all the considered foods in this research. Taking into consideration the healthy diet, the Mediterranean cuisine, the consumers of this cluster eat fish, olive oil and skimmed milk at the lowest proportion when they are compared to other groups and their food expenditures. However the differences in fruits, vegetables and pulses consumption are smaller. This group of consumes follow a balanced diet.

Chart 1. Characteristics of cluster 1
Group: CLUSTER 1 / 3 (Count: 786 Percentage: 63.54)

Variable label	Caracteristic categories	% of category in group	% of category in set	% of group in category	Test-value	Probability	Weight
Education	Primary	90.46	88.44	64.99	2.80	0.003	1094

Characteristic variables	Cluster mean	Overall mean	Cluster Std. deviation	Overall Std. deviation	Test-value	Probability
Age	73.388	73.090	6.012	5.919	2.34	0.010
Income	8774.760	9355.640	4588.430	4919.780	-5.48	0.000
Butter	1.621	3.031	9.246	16.414	-3.99	0.000
Non fatmilk	32.749	40.456	70.526	88.004	-4.06	0.000
Tea	1.683	3.026	10.114	14.883	-4.19	0.000
Beer	13.207	18.942	43.730	60.019	-4.44	0.000
Ice cream	3.351	7.294	16.042	35.358	-5.18	0.000
Pears	14.888	18.705	25.520	32.441	-5.46	0.000
Beans	11.161	16.963	32.117	49.210	-5.47	0.000
Alcoholic beverages	5.737	16.410	36.616	88.678	-5.59	0.000
Poultry	84.530	98.957	102.995	119.764	-5.59	0.000
Pork	49.083	64.556	87.213	128.420	-5.59	0.000
Cocoa	3.654	7.192	17.300	28.654	-5.73	0.000
Wine	36.795	58.557	96.060	174.379	-5.79	0.000
Potatoes	17.569	25.751	34.616	61.352	-6.19	0.000
Juices	5.602	10.221	17.757	32.940	-6.51	0.000
Marmelade	5.386	10.636	24.183	34.554	-7.05	0.000
Banana	15.086	19.767	23.985	30.660	-7.09	0.000
Pasta	7.037	11.281	17.184	25.690	-7.67	0.000
Seafood	31.757	59.352	86.545	163.476	-7.83	0.000
Chocolate	6.074	11.651	20.141	32.818	-7.89	0.000
Margarine	1.287	2.971	5.894	9.804	-7.98	0.000
Spring water	8.099	15.920	24.438	44.437	-8.17	0.000
Olive oil	58.687	92.396	119.576	189.368	-8.26	0.000
Fatmilk	73.092	94.169	95.999	116.851	-8.37	0.000
Citrics	39.771	52.849	49.680	68.732	-8.83	0.000
Rice	8.568	13.334	16.062	23.972	-9.23	0.000
Apples	21.016	29.999	30.883	43.902	-9.50	0.000
Eggs	17.560	24.256	24.856	32.423	-9.59	0.000
Soft drinks	15.962	28.228	37.367	57.533	-9.90	0.000
Yogourth	29.768	44.203	43.017	66.176	-10.12	0.000
Cheese	57.202	83.742	83.260	119.586	-10.30	0.000
Ox. cow. veal	107.037	165.139	172.950	261.316	-10.32	0.000
Coffee	22.464	38.220	47.992	69.835	-10.47	0.000
Bread	183.588	211.337	104.156	117.251	-10.98	0.000
Sugar	10.496	19.819	21.519	36.246	-11.94	0.000
Fish	154.587	222.536	168.448	257.233	-12.26	0.000

Chart 2 depicts the second cluster. This group is defined by its location. The households are located in the north of Spain, capital towns, high density areas y their educational level is higher than the observed in cluster 1. Olders consume more of all the listed foods. It is remarkable that the expenditures in olive oil, fish, and skimmed milk, or yogurt, paramount of a healthy diet, are far much higher than the observed in clusters 1 and 3. They eat a healthy diet.

Chart 2. Characteristics of cluster 2
CLUSTER 2 / 3 (Count = 211 Percentage: 17.05)

Variable label	Caracteristic categories	% of category in group	% of category in set	% of group in category	Test-value	P-value	Weight
Density	High density	59.24	43.25	23.36	5.05	0.000	535
Geographical area	Northwest	24.64	15.68	26.80	3.66	0.000	194
Municipality	Capital town	48.82	39.29	21.19	3.01	0.001	486
Autonomous region	Asturias	9.00	4.61	33.33	2.94	0.002	57
Autonomous region	Cantabria	7.11	3.31	36.59	2.91	0.002	41
Education	Secondary	9.00	5.25	29.23	2.38	0.009	65

Characteristic variables	Cluster mean	Overall mean	Cluster Std. deviation	Overall Std. deviation	Test-value	Probability
Fish	494.932	222.536	396.019	257.233	16.88	0.000
Ox cow veal	391.503	165.139	406.101	261.316	13.81	0.000
Apples	67.256	29.999	66.334	43.902	13.53	0.000
Citrus fruits	109.595	52.849	107.483	68.732	13.16	0.000
Seafood	164.411	59.352	314.632	163.476	10.25	0.000
Pears	37.401	18.705	50.160	32.441	9.19	0.000
Spring water	40.036	15.920	72.404	44.437	8.65	0.000
Yogourth	78.731	44.203	95.521	66.176	8.32	0.000
Banana	34.578	19.767	44.285	30.660	7.70	0.000
Cheese	140.474	83.742	161.793	119.586	7.56	0.000
Poultry	152.955	98.957	172.313	119.764	7.19	0.000
Ice cream	22.197	7.294	72.821	35.358	6.72	0.000
Eggs	37.090	24.256	45.345	32.423	6.31	0.000
Bread	247.428	211.337	107.712	117.251	4.91	0.000
Potatoes	42.324	25.751	96.017	61.352	4.31	0.000
Olive oil	129.789	92.396	198.609	189.368	3.15	0.001
Pork	86.986	64.556	210.380	128.420	2.78	0.003
Non fatmilk	54.224	40.456	94.524	88.004	2.49	0.006
Soft drinks	37.008	28.228	62.895	57.533	2.43	0.007

In cluster 3 is characteristic that the consumers are located in rural and low density areas. The main characteristic in this group is they eat the more unhealthy diet. Older and aging consumers in this group eat filling foods as bread and rice in a greater extent than consumer of cluster 1 and 2 do. Typical food intake in this cluster is harmful fat and grease, as butter and margarine, wine and spirits, fat milk and cheese, white sugar and stimulating drinks as coffee or tea.

This diet, richer in saturated fat and cholesterol, alcoholic drinks and others can affect the blood pressure, arteries health and it is potentially the cause of heart ailments, attacks, collapses or ictus. We can conclude that food habits in this cluster should change. Public authorities should develop social marketing campaigns in order to change the eating habits in this cluster in benefit of no saturated fat, more vegetables, less sugar, coffee and tea.

Chart 3. Characteristics of cluster 3
Group: CLUSTER 3 / 3 (Count: 240 - Percentage: 19.40)

Variable label	Caracteristic categories	% of category in group	% of category in set	% of group in category	Test-value	P-value	Weight
Municipality	Rural areas	42.50	33.63	24.52	3.13	0.001	416
Density	Low density	48.75	40.74	23.21	2.73	0.003	504

Characteristic variables	Cluster mean	Overall mean	Cluster Std. deviation	Overall Std. deviation	Test-value	p-value
Sugar	54.366	19.819	55.853	36.246	16.44	0.000
Coffee	89.740	38.220	101.518	69.835	12.73	0.000
Rice	28.340	13.334	35.782	23.972	10.80	0.000
Margarine	8.891	2.971	15.929	9.804	10.42	0.000
Fatmilk	160.981	94.169	148.093	116.851	9.86	0.000
Soft drinks	60.679	28.228	86.002	57.533	9.73	0.000
Cocoa	23.138	7.192	52.983	28.654	9.60	0.000
Bread	270.486	211.337	134.029	117.251	8.70	0.000
Juices	26.230	10.221	60.347	32.940	8.38	0.000
Marmalade	26.591	10.636	54.540	34.554	7.96	0.000
Chocolat	26.495	11.651	47.412	32.818	7.80	0.000
Pasta	22.429	11.281	36.518	25.690	7.48	0.000
Olive oil	49.919	92.396	303.912	189.368	7.06	0.000
Beans	36.863	16.963	85.564	49.210	6.98	0.000
Wine	122.957	58.557	319.485	174.379	6.37	0.000
Butter	8.854	3.031	31.426	16.414	6.12	0.000
Alcoholic beverages	46.667	16.410	161.626	88.678	5.89	0.000
Eggs	34.904	24.256	34.382	32.423	5.66	0.000
Cheese	120.785	83.742	146.572	119.586	5.34	0.000
Beer	37.346	18.942	96.894	60.019	5.29	0.000
Yogourth	61.122	44.203	80.455	66.176	4.41	0.000
Pork	95.509	64.556	137.823	128.420	4.16	0.000
Tea	6.213	3.026	23.244	14.883	3.69	0.000
Potatoes	37.974	25.751	82.226	61.352	3.44	0.000

CONCLUSION

Throughout this research is based on relevant studies developed by recognized researchers. Empirical tests proved that the diet of aging and older consumers is conditioned by income, gender, education, location and municipality size. Based on these evidences a bundle of hypotheses have been stated and tested using Spanish official data. Sophisticated statistical techniques as principal component analysis and grouping techniques.

The Spanish evidence do not contradicts the observed facts in other countries. In the Spanish case the stated hypothesis cannot be rejected. Older and aging consumers can be clustered intro three groups. In two of them the diet is healthy and balanced, but the total expenditures are different according their income and education level. The third group is located mainly in rural areas. The diet in this case is less healthy, richer in animal and saturated fat, alcoholic and stimulating drinks. A lower consumption of skimmed milk, vegetables, yogurt, olive and sunflower oil also characterizes this group. This diet is potentially the cause of heart collapses, ictus and colon cancer. Public authorities should warn the population the harmful consequences of this diet using social marketing campaigns to benefit healthier diet.

REFERENCES

Bódalo, E. (2003). Aproximación sociológica a las necesidades y al consumo de los mayores. *Revista Española de Investigaciones Sociológicas*, 103, 83-111.

Bone, P.F. (1991). Identifying Mature Segments. *Journal of Services Marketing*. Winter, 47-60.

Burguer, J., Fleischer, J. and Gochfeld, M. (2003). Fish, shellfish and meat meals of the public in Singapore. *Environmental Research*, 92, 254-261.

Coveney, J. and O'Dwyer, L.A. (2009). Effects of mobility and location on food access. Health and Place, 15, 45-55.

Donkin, A., Dowler, E.A., Stevenson, S.J. and Turner, S.A. (1999). Mapping access to food al local level. *British Food of Journal*, 101 (7), 554-564.

Donkin, A.; Johnson, A.; Lilley, J.; Morgan, K.; Neale, R.J.; Page, R.M. and Silburn, R. (1998). Gender and living alone as determinants of fruit and vegetable consumption among the elderly living at home in urban Nottingham. *Appetite*, 30, 39-51.

Entrena, F. (1999). De la alimentación de subsistencia al consumo preferencial: el caso español. *Estudios sobre consumo*, 50, 27-36.

Frewer, L.; Scholderer, J.; Lambert, N. (2003). Consumer acceptance of functional foods: issues for the future. *British Food Journal*, 105 (10), 714-731.

Gil, E. (2004). El "poder gris". Consecuencias culturales y políticas del envejecimiento de la población. *Información Comercial Española*, 815, 219-230.

Gillett, P. L. (1970). A profile of urban in-home shoppers. Journal of Retailing, 49, 38-50.

Grande, I. (1993). Marketing estratégico para la tercera edad. Principios para atender a un segmento creciente. Esic.

Grande, I. (2000). Profiling older consumers. 29 th European Marketing Academy Conference, Rotterdam.

Grande, I. (2002). El consumo de la Tercera Edad. Esic. Madrid.

Hare, C., Kirk, D. and Lang, T. (1999). Identifying the expectations of older food consumers: more than a shopping list of wants. *Journal of Marketing Practice: Applied Marketing Science*, 5 (6/7/8), 212-232.

Hare, C.; Kirk, D. and Lang, T. (2001). The food shopping experience of older consumer in Scotland: critical incidents. *International Journal of Retail and Distribution Management*, 29 (1), 25-40.

Harris, J.M. and Blisard, N. (2002). Food-consumption patterns among elderly age groups. *Journal of Food Distribution Research*, 33 (1), 85-91.

Jauhiainen, J.S. (2008). Will the retiring baby boomers return to rural periphery? *Journal of Rural Studies,* 25 (1), 25-34.

Larsson, K. and Silverstein, M. (2004). The effect of marital and parental status on informal support and service utilization: A study of older Swedes living alone. *Journal of Aging Studies*, 18, 231-244.

Lundkvist, P.; Fjellström, Ch.; Sidenvall, B.; Lumbers, M. and Raats, M. (2010) Management of healthy eating in everyday life among senior Europeans. Appetite, in press. Doi:10.1016/j.appet.2010.09.015.

Marcellini, F.; Giuli, C.; Gagliardi, C. and Papa, R. (2007). Aging in Italy: urban–rural differences. *Archives of Gerontology and Geriatrics*, 44, 243-260.

Mckay, D.L., Houser, R.F., Blumberg, J.B and Goldberg, J.P. (2006). Nutrition information sources vary with education level in a population of older adults. *Journal of the American Dietetic Association*, 106 (7), 1108-1111.

McKie, L. (1999). Older people and food: independence, locality and diet. *British Food Journal,* 101 (7), 528-536.

Moschis, G. (1992). Marketing to older adults: An over view and assessment of present knowledge and practice. *Journal of Consumer Marketing*, 33-41.

Moschis, G. (1994). Consumer behaviour in later life: multidisciplinary contributions and implications for research. Journal of the Academy of Marketing Science, 22, 195-204.

Moss, S.Z.; Moss, M.S.; Kilbride, J.E. and Rubinstein, R.L. (2007). Frail men's perspectives on food and eating. *Journal of Aging Studies*, 21 (4), 314-324.

Ong, F.S., Kitchen, J.P. and Jama, A.T. (2008). Consumption patterns and silver marketing: an analysis of older consumers in Malaysia. *Marketing Intelligence and Planning*, 26 (7), 682-698.

Pieniak, Z.; Verbeke, W.; Olsen, S.O.; Hansen, K.B. and Brunso, K. (2010) Health-related attitudes as a basis for segmenting European fish consumers. Food Policy, 35, 448-455.

Poortinga, W. (2007). The prevalence and clustering of four major lifestyle risk factors in an English adult population. *Preventive Medicine*, 44, 124-128.

Quandt, S.A., Arcudy, T.A. and Bell, R.A. (1998). Self-management of nutritional risk among older adults: A conceptual model and case studies from rural communities. *Journal of Aging Studies*, 12 (4), 351-368.

Rousset, S.; Droit-Volet, S. and Boirie, Y. (2006). Change in protein intake in elderly french people living at home after a nutritional information program targeting protein consumption. *Journal of the American Dietetic Association*, 106 (2), 253-261.

Schewe, C. D. (1988) Marketing to our aging population: Responding to physical changes. *Journal of Consumer Marketing*, 61-73.

Urala, N. and Lähteenmäki, L. (2005) Consumers' changing attitudes towards functional foods. *Food Quality and Preference*.

Verbeke, W. (2004) Consumer acceptance of functional foods: socio-demographic, cognitive and attitudinal determinants. *Food Quality and Preference*.

Wilson, L.C.; Alexander, A. and Lumbers, M. (2004). Food access and dietary variety among older people. *International Journal of Retail and Distribution Management*, 32 (2), 109-122.

Wolfe, D. B. (1997). Older Markets and the new marketing paradigm. *Journal of Consumer Marketing*, 14, 294-303.

Wyne, A. (1999). Nutrition in older people. *Nutrition and Food Science*, 5, 219-233.

Zeithaml, V. and Gilly, M. C. (1987) Characteristics affecting the acceptance of retailing technologies: a comparison of elderly and nonelderly consumers. *Journal of Retailing*, 63 (1), 49-68.

Chapter 7

APPETITE PREFERENCES: INVESTIGATING THE ROLES OF RELATIONSHIP SATISFACTION AND IDEALISTIC THINKING IN FOOD DECISION-MAKING STRATEGIES OF ROMANTIC COUPLES

Jennifer M. Bonds-Raacke
Fort Hays State University, Hays, Kansas, USA

ABSTRACT

Couples who had been dating exclusively for one year or longer were recruited to participate in the study from a public, east coast university. A total of 72 individuals (36 couples) completed a food related decision-making task first independently and then jointly. Participants completed a demographic questionnaire to gather information on gender, age, ethnicity, length of relationship, number of children, and living arrangements. Also, the Evaluation and Nurturing Relationship Issues, Communication and Happiness (ENRICH) Martial Satisfaction Scale (EMS) was modified for dating couples and administered. This scale has two subscales, which measure relationship satisfaction and idealistic thoughts about the relationship.

Hypotheses for the current study were partially supported. First, relationship satisfaction and idealistic thoughts were significantly related to likelihood ratings for eating at specific restaurants. One possible explanation for the current findings is that higher relationship satisfaction scores and lower idealistic thoughts are exhibited by couples who are more comfortable in their respective relationships and have set realistic expectations. Thus, these couples are more likely to demonstrate food preferences when making their likelihood ratings. On the contrary, couples who do not experience these same levels of satisfaction or feel an increased pressure to be the perfect couple, may be less likely to show preferences in their food ratings. Results also indicated that the levels of relationship satisfaction and idealistic thinking did not differ by the joint decision-making strategy of the couple. These results are surprising in that these measures were related to overall joint likelihood ratings. A larger sample of couples utilizing similar decision-making strategies may reveal differences on these measures.

The current study is not without limitations. As previously mentioned, the sample size could be increased to raise the power of the study. Secondly, the researcher was present as the couples were making joint decisions which may have influenced interactions and finally, not all of the couples were members of the clusters demonstrating common decision-making strategies. Although this study provides initial information on relationship measures and food decisions, additional research is needed. In particular, research directed at how couples make decisions about fast food is warranted given its popularity and health risks. Future research is also needed to explore how the stage of the romantic relationship influences food decisions and relationship domains.

INTRODUCTION

The importance of food during the dating stage of romantic relationships has been noted by many scholars (e.g., Rappoport, 2003; Sobal, Bove, and Rauschenbach, 2002). In fact, romantic relationships develop and progress in intimacy over shared meals (Rappoport, 2003). Shared meals continue to be of importance as individuals move from the dating stage of the relationship to marriage (Dianton, 1998; Marshall and Anderson, 2002) with food used during the wedding ceremony to communicate values and heritage (Rappoport, 2003). Some level of compromise regarding the food consumed during shared meals will be needed (Bove, Sobal, and Rauschenbach, 2003; Kozak, 2010) to avoid conflict. However, couples can attain many benefits from regularly sharing a meal such as reducing work related stress (Jacob, Allen, Hill, Mead, and Ferris, 2008). Thus, eating behavior, and food in general, plays an important role in all stages of romantic relationships.

This established link between food and romantic relationships raises an important question. Namely, to what extent are eating behaviors, and consequently body size, impacting other components of the romantic relationship? Researchers have found that in the early stages of a relationship, the weight of an individual is related to many factors. First, weight is related to the likelihood of dating for women. Specifically, overweight women are less likely to be dating than their peers of normal weight (Sheets and Ajmere, 2005). The weight of an individual is also related to partner selection. When selecting partners, women are more likely to demonstrate a preference for men of a similar body size to themselves, while men are more likely to demonstrate a preference for women of a smaller body size (Aruguete, Edman, and Yates, 2009). With regard to women, research documents a discrepancy between current weight and idealized wedding weights (Neighbors and Sobal, 2008). Finally, in younger couples, research has found evidence of matching by weight (Schafer and Keith, 1990).

As a relationship progresses, food continues to be linked to the relationship differently for men and women in the areas of dieting, weight, and body image. To begin, dieting patterns differ between men and women. For men, higher relationship satisfaction leads to higher levels of body satisfaction and less dieting for their partners. For women, on the other hand, lower relationship satisfaction is linked to the decision to engage in dieting behaviors (Friedman, Dixon, Brownell, Whisman, and Wilfley, 1999; Markey, Markey, and Birch 2001) and higher self-esteem leads to higher levels of dieting for their partners (Boyes, Flecther, and Latner, 2007). Women, in general, also monitor the dieting of their partners more than men (Markey, Gomel, and Markey, 2008). Next, weight influences men and women in different ways. For example, relationship functioning and weight are negatively related for women, whereas relationship functioning and weight are not significantly related for men (Boyes and Latner, 2009). This discrepancy is similar to that of Sheets and Ajmere (2005) who found that weight and relationship satisfaction are negatively correlated for women and positively correlated for men. Even marital change (e.g., entering into marriage, divorce) impacts men's and women's weight in different ways (Sobal, Rauschenbach, and Frongillo, 2003). Third, body image also varies between the sexes, with the wife's body image explaining a larger portion of the variance in martial satisfaction (Meltzer and McNulty, 2010).

Although there are documented differences between men and women in terms of the role that eating plays in the relationship, there are also similarities. For example, both men and women will regulate the eating behaviors of their partners if their partners have relatively high BMIs (Markey, et al., 2008). Research also finds that spouses influence one another in positive or negative ways when making healthy food choices (Markey, et al., 2001; Schafer, Keith, and Schafer, 2000). It is important to note and understand the positive influences that spouses can have on one another to negate negative factors including: (a) the nutritional problems associated with fast food behaviors (Larson, Neumark-Sztainer, Story, Wall, Harnack, and Eisenberg, 2008), the demands of work and family that can lead to unhealthy eating (Lallukka, et al., 2010), the pressure that women face to provide healthy meals for the entire family without support from spouses (Madden and Chamberlain, 2010), and the amount of money spent yearly on prepared foods (Kroshus, 2008). Yet, one of the most salient reasons to better understand how spouses can have a positive influence on food decisions is the finding that couples have concordant health statuses (Meyler, Stimpson, and Peek, 2007). Research has examined the extent to which couples have concordant health status on variables including: dietary intake, smoking, alcohol, illegal drug use, and lifestyle. Physical activity and nutrition programs have been successful at improving healthy behaviors in couples (Burke, Giangiulio, Gillam, Beilin, and Houghton, 2003) and combat marital obligations that might compete with physical activity (Craig and Truswell, 1990). It has been recommended that future nutritional programs explore food choice scripts. These scripts can provide needed information on what behaviors and cognitions individuals engage in during the evening meal (Blake, Bisogni, Sobal, Jastran, and Devine, 2008), which can be used to help prepare individuals to make healthier decisions rather than decisions made out of habit.

To provide additional insights into how food impacts romantic relationships, food related decisions by couples have been examined. Szybillo, Sosanie, and Tenebein (1977) recognized the importance many years ago to the food industry of understanding how married couples make decisions to eat out at different types of restaurants. In order to obtain information, the researchers interviewed married couples to determine who in the family made decisions about eating out at restaurants. Results indicated that both husbands and wives were involved in the decision to eat at conventional restaurants. Recently, Amiraian and Sobal (2009) investigated how the type of restaurant selected for dining was influenced by the stage of the relationship. For example, participants indicated that fast food restaurants were viewed as the least appropriate place to eat on a date when compared to casual / family restaurants, upscale restaurants, and in the home. Yet, eating at fast food restaurants was more acceptable in long-term relationships than on a first date. Bonds-Raacke investigated how married couples (2006) and extended dating couples (2008) made decisions about eating at restaurants. In both experiments, a decision task regarding eating at restaurants was completed independently by each member of the couple and then collectively. Results indicated that dating couples utilized more decision-making strategies than married couples did. For example, married couples used the following three decision-making strategies: the familiarity strategy, the flexible strategy, and the genre based strategy. However, extended dating couples exhibited five decision-making strategies: the familiarity strategy, the flexible strategy, the genre and familiarity strategy, the seafood genre based strategy, and the Italian genre based strategy. In addition, collective decisions about eating out more frequently resembled the male's independent decisions in married couples, whereas collective strategies more frequently resembled the female's independent decisions in extended dating couples. These results support previous work by Brown and Miller (2002) who found that traditional couples made food decisions consistent with the husband's food preferences.

The purpose of the current study was to further investigate how food decisions impact couples in romantic relationships. Specifically, this study sought to examine how food decisions were related to self-reported measures of relationship satisfaction and idealistic thoughts about romantic relationships. Thus, two hypotheses were formed.

- H_1 In the first hypothesis, it was predicated that relationship satisfaction and idealistic thoughts would be related to willingness to eat at specific restaurants genres. This hypothesis was formed from previous research such as that by Amiraian and Sobal (2009) demonstrating that stage of romantic relationship is related to selected places to eat. It was further predicted that couples with higher levels of relationship satisfaction would indicate more preferences in general and less of a desire to eat at traditional "dating" restaurant genres.
- H_2 It was also predicted that levels of relationship satisfaction and idealistic thoughts would differ by the joint decision-making strategies employed by the couples. This prediction was formed with previous research in mind that identified decision-making strategies of couples in romantic relationships. In order to examine this hypothesis, the joint decision-making strategies identified by Bonds-Raacke (2008) were utilized. It was hypothesized that couples using the flexible decision-making strategy would have higher levels of relationship satisfaction and lower levels of idealistic distortions.

METHOD

A total of 72 individuals (36 couples) were recruited and participated from Introduction to Psychology courses at a public, east cost university. For couples to be considered as extended dating couples, they needed to meet the requirement of dating the same person for a minimum period of one year or longer (as used in previous research; Bonds-Raacke, Bearden, Carriere, Anderson, and Nicks, 2001). Students currently enrolled in Introduction to Psychology received partial course credit for their participation. Of the participants, 38% were Caucasian, 29% were Native-American, 25% were African-American, 4% were Hispanic, and 4% were multiracial. In addition, couples had been dating for an average of 23 months (SD = 14) and only a small percentage had children (9) or currently cohabited (11).

A 3 (type of restaurant: steakhouse, seafood, and Italian) X 2 (familiarity with restaurant: well known and not well known) within-subjects design was utilized. Thus, participants viewed the following 6 restaurant menus that were formatted in the same manner: seafood restaurant that was well known (*Red Lobster*), seafood restaurant that was not well known (*McGrath's Fish House*), Italian restaurant that was well known (*The Olive Garden*), Italian restaurant that was not well known (*Biaggi's*), steakhouse that was well known (*Outback Steakhouse*), and steakhouse that was not well known (*Cask 'n Cleaver*). Type of restaurant and familiarity with restaurant was determined prior to the study through a pilot test on the sample population.

Upon arriving for the study, the members of the couple were separated into different rooms. One member of the couple completed two surveys. The first survey was a demographic survey to gather information on gender, age, ethnicity, length of relationship, number of children if any, and living arrangements. The second survey was the Evaluation and Nurturing Relationship Issues, Communication and Happiness (ENRICH) Martial Satisfaction Scale (EMS) determined by prior research to be a valid and reliable measure (Fowers and Olson, 1993) and modified for dating couples for the present experiment. This scale has two subscales which measure marital satisfaction (MS) and idealistic distortions (ID) (Fournier, Olson, and Druckman, 1983). Specifically, the scale has 15 items, with 10 items surveying marital status and 5 items correcting for cognitive distortions (i.e., idealistic distortions). Participants responded on a scale ranging from 1 to 5, with 1 indicating strongly disagree and 5 indicating strongly agree. Example statements include: "my partner and I understand each other completely" and "our relationship is a perfect success."

While the one member of the couple completed the previously described surveys, the other member of the couple viewed the 6 sample restaurants menus and indicated how likely they would be to eat at each of the restaurants on his or her birthday. The members of the couple then switched rooms so that both members of the couple viewed the sample restaurant menus giving independent likelihood ratings for each and completed the two surveys. Next, the couple was brought back together for a collective task. At this time, the couple was asked to imagine that only the two of them were going out to dinner and to indicate how likely they would be to eat at each of the restaurants. During the collective task, menus were only provided if participants requested them. At the end of the study, participants were debriefed and given contact information of the researcher should questions arise or they desired to know the overall results of the experiment.

RESULTS

To begin, analyses were conducted to test the first hypothesis. Specifically, correlations were conducted to determine if relationship satisfaction and idealistic thoughts would be related to willingness to eat at specific restaurants genres (i.e., seafood, steakhouse, and Italian). Results indicated that idealistic scores were positively correlated with willingness to eat at a steakhouse, r (N = 34) = .35, p <.05. In addition, relationship satisfaction scores were negatively correlated with willingness to eat at an Italian restaurant, r (N = 24) = -.35, p <.05.

To test the second hypothesis, the five common decision-making strategies obtained using cluster analysis from Bonds-Raacke (2008) were used to determine if differences in relationship satisfaction and idealistic distortions existed among couples. Thus, five clusters were utilized with 3 couples in cluster 1, 4 couples in cluster 2, 3 couples in cluster 4, 6 couples in cluster 5, and 2 couples in cluster 6. To begin, scores from both partners were summed to provide each couple with one score on the MS and the ID sub-scales. Next, a MANOVA was conducted to determine if there were differences in relationship satisfaction and idealistic distortion based on the type of decision-making strategy the extended dating couples employed. Results indicated no differences in relationship satisfaction and idealistic distortion based on decision-making strategy employed, $F(10, 34) = .85$, $p = .59$, $\eta^2 = .20$, power = .36. Mean scores on the idealistic distortion scale per cluster were as follows: 40.67 (cluster 1), 43.00 (cluster 2), 38.00 (cluster 4), 38.67 (cluster 5), and 41.50 (cluster 6). For relationship satisfaction, the mean scores were as follows: 82.00 (cluster 1), 85.75 (cluster 2), 79.00 (cluster 4), 76.50 (cluster 5), and 82.50 (cluster 6). For both scales, higher scores indicate higher levels on each measure.

Conclusion

Eating is a complex human behavior. Many factors such as familiarity with co-eaters (Salvy, Vartanian, Coelho, Jarrin, and Pliner, 2008) and sex of co-eaters (Hermans, Herman, Larsen, and Engels, 2010) influence food related behaviors and decisions. One interesting link is that between eating and romantic relationships (e.g., Sobal, et al., 2002; Sobal et al, 2003). The purpose of the current experiment was to further explore how components in romantic relationships such as relationship satisfaction and idealistic distortions related to joint or collective food decisions. Hypotheses for the current study were partially supported. First, relationship satisfaction and idealistic thoughts were significantly related to likelihood ratings for eating at specific restaurants. Specifically, willingness to eat at an Italian restaurant was negatively correlated with scores on the relationship satisfaction scale and willingness to eat at a steakhouse was positively correlated with scores on the idealistic distortion scale. One possible explanation for the current findings is that couples with a higher relationship satisfaction feel less of a desire, or need, to eat at restaurants with a traditional date genre (Italian). Conversely, couples who had higher idealistic thoughts were more likely to defer to the man's preference, which according to previous research by Bonds-Raacke (2006, 2008) would be the steakhouse genre. It could therefore be reasoned that higher relationship satisfaction scores and lower idealistic thoughts are exhibited by couples who are more comfortable in their respective relationships and have set realistic expectations. Thus, these couples are more likely to demonstrate food preferences when making their likelihood ratings. On the contrary, couples who do not experience these same levels of satisfaction or feel an increased pressure to be the perfect couple, may be less likely to show preferences in their food ratings. As predicted, these findings are consistent with previous research. First, genre preferences by couples is similar to Amiraian and Sobal (2009) who found that the type of restaurant selected for dining was influenced by the stage of the relationship. Second, the collective nature of the task emphasizes the results of Szybillo et al. (1977) that both members of the couple are involved in decisions to eat at conventional restaurants.

The second hypothesis, that scores on the relationship satisfaction scale and idealistic distortion scale would differ by type of decision-making strategy utilized, was not supported. In other words, the level of satisfaction within the relationship, as well as the level at which couples perceive their relationship to be functioning, seem to not be influenced by the way in which couples arrive at decisions jointly. These results are surprising in that these measures were related to overall joint likelihood ratings. A larger sample of couples utilizing similar decision-making strategies may reveal differences on these measures. Relationship satisfaction is associated with other food related variables such as weight (Sheets and Ajmere, 2005), dieting (Friedman et al, 1999), and body image (Meltzer and McNulty, 2010). Thus, it would be surprising if decision-making strategies are not also related. On the other hand, it could be that these specific relationship components are not influenced by decision-making strategies. Gender roles, education level, and socioeconomic status have been found to also not differ by decision-making strategies (Bonds-Raacke, 2006). Replication of the current experiment, while controlling for the limitations addressed below, is needed to bring clarity to this issue.

The current study is not without limitations. Limitation of the current study include: the researcher was present as the couples were making their independent and joint decisions, the task could have seemed artificial for couples that had children, and not all of the couples (N = 10) were members of the clusters demonstrating common decision-making strategies. The main concern for the present study is the low power obtained. However, the study is exploratory in nature and has a very small sample size. A power analysis using a statistical program indicated that a sample size of 30 participants per decision-making strategy would be needed to achieve a power of .80. Thus, power could be significantly increased by adding to the sample size and such an addition for this study with a small number of participants would have a great influence (Keppel and Zedeck, 2000). In this case, reporting inconclusive results aids in furthering the literature in the area by providing a starting point for research on the topic. Some have even argued that the practice of only reporting significant results in journals leads to an increase in the number of type I errors (Baken, 1966).

Future research in this area is needed. First, the relationships between the stage of the romantic relationship, relationship satisfaction, idealistic thoughts, and decision-making strategies need to be explored. One would expect that couples new to the relationship would have higher levels of idealistic thoughts and consequently employ unique decision-making strategies. Second, how couples make joint decisions to consume fast food, with negative health consequences, needs to better understand so healthier behaviors can be promoted.

REFERENCES

Amiraian, D., and Sobal, J. (2009). Dating and eating. How university students select eating settings. *Appetite, 52,* 226-229.

Aruguete, M. S., Edman, J. L., and Yates, A. (2009). Romantic interest in obese college students. *Eating Behaviors, 10,* 143-145.

Baken, D. (1996). The test of significance in psychological research. *Psychological Bulletin, 66* (6), 423-437.

Blake, C. E., Bisogni, C. A., Sobal, J., Jastran, M., and Devinee, C. M. (2008). How adults construct evening meals. Scripts for food choice. *Appetite, 51,* 654–662.

Bonds-Raacke, J. M. (2006). Using cluster analysis to examine husband-wife decision-making. *The Psychological Record, 56* (4), 521-550.

Bonds-Raacke, J. M. (2008). Extended dating couples decision-making strategies about eating: A comparison to married couples. *Appetite, 51* (1), 198-201.

Bonds-Raacke, J. M., Bearden, E. S., Carriere, N. J., Anderson, E. M., and Nicks, S. D. (2001). Engaging distortions: Are we idealizing marriage? *The Journal of Psychology: Interdisciplinary and Applied, 135* (2), 179-184.

Bove, C. F., Sobal, J., and Rauschenbach, B. S. (2003). Food choices among newly married couples: Convergence, conflict, individualism, and projects. *Appetite, 40*, 25-41.

Boyes, A. D., Fletcher, G. J. O., and Latner, J. D. (2007). Male and female body image and dieting in the context of intimate relationships. *Journal of Family Psychology, 21* (4), 764-768.

Boyes, A. D., and Latner, J. D. (2009). Weight stigma in existing romantic relationships. *Journal of Sex and Marital Therapy, 35,* 282-293.

Brown, J. L., and Miller D. (2002). Couples' gender role preferences and management of family food preferences. *Journal of Nutrition Education and Behavior, 34*, 215-223.

Burke, V., Giangiulioa, N., Gillama, H. F., Beilina, L. J., and Houghtonc, J. (2003). Physical activity and nutrition programs for couples: A randomized controlled trial. *Journal of Clinical Epidemiology, 56,* 421–432.

Craig, P. L., and Truswell, A. S. (1990). Dynamics of food habits of newly married couples: Weight and exercise patterns. *Australian Journal of Nutrition and Dietetics, 47*, 42–46.

Dianton, M. (1998). Everyday interaction in marital relationships: Variations in relative importance and event duration. *Communication Reports, 11*, 101-109.

Fournier, D. G., Olson, D. H., and Druckman, J. M. (1983). Assessing marital and premarital relationships: The PREPARE/ENRICH inventories. In E. E. Filsinger (Ed.), *Marriage and family assessment* (pp.229-250). Newbury Park, CA: Sage.

Fowers, B. J., and Olson, D. H. (1993). ENRICH martial satisfaction scale: A brief research and clinical tool. *Journal of Family Psychology, 72,* 176-185.

Friedman, M. A., Dixon, A. E., Brownell, K. D., Whisman, M. A., and Wilfley, D. E. (1999). Marital status, marital satisfaction, and body image dissatisfaction. *International Journal of Eating Disorders, 26,* 81-85.

Hermans, R. C. J., Herman, C. P., Larsen, J. K., and Engels, R. C. M. E. (2010). Social modeling effects on snack intake among young men. The role of hunger. *Appetite, 54,* 378-383.

Jacob, J. I., Allen, S., Hill, E. J., Mead, N. L., and Ferris, M. (2008). Work interference with dinnertime as a mediator and moderator between work hours and work and family outcomes. *Family and Consumer Sciences Research Journal, 36*, 310-327.

Keppel, G., and Zedeck, S. (2000). *Data analysis for research designs.* New York: W. H. Freeman.

Kozak, M. (2010). Holiday taking decisions—The role of spouses. *Tourism Management, 31,* 489-494.

Kroshus, E. (2008). Gender, marital status, and commercially prepared food expenditure. *Journal of Nutrition Education and Behavior, 40,* 355-360.

Lallukka, T., Chandola, T., Roos, E., Cable, N., Sekine, M., Kagamimori, S., Tatsuse, T., Marmot, M., and Lahelma, E. (2010). Work–family conflicts and health behaviors among British, Finnish, and Japanese employees. *International Journal of Behavioral Medicine, 17,* 134-142.

Larson, N. I., Neumark-Sztainer, D. R., Story, M. T., Wall, M. M., Harnack, L. J., and Eisenberg, M. E. (2008). Fast food intake: Longitudinal trends during the transition to young adulthood and correlates of intake. *Journal of Adolescent Health, 43*, 79-86.

Madden, H., and Chamberlain, K. (2010). Nutritional health, subjectivity and resistance: Women's accounts of dietary practices. *Health: An Interdisciplinary Journal for the Social Study of Health, Illness and Medicine, 14,* 292-309.

Markey, C. N., Gomel, J. N., and Markey, P. M. (2008). Romantic relationships and eating regulation: An investigation of partners' attempts to control each others' eating behaviors. *Journal of Health Psychology, 13,* 422-432.

Markey, C. N., Markey, P. M., and Birch, L. L. (2001). Interpersonal predictors of dieting practices among married couples. *Journal of Family Psychology, 15,* 464-475.

Marshall, D. W., and Anderson, A. S. (2002). Proper meals in transition: Young married couples on the nature of eating together. *Appetite, 39,* 193-206.

Meltzer, A. L., and McNulty, J. K. (2010). Body image and marital satisfaction: Evidence for the mediating role of sexual frequency and sexual satisfaction. *Journal of Family Psychology, 24,* 156-164.

Meyler, D., Stimpson, J. P., and Peek, M. K. (2007). Health concordance within couples: A systematic review. *Social Science and Medicine, 64,* 2297–2310.

Neighbors, L. A., and Sobal, J. (2008). Weight and weddings: Women's weight ideals and weight management behaviors for their wedding day. *Appetite, 50,* 550-554.

Rappoport, L. (2003). *How we eat: Appetite, culture, and the psychology of food.* Toronto: E. C. W. Press.

Salvy, S-J., Vartanian, L. R., Coelho, J. S., Jarrin, D., and Pliner, P. P. (2008). The role of familiarity on modeling of eating and food consumption in children. *Appetite, 50,* 514-518.

Schafer, R. B., and Keith, P. M. (1990). Matching by weight in married couples: A life cycle perspective. *The Journal of Social Psychology, 130,* 657-664.

Schafer, R. B., Keith, P. M., and Schafer, E. (2000). Marital stress, psychological distress, and healthy dietary behavior: A longitudinal analysis. *Journal of Applied Social Psychology, 20,* 1639-1656.

Sheets, V., and Ajmere, K. (2005). Are romantic partners a source of college students' weight concern? *Eating Behaviors, 6,* 1-9.

Sobal, J., Bove, C. F., and Rauschenbach, B. S. (2002). Commensal careers at entry into marriage: Establishing commensal units and managing commensal circles. *Sociological Review, 50,* 378-397.

Sobal, J., Rauschenbach, B., and Frongillo, E. A. (2003). Marital status changes and body weight changes: A US longitudinal analysis. *Social Science and Medicine, 56,* 1543–1555.

Szybillo, G. J., Sosanie, A. K., and Tenebein, A. (1977). Should children be seen but not heard? *Journal of Advertising Research, 17,* 7-13.

In: Appetite: Regulation, Role in Disease and Control
Editor: Steven R. Mitchell, pp. 135-151
ISBN 978-1-61209-842-5
© 2011 Nova Science Publishers, Inc.

Chapter 8

DISEASE-ASSOCIATED ANOREXIA AS PART OF THE ANOREXIA-CACHEXIA SYNDROME: POTENTIAL ETIOLOGIES AND INTERVENTIONS

Mark D. DeBoer

University of Virginia School of Medicine, Charlottesville, VA, USA

SUMMARY

The most common pathological form of anorexia is seen as part of the anorexia-cachexia syndrome. The anorexia-cachexia syndrome results in a devastating degree of body wasting that worsens quality of life and survival for patients suffering from already dire and restrictive diseases such as cancer, chronic kidney disease and chronic heart failure. The common features of anorexia-cachexia in these disease states and the common feature of systemic inflammation suggest shared pathophysiologic roots of cachexia in these conditions. However, previous attempts to treat anorexia-cachexia via anti-inflammatory interventions and multiple other means have not proven effective, and no unifying treatment has emerged that is effective in treating anorexia-cachexia in multiple disease states. Basic science investigations have revealed that inflammation-induced activation of the central melanocortin system is one likely means of producing anorexia and lean body wasting in this syndrome. Similarly, basic science approaches to blocking melanocortin activity appeared promising by demonstrating improvement of food intake and weight retention in anorexia-cachexia, though unfortunately data regarding human treatment is still lacking. Finally, a new treatment approach via administration of ghrelin or ghrelin agonists appears to be a promising means of treatment, as suggested by both basic science and early human experiments, though much more investigation is needed. The hope of all investigators and clinicians in the field is that successful treatment of the symptoms of anorexia-cachexia will lead to an improvement in quality of life and survival among all patients suffering from this disease.

INTRODUCTION

The anorexia-cachexia syndrome refers to a state of wasting that afflicts patients with multiple different underlying diseases and that has been recognized since antiquity for its dire effects on prognosis. The term cachexia itself is derived from the Greek "kakos" (bad) and "hexis" (condition), and indeed the syndrome of lost body mass was described by Hippocrates, who observed, "...the shoulders, clavicles, chest and thighs melt away. This illness is fatal..." Despite this long-standing nature of our recognition of this disorder, successful treatment has remained elusive. However, as the entity of anorexia-cachexia has gained recognition over the past decade new treatment modalities have continued to be introduced in an attempt to improve the destructive symptoms seen in this disease.

The anorexia-cachexia syndrome involves loss of appetite, loss of lean and fat mass, and increased energy expenditure, symptoms that occur with remarkable similarity among patients with a variety of underlying disease processes including cancer,[1] renal failure, [2] and heart failure. [3] Given the catabolic nature of the syndrome, perhaps the most perplexing symptom is the loss of appetite, which occurs at a time when the body would logically require increased energy supply as it utilizes muscle and fat stores. Additionally, given the pleasure that most individuals derive from food consumption, the anorexia associated with cachexia also contributes to decreases in quality of life. Not surprisingly, then, many of the newer proposed treatments for cachexia focus on increasing appetite and food intake.

As we shall see, in addition to sharing common symptoms of anorexia-cachexia, the underlying diseases that involve this syndrome also bear other similarities with respect to each other, including the production of systemic inflammation. This is seen by increases in acute phase reactants and pro-inflammatory cytokines in the setting of cancer, renal failure and heart failure. This systemic inflammation is felt to be part of the underlying pathophysiology resulting in anorexia-cachexia. Recent work has demonstrated that inflammation acts on the brain to stimulate important appetite-regulating centers including the central melanocortin system in the hypothalamus. Thus, many additional interventions have focused on decreasing inflammation as a means of improving the cachexia.

We will review here the data on clinical symptoms of anorexia-cachexia caused by three common underlying conditions: cancer, chronic kidney disease, and chronic heart failure. We will also review data regarding the inflammatory processes increased by these diseases and evidence from trials for potential therapeutic agents to treat cachexia in these settings, revealing an overall impression that current treatment modalities have been for the most part ineffective. We will end by reviewing promising data on the use of two potential treatments for anorexia-cachexia: antagonism of the melanocortin system and appetite stimulation via use of ghrelin-receptor agonists.

I. UNDERLYING DISEASE STATES AND EARLY TREATMENT APPROACHES

Cancer

Clinical Features

Anorexia-cachexia is a common feature of multiple malignancies, affecting up to 85% of patients with certain types of cancer and contributing to over 20% of all cancer deaths. [1, 4, 5] The weight loss experienced by patients can be severe, including loss of up to 75% of muscle mass [6] However, even subtle amounts of weight loss and anorexia are associated with a poorer prognosis, a worsened response to chemotherapy and increased morbidity. [4, 6, 7] Additionally, the loss of appetite as a feature is an ominous sign among malignancies: one survey of patients with terminal cancer found the presence of nausea or emesis was associated with a 68% decrease in survival [8]. Despite this weight loss, patients with cancer cachexia frequently exhibit a paradoxic increase in resting energy expenditure. [9, 10] The sum of these issues is that cancer patients with cachexia have a substantial decrease in quality of life. [11, 12]

Not surprisingly, cancer cachexia is pleomorphic in etiology with multiple contributing causes including tumor production of anorexia-cachexia-related factors and host responses to the tumor burden [1]. One mechanism for wasting in cancer cachexia appears to be via tumor release of specific cachectogenic agents including lipid mobilizing factor (LMF), which was originally isolated from the urine of patients with anorexia-cachexia [13, 14]. LMF stimulates lipolysis and increases uncoupling proteins that contribute to increased metabolic rate. Despite a strong implication in the loss of lean body mass, LMF has not been linked to the loss of appetite related to cancer cachexia [1].

One common factor that has been implicated in the loss of appetite in cancer is the presence of pro-inflammatory cytokines including IL-1β, IL-6 and TNF-α. [11] These have been demonstrated to be produced by tumor cells in tissue culture as well as in vivo, suggesting a possible survival advantage to the tumor from increased local mobilization of nutrients [15, 16]. Additionally, the host response to tumor presence involves production of acute phase proteins (APP) including C-reactive protein (CRP) that are associated with increased levels of pro-inflammatory cytokines. Up to 50% of cancer patients have elevated APP at diagnosis and the associated increase in cytokines is strongly implicated in producing anorexia [1, 17]. The importance of APP in tumor prognosis was demonstrated in a study of patients with pancreatic cancer in which elevated CRP at diagnosis predicted a 78% reduction in survival time [17]. Among patients with other gastrointestinal malignancies, CRP was better than tumor staging at predicting survival one year after surgery [16]. This production of inflammation is important because one means by which inflammation suppresses appetite in cancer cachexia and other anorexia-cachexia syndromes has been shown to be via direct stimulation of appetite-regulating centers in the hypothalamus and brainstem, including the central melanocortin system, as will be discussed later.

Anti-Inflammatory Treatment

Because of the prominent feature of inflammation in cancer cachexia, many attempts to treat the associated wasting have focused on decreasing the inflammatory state. Non-steroidal anti-inflammatory agents and monoclonal antibodies against specific pro-inflammatory cytokines have produced minor improvements in decreasing serum markers of APP response but have not produced significant improvements in weight. For example, one randomized trial tested the effect of providing indomethacin, prednisone or placebo to 135 patients with terminal solid tumor malignancies. In this trial, indomethacin treatment failed to increase weight, and though prednisone did result in a significant weight gain, other studies have shown a high rate of corticosteroid toxicity that ultimately had a negative impact on quality of life [18, 19]. Thus far, no NSAID or corticosteroid treatment has produced significant improvements in retaining or increasing lean body mass in cachectic patients.

Another treatment chosen for its anti-inflammatory characteristics is eicosapentanoic acid (EPA), which is an essential polyunsaturated fatty acid found in fish oil. EPA has been shown to decrease levels of IL-6 [20, 21]. Initially it appeared that EPA might increase weight gain in cancer, such as in a trial in an unrandomized trial among patients with pancreatic cancer. [22] More recently, however, other randomized trials of EPA vs. placebo failed to produce clinically significant differences in weight or lean body mass over an 8 week time frames. [23, 24]

Megestrol Acetate

Megestrol acetate, a synthetic prostaglandin analogue, also initially offered much promise as a treatment modality for cancer cachexia. Administration of megestrol acetate has been shown in multiple studies and a recent Cochran review to increase food intake in patients with anorexia-cachexia through an unknown mechanism. [25] Unfortunately, the weight gain observed following megestrol acetate treatment has been demonstrated to be due primarily to increased water and fat content without significant changes in lean body mass. [26-28] Also, patients taking megestrol acetate did not have an increase in quality of life or an improvement in cancer outcomes, deflating many of the initial hopes. Other failed treatments included cyproheptidine and dronabinol, both of which failed to prevent weight loss or perform better than megestrol acetate.[29, 30]

Need for Effective Therapies in Cancer Cachexia

Thus, as will become a theme among the common anorexia-cachexia syndromes, none of the treatments studied have had an impressive enough effect on weight, quality of life or survival to transfer to widespread use. In such a common and emotional disease pattern, the introduction of an *effective* treatment would be likely to be employed in widespread use and have major effects on patients suffering from cancer cachexia.

Chronic Kidney Disease

Clinical Features

Significant weight loss—predominantly in the form of protein energy imbalance—is also a major feature of chronic kidney disease (CKD), affecting up to 64% of patients on hemodialysis. [31] In the setting of CKD this syndrome is sometimes incorrectly referred to as "malnutrition," which is misleading because it implies that the syndrome can be resolved simply by improving the diet. [32, 33] As in cancer cachexia, the anorexia and decreased protein intake of chronic renal failure are associated with increased metabolic demand. [34] Increased resting energy expenditure (REE) is common in patients on dialysis and in one prospective study, higher REE was associated with greater mortality in patients on peritoneal dialysis. [35]

The appetite and metabolic changes associated with CKD have been attributed to a wide variety of causes including uremia, acidosis and high levels of leptin (due to impaired renal clearance). [33, 34, 36] As is the case with cancer cachexia, the anorexia-cachexia of CRF is strongly linked to increased inflammatory markers, though the cause of the increased inflammation in CKD is not entirely clear. [32] Inflammatory markers such as c-reactive protein (CRP) are highly associated with clinical features of protein energy imbalance, increased metabolic rate and poor prognosis. [37] A study of 128 patients on hemodialysis who were followed prospectively for 36 months found that compared to survivors patients who died over the 3 years were approximately twice as likely (85% vs. 44%) to have had malnutrition and were more than three times as likely (44% vs. 13%) to have a highly elevated c-reactive protein (CRP). [38] Both elevated CRP and malnutrition were likely to coincide with heart disease, and each is an independent risk factor for mortality.

Treatment Approaches

Approaches to treating anorexia-cachexia of CKD have differed somewhat from cancer cachexia, likely owing to the differences in the underlying diseases. Unlike the cancer field, anti-inflammatory treatment for CKD has not yet been studied extensively, though pilot studies for such an intervention are now underway. One unblinded trial of omega 3 fatty acids failed to reduce markers of inflammation. [39]

Pharmacologic treatment of wasting in CKD has thus far focused on increasing lean body mass via anabolic compounds. Two trials used recombinant human growth hormone for adults who had lost weight on dialysis, since there is some evidence that adults and children with renal failure exhibit growth hormone resistance. These trials were performed as double-blinded, placebo-controlled studies over a 6 month time course. Growth hormone treatment resulted in 3-6 kg gains in lean body mass accompanied by a 3-6 kg decreases in fat mass. [40, 41] Neither of these trials evaluated changes in appetite or sense of well-being.

Another randomized trial used the anabolic steroid nandrolone or placebo for 6 months among 29 subjects on hemo- or peritoneal-dialysis. [42] Nandrolone produced a 4.5 kg gain in lean body mass (versus 2 kg gain for placebo) with a 2.5 kg loss in fat mass (vs. 0.5 kg loss for placebo). Quality of life was improved as indicated by decreased fatigue in the nandrolone group vs. placebo but again no comment was made regarding the effects of treatment on appetite. These results clearly are promising, though one limitation of nandrolone treatment is that it can only be used in male patients, since women would experience excessive virilization during treatment.

As with cancer cachexia, treatment with megestrol acetate has been attempted in a double-blined, crossover study of patients with CKD on hemodialysis. This study revealed a significant amount of side effects during treatment with megestrol acetate vs. placebo. As was the case in cancer cachexia, megestrol acetate failed to improve retention of lean body mass. [43]

Thus, cachexia caused by chronic kidney disease has had some improvement in identifying potential treatments—including growth hormone injections and an anabolic steroid—but neither with any reported improvement in appetite.

Heart Failure

Clinical Features

Chronic heart failure (CHF) caused by prior myocardial infarctions or dilated cardiomyopathy is seen in 1-2% of the population of developed countries. [44, 45] As is the case with cancer and chronic kidney disease patients, many of these patients begin to exhibit significant weight loss and anorexia, frequently referred to as cardiac cachexia, affecting approximately 15% of this population. [46] The weight loss observed in this group involves significant losses of lean and adipose tissue (18% and 37% respectively, compared to non-cachectic patients with CHF) and this loss of body mass is an independent risk factor for mortality with a hazard ratio of 3.73 over an 18 month period. [46, 47] Interestingly, whereas non-cachectic patients with CHF exhibit increase in resting metabolic rate vs. controls, CHF patients with cachexia exhibit a decreased resting metabolic rate, marking a difference between anorexia-cachexia in CHF and cancer or chronic kidney disease. [48, 49]

The exact etiology behind the anorexia-cachexia seen in CHF is again uncertain, and the importance of adequate perfusion to many normal body processes further complicates the process. Anorexia in CHF can be related to dyspnea and fatigue, as well as to intestinal edema and resultant nausea. [50] Fat malabsorption further contributes to decreased calorie influx. [51] Also, anorexia in CHF can be associated with some of the treatments for CHF such as due to side effects of medications such as digoxin and ACE inhibitors or due to lower palatability of a sodium-restricted diet. [50]

Finally, as was the case for anorexia-cachexia caused by cancer and chronic kidney disease, a constant feature in CHF cachexia is the presence of inflammatory markers. Patients with CHF cachexia exhibit a 2-2.5 fold increase in TNF-α and IL-6 compared to patients with non-cardiac CHF. This increase in inflammation is the strongest predictor for prior weight loss. [52-54] Serum levels of TNF-α and IL-6 are also independent risk factors for survival in CHF patients. [55, 56] The increase in cytokines is postulated to be due to several sources including release of TNF-α by the failing myocardium, release of endotoxin through an edematous bowel wall or production of inflammatory factors from hypoxic tissue. [50] As is observed for patients with anorexia secondary to CRF, patients with CHF-induced anorexia-cachexia exhibit a growth hormone resistance, which is associated with increased levels of TNF-α. [57]

Treatment Approaches

Many of the treatments that have been shown to help in anorexia-cachexia associated with CHF are aimed at treating the underlying disease. Short term trials of the positive inotrope levosimendan resulted in decreased levels of IL-6, though it is not known if this resulted in a change in lean body mass. [58] Use of angiotensin-converting enzyme (ACE) inhibitors in a large (817 subject) trial showed a decreased risk of weight loss vs placebo (hazard ratio 0.8) over a 4 year study period. [59] The effect of ACE inhibitors was likely partially due to improved disease but may also have produced effects through decreasing the effects of angiotensin II on IGF-1. [60]

Lastly, anti-inflammatory treatment has thus far proven ineffective in the setting of CHF. For example, a TNF-α receptor fusion protein (eternacept) was designed to decrease bioavailable TNF-α, but it produced no difference in outcome from placebo in a large trial. In another trial, adminstration of a TNF-α antibody resulted in increased mortality in the treatment group. [50] Furthermore, long-term use of non-steroidal anti-inflammatory COX-2 inhibitors caused an increase in cardiac events. One anti-inflammatory trial that did prove successful from a cardiac standpoint involved the use of a procedure known as Celacade™, in which autologous blood is exposed to oxidative stress at an increased temperature and then re-administered intramuscularly. This is known to decrease pro-inflammatory cytokine levels possibly via increases in anti-inflammatory mediators. A randomized, double blinded trial of this failed to change serum levels of cytokines but did result in an improvement in mortality.[61] No comment was made on changes in appetite, weight or lean body mass during this trial.

Summary of Cachexia Associated with Cancer, CRF and CHF

There are many similarities in the syndrome of anorexia-cachexia caused by these diverse disease processes. In each of these conditions anorexia-cachexia consists of wasting of lean body mass with a paradoxical decrease in appetite and an association with worsened prognosis. In each of these disorders there appears to be a link to elevated inflammatory markers or cytokines are in turn thought to play a role in the pathophysiology and illness symptoms. Nutritional support alone does not appear to improve the symptoms of anorexia-cachexia caused by any of these diseases and pharmacologic interventions have failed to produce demonstrable gains in appetite, lean body mass and quality of life.

II. TARGETED APPETITE INTERVENTIONS IN THE TREATMENT OF CACHEXIA

Central Melanocortin System

In addition to the targeting of inflammatory pathways for the treatment of anorexia-cachexia, much of the recent focus has been on affecting appetite regulating centers in the brainstem and hypothalamus. The best-described of these centers is the central melanocortin system, the main nucleus of which is in the arcuate nucleus of the hypothalamus. [62] The importance of the central melanocortin system first came to widespread recognition with the description of the agouti mouse, which exhibited hyperphagia and morbid obesity due to over-expression of agouti, an endogenous inhibitor of the melanocortin system. [63] Since that time, the melanocortin system has been well-described as consisting of two classes of neurons: anorexigenic and orexigenic. The anorexigenic neurons produce pro-opiomelanocortin (POMC), which is a long precursor peptide that is cleaved to produce α-MSH. α-MSH then binds to and activates specific melanocortin receptors on a variety of second-order neurons in the hypothalamus and brainstem (see Figure 1). [64] The action of α-MSH on these receptors—including the melanocortin 3 receptor (MC3-R) and melanocortin-4 receptor (MC4-R)—produces a tonic restraint on feeding activity. That is to say that activation of the central melanocortin system causes a decrease in appetite.

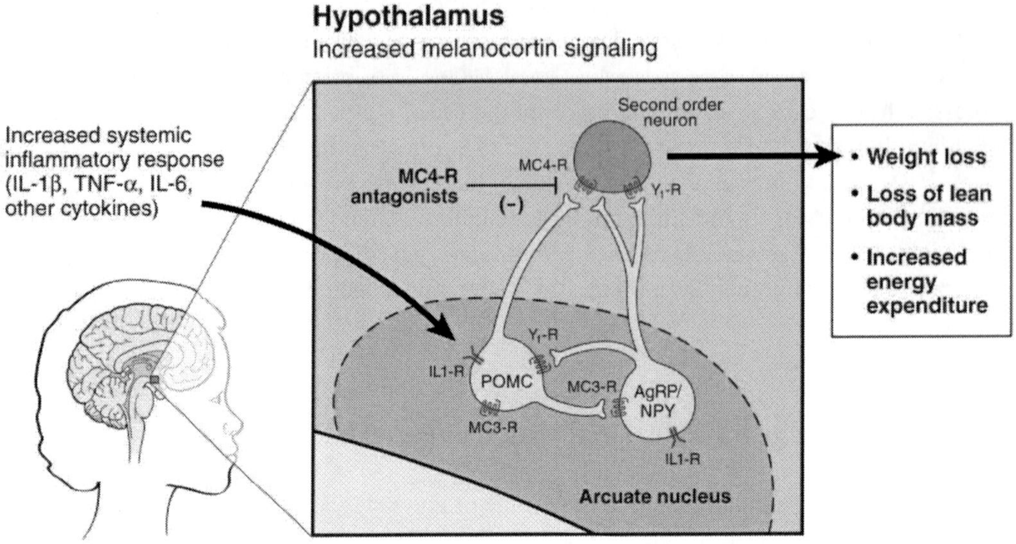

Figure 1. Model of the effects of inflammation produced during anorexia-cachexia on activity to the central melanocortin system. Inflammatory cytokines such as that are produced by the underlying disease activate cytokine receptors on neurons in the arcuate nucleus of the hypothalamus (such as IL-1β binding to the IL-1 receptor in the figure). When this occurs on neurons expressing pro-opiomelanocortin (POMC), this leads to an increase in anorexigenic signaling via stimulation of MC4 receptors on second-order neurons. Conversely, when IL-1β binds to neurons that produce Agouti-related peptide (AgRP) and neuropeptide Y (NPY) this leads to a decrease in orexigenic signaling by NPY via the NPY Y1 receptor and by AgRP acting as an antagonist of MC4 receptors on second-order neurons. The response of second order neurons produces signals that lead to anorexia-cachexia. Blockade of MC4 receptors on second-order neurons attenuates the increased anorexigenic signals and improves the symptoms of anorexia-cachexia. From reference 64, used by permission.

By contrast the orexigenic neurons in the arcuate nucleus produce both neuropeptide-Y (NPY) and agouti-related peptide (AgRP), both of which act on second-order neurons to result in an increase in feeding behavior. What is unique about the melanocortin system is that AgRP acts on the same MC3-R and MC4-R receptors as does α-MSH but AgRP acts as an antagonist and thus produces an increase in feeding behavior. Thus, inhibition of the melanocortin system causes an increase in appetite. These pathways of the central melanocortin system lead to another interesting feature of the system in that mutations in the MC4-R receptor in humans result in early onset obesity and increased lean mass. In fact these MC-4R mutations are the most common monogenic cause of severe obesity, though they also lead to an increase in lean body mass as well. [65]

The demonstration that melanocortin inhibition causes an increased appetite immediately made the melanocortin system a logical target for pharmacologic interventions to treat cachexia. [66, 67] These efforts became an even more logical step when it was demonstrated that the anorexigenic output by the melanocortin system was mediated by direct stimulation by central inflammation—particularly mediated by IL-1β—on neurons that express POMC in the arcuate nucleus. [68] This sets up the link between underlying anorexia-cachexia-associated conditions and activation of the central melanocortin system. As discussed previously, each of the conditions that result in anorexia-cachexia also involves the up-regulation of inflammatory mediators. Also, for the case of cancer cachexia and chronic renal failure, it has been demonstrated that increases in inflammation cause decreased expression of AgRP and/or increased expression of POMC in the hypothalamus. [69, 70]

Thus, it appears that a common path for varying conditions resulting in anorexia-cachexia is activation of the melanocortin system via increased inflammation. This increase in melanocortin activity by inflammation is at least in part at the level of the neurons expressing POMC and thus upstream of second-order neurons expressing MC4-R. Importantly, the sequence of these events leaves open the possibility of inhibiting the MC4-R—via use of genetic knock out animals or through administration of AgRP or small molecule antagonists—as a means of ameliorating the effects of increased inflammation on melanocortin tone.

It is not surprising, then, that animal models of anorexia-cachexia have consistently shown improvements in appetite and weight-gain following inhibition of the melanocortin system. The approaches that have been tested have employed models of anorexia-cachexia produced via multiple underlying stimuli in rodents, including multiple types of implanted tumors and models of chronic kidney disease. [67, 71-80] When left untreated, these models of anorexia-cachexia result in decreased appetite and weight loss, ranging from a decrease in food intake of 50%-80% vs. controls and loss of lean mass of 5%-10% vs. controls. Melanocortin inhibition was initially studied by using knock-out mice that are unable to express MC4-R and thus lack the constant anorexigenic tone placed on second-order neurons. Once this approach toward melanocortin antagonism was shown to ameliorate the decrease in appetite and weight loss among laboratory animals, administration of AgRH and multiple different small molecule antagonists of the MC-4R have been employed with success. [67, 71-80]

The success of melanocortin antagonists in laboratory models of anorexia-cachexia lead to optimism that these would produce impressive clinical results as well. Unfortunately, as of the date of this publication, no clinical trial information has been released—positive or negative—regarding the use of melanocortin antagonists in the treatment of anorexia-cachexia in humans. [81] This raises strong suspicions that treatment with these molecules is either inefficacious in humans or involves excessive risk or side effects. It is unclear when we will have answers to these questions.

Ghrelin Treatment

Another new avenue of treatment for anorexia-cachexia involves the endogenous hormone ghrelin. Ghrelin was originally discovered because of its ability to stimulate growth hormone release via activity on the growth-hormone-secretagogue-1a (GHS-1a) receptor on growth hormone secreting cells in the pituitary. [82] However, after its discovery it became clear that a much more striking property of ghrelin was to stimulate food intake. Ghrelin is the only known circulating orexigenic hormone and is released principally by the stomach in response to time after a meal. Following meal ingestion, ghrelin levels in the serum then drop back to basal amounts and begin to rise again until the next meal. [83] Ghrelin is thus felt to be a meal-initiating signal. Another interesting feature of ghrelin is that serum levels increase in individuals following weight loss, paralleling an increased perception of hunger. [83] As with the central melanocortin system, the properties of increasing appetite made ghrelin a logical tool to test in anorexia-cachexia intervention. [84]

Interestingly, treatment with ghrelin may end up being the means by which melanocortin inhibition is achieved in clinical settings. This is because one of ghrelin's mechanisms of action is via stimulation of GHS-1a receptor in the hypothalamus. [85] In normal physiology, ghrelin acts on these receptors in the arcuate nucleus to increase expression and release of AgRP and NPY. [86] The same is also true when ghrelin is used as a treatment during an animal model of cancer cachexia, in which animals reviewing ghrelin exhibit an increase in AgRP and NPY expression as well as increased food intake and lean body mass retention vs. controls. [69] Thus, one means by which ghrelin improves food intake in anorexia-cachexia is via inhibition of the central melanocortin system.

Another intriguing property of ghrelin is that the GHS-1a receptors are expressed on leukocytes, and ghrelin treatment has been shown to decrease release of immune mediators. This was shown in a mouse model of arthritis in which ghrelin treatment caused a decrease in paw swelling. [87] Additionally, pre-treatment with ghrelin caused a decrease in lipopolysaccharide-induced cytokine release from isolated macrophages. In a rat model of chronic kidney disease, ghrelin treatment caused an overall decrease in systemic inflammatory cytokines,[88] and a growing body of reports confirm other anti-inflammatory effects. [89-91] These anti-inflammatory effects of ghrelin may be another means by which ghrelin decreases melanocortin activity and improves appetite in the setting of anorexia-cachexia.

As was demonstrated with melanocortin antagonists, ghrelin has been shown to be efficacious in improving food intake and improving retention of lean body mass in a great variety of models of anorexia-cachexia, including that caused by cancer, chronic renal failure and chronic heart failure. [69, 88, 92-95] These experiments have consistently demonstrated improvements in food intake (increases of 20%-56% vs. placebo), weight gain (300%-2200% over placebo) and lean body mass retention (changes of -1%-+26% following ghrelin treatment vs. changes of -12.6% - +2.8% with placebo).

More significantly, ghrelin treatment has also been shown to be efficacious in short-term trials on humans with anorexia-cachexia as well. Double-blinded cross-over studies of single doses of ghrelin given intravenously to patients with cancer cachexia resulted in 31-56% increases in food intake following administration. [96, 97] Among patients with renal failure, a cross-over trial demonstrated that a single dose of ghrelin given subcutaneously increased food intake by 57% over placebo. And on a more long-term basis, ghrelin infusions were administered to in separate studies to patients with anorexia-cachexia related to either chronic heart failure or chronic obstructive pulmonary disease. [98, 99] In both of these studies, patients received twice-daily infusions of ghrelin over a 3 week course, resulting in 8-9% increases in food intake, 1.6-2% increases in weight and 1.8-2% increases in lean body mass.

One draw back of all of the above studies is that they utilized ghrelin itself, as opposed to a small-molecule agonist. The acylated (active) ghrelin molecule has a half life of approximately 30 minutes in the serum and requires IV or subcutaneous administration. [100] The potential to design GHS-1a agonists with longer serum half-lives and oral bioavailability has stimulated the development of multiple synthetic ghrelin analogues. The only one of these to be reported in clinical use was RC-1291, an orally-bioavailable GHS-1a agonist that was administered to patients with cancer cachexia during a 12-week trial, resulting in a 0.6% increase in weight vs. a 1.45% weight loss among patients treated with placebo.[101] Several other such compounds have had efficacy demonstrated in animal models of anorexia-cachexia but have yet to be reported in human application.

Thus, treatment with ghrelin and other GHS-1a agonists represents an emerging avenue in the field of anorexia-cachexia, with hope that its use will prove effective in the treatment of anorexia-cachexia caused by a host of underlying etiologies. An important issue for consideration as ghrelin agonists are tested is whether the stimulation of growth hormone by ghrelin will prove problematic to patients with tumors. Also, there has been some suggestion of uncomfortable gastrointestinal side effects with ghrelin administration to humans which will have to looked at carefully as these studies proceed. [84, 97] Finally, long-term studies will be necessary to see whether the short-term effects of ghrelin on appetite and weight gain will be sustained with long-term use. A major hope in the field of anorexia-cachexia is that medications that prove effective in treating the symptoms of anorexia-cachexia—particularly improving appetite, retention of lean and fat mass, and improved quality of life—will also improve the treatment and survival of the underlying disease. This consideration will be important in the analysis of any new compounds proposed as new treatments for anorexia-cachexia.

CONCLUSION

In conclusion, anorexia-cachexia is a devastating syndrome of body wasting that worsens quality of life and survival for patients suffering from already dire and restrictive diseases such as cancer, chronic kidney disease and chronic heart failure. The common features of anorexia-cachexia in these disease states and the common feature of systemic inflammation suggest shared pathophysiologic roots. However, previous attempts to treat anorexia-cachexia via anti-inflammatory interventions have not proven effective, and no unifying treatment has emerged that is effective in treating anorexia-cachexia in multiple disease states. Basic science investigations have revealed that inflammation-induced activation of the central melanocortin system is one likely means of producing anorexia and lean body wasting in this syndrome. Similarly, basic science approaches to blocking melanocortin activity appeared promising by demonstrating improvement of food intake and weight retention in anorexia-cachexia, though unfortunately data regarding human treatment is still lacking. Finally, a new treatment approach via administration of ghrelin or ghrelin agonists appears to be a promising means of treatment, as suggested by both basic science and early human experiments, though much more investigation is needed. The hope of all investigators and clinicians in the field is that successful treatment of the symptoms of anorexia-cachexia will lead to an improvement in quality of life and survival among all patients suffering from this disease.

REFERENCES

[1] Tisdale MJ. Cachexia in cancer patients. *Nat Rev Cancer.* Nov 2002;2(11):862-871.
[2] Mak RH, Cheung W. Therapeutic strategy for cachexia in chronic kidney disease. *Curr Opin Nephrol Hypertens.* Nov 2007;16(6):542-546.
[3] von Haehling S, Doehner W, Anker SD. Nutrition, metabolism, and the complex pathophysiology of cachexia in chronic heart failure. *Cardiovasc Res.* Jan 15 2007;73(2):298-309.

[4] Dewys WD, Begg C, Lavin PT, et al. Prognostic effect of weight loss prior to chemotherapy in cancer patients. Eastern Cooperative Oncology Group. *Am J Med.* Oct 1980;69(4):491-497.

[5] Tan BH, Fearon KC. Cachexia: prevalence and impact in medicine. *Curr Opin Clin Nutr Metab Care.* Jul 2008;11(4):400-407.

[6] Fearon KC. The Sir David Cuthbertson Medal Lecture 1991. The mechanisms and treatment of weight loss in cancer. *Proc Nutr Soc.* Aug 1992;51(2):251-265.

[7] Barber MD, Ross JA, Fearon KC. Changes in nutritional, functional, and inflammatory markers in advanced pancreatic cancer. *Nutr Cancer.* 1999;35(2):106-110.

[8] Vigano A, Donaldson N, Higginson IJ, Bruera E, Mahmud S, Suarez-Almazor M. Quality of life and survival prediction in terminal cancer patients: a multicenter study. *Cancer.* Sep 1 2004;101(5):1090-1098.

[9] Bosaeus I, Daneryd P, Lundholm K. Dietary intake, resting energy expenditure, weight loss and survival in cancer patients. *J Nutr.* Nov 2002;132(11 Suppl):3465S-3466S.

[10] Falconer JS, Fearon KC, Plester CE, Ross JA, Carter DC. Cytokines, the acute-phase response, and resting energy expenditure in cachectic patients with pancreatic cancer. *Ann Surg.* Apr 1994;219(4):325-331.

[11] Richey LM, George JR, Couch ME, et al. Defining cancer cachexia in head and neck squamous cell carcinoma. *Clin Cancer Res.* Nov 15 2007;13(22 Pt 1):6561-6567.

[12] Fearon KC. Cancer cachexia: developing multimodal therapy for a multidimensional problem. *Eur J Cancer.* May 2008;44(8):1124-1132.

[13] Todorov P, Cariuk P, McDevitt T, Coles B, Fearon K, Tisdale M. Characterization of a cancer cachectic factor. *Nature.* Feb 22 1996;379(6567):739-742.

[14] Hirai K, Hussey HJ, Barber MD, Price SA, Tisdale MJ. Biological evaluation of a lipid-mobilizing factor isolated from the urine of cancer patients. *Cancer Res.* Jun 1 1998;58(11):2359-2365.

[15] Wigmore SJ RJ, Fearon KCH et al. IL-8 and IL-6 are produced constitutively by human pancreatic cancer cell lines. *Gut.* 1994;35(Suppl 5):539.

[16] Deans C, Wigmore SJ. Systemic inflammation, cachexia and prognosis in patients with cancer. *Curr Opin Clin Nutr Metab Care.* May 2005;8(3):265-269.

[17] Falconer JS, Fearon KC, Ross JA, et al. Acute-phase protein response and survival duration of patients with pancreatic cancer. *Cancer.* Apr 15 1995;75(8):2077-2082.

[18] Lundholm K, Gelin J, Hyltander A, et al. Anti-inflammatory treatment may prolong survival in undernourished patients with metastatic solid tumors. *Cancer Res.* Nov 1 1994;54(21):5602-5606.

[19] Loprinzi CL, Kugler JW, Sloan JA, et al. Randomized comparison of megestrol acetate versus dexamethasone versus fluoxymesterone for the treatment of cancer anorexia/cachexia. *J Clin Oncol.* Oct 1999;17(10):3299-3306.

[20] Wigmore SJ, Fearon KC, Maingay JP, Ross JA. Down-regulation of the acute-phase response in patients with pancreatic cancer cachexia receiving oral eicosapentaenoic acid is mediated via suppression of interleukin-6. *Clin Sci (Lond).* Feb 1997;92(2):215-221.

[21] Smith HJ, Lorite MJ, Tisdale MJ. Effect of a cancer cachectic factor on protein synthesis/degradation in murine C2C12 myoblasts: modulation by eicosapentaenoic acid. *Cancer Res.* Nov 1 1999;59(21):5507-5513.

[22] Barber MD, Ross JA, Voss AC, Tisdale MJ, Fearon KC. The effect of an oral nutritional supplement enriched with fish oil on weight-loss in patients with pancreatic cancer. *Br J Cancer.* Sep 1999;81(1):80-86.

[23] Fearon KC, Barber MD, Moses AG, et al. Double-blind, placebo-controlled, randomized study of eicosapentaenoic acid diester in patients with cancer cachexia. *J Clin Oncol.* Jul 20 2006;24(21):3401-3407.

[24] Fearon KC, Von Meyenfeldt MF, Moses AG, et al. Effect of a protein and energy dense N-3 fatty acid enriched oral supplement on loss of weight and lean tissue in cancer cachexia: a randomised double blind trial. *Gut.* Oct 2003;52(10):1479-1486.

[25] Berenstein EG, Ortiz Z. Megestrol acetate for the treatment of anorexia-cachexia syndrome. *Cochrane Database Syst Rev.* 2005(2):CD004310.

[26] Loprinzi CL, Schaid DJ, Dose AM, Burnham NL, Jensen MD. Body-composition changes in patients who gain weight while receiving megestrol acetate. *J Clin Oncol.* Jan 1993;11(1):152-154.

[27] Simons JP, Schols AM, Hoefnagels JM, Westerterp KR, ten Velde GP, Wouters EF. Effects of medroxyprogesterone acetate on food intake, body composition, and resting energy expenditure in patients with advanced, nonhormone-sensitive cancer: a randomized, placebo-controlled trial. *Cancer.* Feb 1 1998;82(3):553-560.

[28] Strang P. The effect of megestrol acetate on anorexia, weight loss and cachexia in cancer and AIDS patients (review). *Anticancer Res.* Jan-Feb 1997;17(1B):657-662.

[29] Kardinal CG, Loprinzi CL, Schaid DJ, et al. A controlled trial of cyproheptadine in cancer patients with anorexia and/or cachexia. *Cancer.* Jun 15 1990;65(12):2657-2662.

[30] Jatoi A, Windschitl HE, Loprinzi CL, et al. Dronabinol versus megestrol acetate versus combination therapy for cancer-associated anorexia: a North Central Cancer Treatment Group study. *J Clin Oncol.* Jan 15 2002;20(2):567-573.

[31] Qureshi AR, Alvestrand A, Danielsson A, et al. Factors predicting malnutrition in hemodialysis patients: a cross-sectional study. *Kidney Int.* Mar 1998;53(3):773-782.

[32] Mak RH, Cheung W, Cone RD, Marks DL. Orexigenic and anorexigenic mechanisms in the control of nutrition in chronic kidney disease. *Pediatr Nephrol.* Mar 2005;20(3):427-431.

[33] Mitch WE. Robert H Herman Memorial Award in Clinical Nutrition Lecture, 1997. Mechanisms causing loss of lean body mass in kidney disease. *Am J Clin Nutr.* Mar 1998;67(3):359-366.

[34] Bergstrom J. Why are dialysis patients malnourished? *Am J Kidney Dis.* Jul 1995;26(1):229-241.

[35] Wang AY, Sea MM, Tang N, et al. Resting energy expenditure and subsequent mortality risk in peritoneal dialysis patients. *J Am Soc Nephrol.* Dec 2004;15(12):3134-3143.

[36] Heimburger O, Lonnqvist F, Danielsson A, Nordenstrom J, Stenvinkel P. Serum immunoreactive leptin concentration and its relation to the body fat content in chronic renal failure. *J Am Soc Nephrol.* Sep 1997;8(9):1423-1430.

[37] Kaysen GA, Rathore V, Shearer GC, Depner TA. Mechanisms of hypoalbuminemia in hemodialysis patients. *Kidney Int.* Aug 1995;48(2):510-516.

[38] Qureshi AR, Alvestrand A, Divino-Filho JC, et al. Inflammation, malnutrition, and cardiac disease as predictors of mortality in hemodialysis patients. *J Am Soc Nephrol.* Jan 2002;13 Suppl 1:S28-36.

[39] Fiedler R, Mall M, Wand C, Osten B. Short-term administration of omega-3 fatty acids in hemodialysis patients with balanced lipid metabolism. *J Ren Nutr.* Apr 2005;15(2):253-256.

[40] Johannsson G, Bengtsson BA, Ahlmen J. Double-blind, placebo-controlled study of growth hormone treatment in elderly patients undergoing chronic hemodialysis: anabolic effect and functional improvement. *Am J Kidney Dis.* Apr 1999;33(4):709-

[41] Hansen TB, Gram J, Jensen PB, et al. Influence of growth hormone on whole body and regional soft tissue composition in adult patients on hemodialysis. A double-blind, randomized, placebo-controlled study. *Clin Nephrol.* Feb 2000;53(2):99-107.

[42] Johansen KL, Mulligan K, Schambelan M. Anabolic effects of nandrolone decanoate in patients receiving dialysis: a randomized controlled trial. *Jama.* Apr 14 1999;281(14):1275-1281.

[43] Boccanfuso JA, Hutton M, McAllister B. The effects of megestrol acetate on nutritional parameters in a dialysis population. *J Ren Nutr.* Jan 2000;10(1):36-43.

[44] Ho KK, Pinsky JL, Kannel WB, Levy D. The epidemiology of heart failure: the Framingham Study. *J Am Coll Cardiol.* Oct 1993;22(4 Suppl A):6A-13A.

[45] Cowie MR, Mosterd A, Wood DA, et al. The epidemiology of heart failure. *Eur Heart J.* Feb 1997;18(2):208-225.

[46] Anker SD, Swan JW, Volterrani M, et al. The influence of muscle mass, strength, fatigability and blood flow on exercise capacity in cachectic and non-cachectic patients with chronic heart failure. *Eur Heart J.* Feb 1997;18(2):259-269.

[47] Anker SD, Ponikowski P, Varney S, et al. Wasting as independent risk factor for mortality in chronic heart failure. *Lancet.* Apr 12 1997;349(9058):1050-1053.

[48] Poehlman ET, Scheffers J, Gottlieb SS, Fisher ML, Vaitekevicius P. Increased resting metabolic rate in patients with congestive heart failure. *Ann Intern Med.* Dec 1 1994;121(11):860-862.

[49] Toth MJ, Gottlieb SS, Goran MI, Fisher ML, Poehlman ET. Daily energy expenditure in free-living heart failure patients. *Am J Physiol.* Mar 1997;272(3 Pt 1):E469-475.

[50] Anker SD, Sharma R. The syndrome of cardiac cachexia. *Int J Cardiol.* Sep 2002;85(1):51-66.

[51] King D, Smith ML, Chapman TJ, Stockdale HR, Lye M. Fat malabsorption in elderly patients with cardiac cachexia. *Age Ageing.* Mar 1996;25(2):144-149.

[52] Levine B, Kalman J, Mayer L, Fillit HM, Packer M. Elevated circulating levels of tumor necrosis factor in severe chronic heart failure. *N Engl J Med.* Jul 26 1990;323(4):236-241.

[53] Anker SD, Chua TP, Ponikowski P, et al. Hormonal changes and catabolic/anabolic imbalance in chronic heart failure and their importance for cardiac cachexia. *Circulation.* Jul 15 1997;96(2):526-534.

[54] Torre-Amione G, Kapadia S, Benedict C, Oral H, Young JB, Mann DL. Proinflammatory cytokine levels in patients with depressed left ventricular ejection fraction: a report from the Studies of Left Ventricular Dysfunction (SOLVD). *J Am Coll Cardiol.* Apr 1996;27(5):1201-1206.

[55] Deswal A, Petersen NJ, Feldman AM, Young JB, White BG, Mann DL. Cytokines and cytokine receptors in advanced heart failure: an analysis of the cytokine database from the Vesnarinone trial (VEST). *Circulation.* Apr 24 2001;103(16):2055-2059.

[56] Rauchhaus M, Doehner W, Francis DP, et al. Plasma cytokine parameters and mortality in patients with chronic heart failure. *Circulation.* Dec 19 2000;102(25):3060-3067.

[57] Niebauer J, Pflaum CD, Clark AL, et al. Deficient insulin-like growth factor I in chronic heart failure predicts altered body composition, anabolic deficiency, cytokine and neurohormonal activation. *J Am Coll Cardiol.* Aug 1998;32(2):393-397.

[58] Parissis JT, Panou F, Farmakis D, et al. Effects of levosimendan on markers of left ventricular diastolic function and neurohormonal activation in patients with advanced heart failure. *Am J Cardiol.* Aug 1 2005;96(3):423-426.

[59] Anker SD, Negassa A, Coats AJ, et al. Prognostic importance of weight loss in chronic heart failure and the effect of treatment with angiotensin-converting-enzyme inhibitors: an observational study. *Lancet.* Mar 29 2003;361(9363):1077-1083.

[60] Brink M, Wellen J, Delafontaine P. Angiotensin II causes weight loss and decreases circulating insulin-like growth factor I in rats through a pressor-independent mechanism. *J Clin Invest.* Jun 1 1996;97(11):2509-2516.

[61] Torre-Amione G, Sestier F, Radovancevic B, Young J. Broad modulation of tissue responses (immune activation) by celacade may favorably influence pathologic processes associated with heart failure progression. *Am J Cardiol.* Jun 6 2005;95(11A):30C-37C; discussion 38C-40C.

[62] Cone RD. Anatomy and regulation of the central melanocortin system. *Nat Neurosci.* May 2005;8(5):571-578.

[63] Ollmann MM, Wilson BD, Yang YK, et al. Antagonism of central melanocortin receptors in vitro and in vivo by agouti-related protein. *Science.* 1997;278(5335):135-138.

[64] DeBoer MD, Marks DL. Cachexia: lessons from melanocortin antagonism. *Trends Endocrinol Metab.* Jul 2006;17(5):199-204.

[65] Farooqi IS, Keogh JM, Yeo GS, Lank EJ, Cheetham T, O'Rahilly S. Clinical spectrum of obesity and mutations in the melanocortin 4 receptor gene. *N Engl J Med.* Mar 20 2003;348(12):1085-1095.

[66] DeBoer MD, Marks DL. Therapy insight: Use of melanocortin antagonists in the treatment of cachexia in chronic disease. *Nat Clin Pract Endocrinol Metab.* Aug 2006;2(8):459-466.

[67] Marks DL, Ling N, Cone RD. Role of the Central Melanocortin System in Cachexia. *Cancer Res.* 2001;61(4):1432-1438.

[68] Scarlett JM, Jobst EE, Enriori PJ, et al. Regulation of Central Melanocortin Signaling by Interleukin-1{beta}. *Endocrinology.* Sep 2007;148(9):4217-4225.

[69] DeBoer MD, Zhu XX, Levasseur P, et al. Ghrelin treatment causes increased food intake and retention of lean body mass in a rat model of cancer cachexia. *Endocrinology.* Jun 2007;148(6):3004-3012.

[70] Marks DL, Cone RD. Central melanocortins and the regulation of weight during acute and chronic disease. *Recent Prog Horm Res.* 2001;56:359-375.

[71] Chen C, Tucci FC, Jiang W, et al. Pharmacological and pharmacokinetic characterization of 2-piperazine-alpha-isopropyl benzylamine derivatives as melanocortin-4 receptor antagonists. *Bioorg Med Chem.* May 15 2008;16(10):5606-5618.

[72] Cheung W, Yu PX, Little BM, Cone RD, Marks DL, Mak RH. Role of leptin and melanocortin signaling in uremia-associated cachexia. *J Clin Invest.* Jun 2005;115(6):1659-1665.

[73] Cheung WW, Kuo HJ, Markison S, et al. Peripheral administration of the melanocortin-4 receptor antagonist NBI-12i ameliorates uremia-associated cachexia in mice. *J Am Soc Nephrol.* Sep 2007;18(9):2517-2524.

[74] Cheung WW, Rosengren S, Boyle DL, Mak RH. Modulation of melanocortin signaling ameliorates uremic cachexia. *Kidney Int.* Jul 2008;74(2):180-186.

[75] Joppa MA, Gogas KR, Foster AC, Markison S. Central infusion of the melanocortin receptor antagonist agouti-related peptide (AgRP(83-132)) prevents cachexia-related symptoms induced by radiation and colon-26 tumors in mice. *Peptides.* Jan 2 2007.

[76] Markison S, Foster AC, Chen C, et al. The regulation of feeding and metabolic rate and the prevention of murine cancer cachexia with a small-molecule melanocortin-4 receptor antagonist. *Endocrinology.* Jun 2005;146(6):2766-2773.

[77] Marks DL, Butler AA, Turner R, Brookhart GB, Cone RD. Differential role of melanocortin receptor subtypes in cachexia. *Endocrinology.* 2003;144(4):1513-1523.

[78] Nicholson JR, Kohler G, Schaerer F, Senn C, Weyermann P, Hofbauer KG. Peripheral administration of a melanocortin 4-receptor inverse agonist prevents loss of lean body mass in tumor-bearing mice. *J Pharmacol Exp Ther.* May 2006;317(2):771-777.

[79] Vos TJ, Caracoti A, Che JL, et al. Identification of 2-[2-[2-(5-bromo-2-methoxyphenyl)-ethyl]-3-fluorophenyl]-4,5-dihydro-1H-imidazole (ML00253764), a small molecule melanocortin 4 receptor antagonist that effectively reduces tumor-induced weight loss in a mouse model. *J Med Chem.* Mar 25 2004;47(7):1602-1604.

[80] Wisse BE, Frayo RS, Schwartz MW, Cummings DE. Reversal of cancer anorexia by blockade of central melanocortin receptors in rats. *Endocrinology.* 2001;142(8):3292-3301.

[81] DeBoer MD. Melanocortin interventions in cachexia: how soon from bench to bedside? *Curr Opin Clin Nutr Metab Care.* Jul 2007;10(4):457-462.

[82] Kojima M, Hosoda H, Date Y, Nakazato M, Matsuo H, Kangawa K. Ghrelin is a growth-hormone-releasing acylated peptide from stomach. *Nature.* Dec 9 1999;402(6762):656-660.

[83] Cummings DE, Weigle DS, Frayo RS, et al. Plasma ghrelin levels after diet-induced weight loss or gastric bypass surgery. *N Engl J Med.* May 23 2002;346(21):1623-1630.

[84] DeBoer MD. Emergence of ghrelin as a treatment for cachexia syndromes. *Nutrition.* Sep 2008;24(9):806-814.

[85] Willesen MG, Kristensen P, Romer J. Co-localization of growth hormone secretagogue receptor and NPY mRNA in the arcuate nucleus of the rat. *Neuroendocrinology.* Nov 1999;70(5):306-316.

[86] Chen HY, Trumbauer ME, Chen AS, et al. Orexigenic action of peripheral ghrelin is mediated by neuropeptide Y and agouti-related protein. *Endocrinology.* Jun 2004;145(6):2607-2612.

[87] Granado M, Priego T, Martin AI, Villanua MA, Lopez-Calderon A. Anti-inflammatory effect of the ghrelin agonist growth hormone-releasing peptide-2 (GHRP-2) in arthritic rats. *Am J Physiol Endocrinol Metab.* Mar 2005;288(3):E486-492.

[88] DeBoer MD, Zhu X, Levasseur PR, et al. Ghrelin treatment of chronic kidney disease: improvements in lean body mass and cytokine profile. *Endocrinology.* Feb 2008;149(2):827-835.

[89] Gonzalez-Rey E, Delgado M. Anti-inflammatory neuropeptide receptors: new therapeutic targets for immune disorders? *Trends Pharmacol Sci.* Sep 2007;28(9):482-491.

[90] Chorny A, Anderson P, Gonzalez-Rey E, Delgado M. Ghrelin protects against experimental sepsis by inhibiting high-mobility group box 1 release and by killing bacteria. *J Immunol.* Jun 15 2008;180(12):8369-8377.

[91] Kodama T, Ashitani J, Matsumoto N, Kangawa K, Nakazato M. Ghrelin treatment suppresses neutrophil-dominant inflammation in airways of patients with chronic respiratory infection. *Pulm Pharmacol Ther.* 2008;21(5):774-779.

[92] Hanada T, Toshinai K, Kajimura N, et al. Anti-cachectic effect of ghrelin in nude mice bearing human melanoma cells. *Biochem Biophys Res Commun.* Feb 7

[93] Nagaya N, Uematsu M, Kojima M, et al. Chronic administration of ghrelin improves left ventricular dysfunction and attenuates development of cardiac cachexia in rats with heart failure. *Circulation.* Sep 18 2001;104(12):1430-1435.

[94] Wang W, Andersson M, Iresjo BM, Lonnroth C, Lundholm K. Effects of ghrelin on anorexia in tumor-bearing mice with eicosanoid-related cachexia. *Int J Oncol.* Jun 2006;28(6):1393-1400.

[95] Xu XB, Pang JJ, Cao JM, et al. GH-releasing peptides improve cardiac dysfunction and cachexia and suppress stress-related hormones and cardiomyocyte apoptosis in rats with heart failure. *Am J Physiol Heart Circ Physiol.* Oct 2005;289(4):H1643-1651.

[96] Neary NM, Small CJ, Wren AM, et al. Ghrelin increases energy intake in cancer patients with impaired appetite: acute, randomized, placebo-controlled trial. *J Clin Endocrinol Metab.* Jun 2004;89(6):2832-2836.

[97] Strasser F, Lutz TA, Maeder MT, et al. Safety, tolerability and pharmacokinetics of intravenous ghrelin for cancer-related anorexia/cachexia: a randomised, placebo-controlled, double-blind, double-crossover study. *Br J Cancer.* Jan 29 2008;98(2):300-308.

[98] Nagaya N, Itoh T, Murakami S, et al. Treatment of cachexia with ghrelin in patients with COPD. *Chest.* Sep 2005;128(3):1187-1193.

[99] Nagaya N, Moriya J, Yasumura Y, et al. Effects of ghrelin administration on left ventricular function, exercise capacity, and muscle wasting in patients with chronic heart failure. *Circulation.* Dec 14 2004;110(24):3674-3679.

[100] Akamizu T, Takaya K, Irako T, et al. Pharmacokinetics, safety, and endocrine and appetite effects of ghrelin administration in young healthy subjects. *Eur J Endocrinol.* Apr 2004;150(4):447-455.

[101] Garcia JM BR, Graham, C, Kumor K, Polvino W. A Phase II, randomized, placebo-controlled, double blind study of the efficacy and safety of RC-1291 for the treatment of cancer-cachexia. Abstract 2007 American Society of Clinical Oncology (ASCO) Meeting, Chicago, IL. *Journal of Clinical Oncology.* 2007;Supp. Vol 25 (No18S).

Chapter 9

REGULATION OF CHILDREN'S FOOD INTAKE

Gie Liem
School of Exercise and Nutrition Sciences, Sensory Science Group, Deakin University,
Burwood, Australia

INTRODUCTION

The alarming increase of child obesity in many parts of the world suggests that children consume more energy than they need [1]. Insights into how children regulate their food intake will enable health professionals and parents to develop strategies to improve the balance between energy intake and energy expenditure.

From a biological point of view food intake is regulated by demand. When there is a shortage of energy, food intake needs to be increased. When there is enough energy consumed, food intake needs to be limited or terminated. The increase of obesity in the past decades clearly shows a mismatch between energy intake and energy expenditure in an obeseogenic environment [2]. It has been suggested that the human body is better able to protect itself from energy deprivation, than it is from over consumption of energy [3]. It has been argued that humans' body and brain is not able to handle today's food environment, where an overflow of highly palatable foods are available and easy accessible without severe hunting or gathering efforts [4].

The current chapter will provide a brief overview of the scientific evidence regarding children's ability to effectively regulate their energy intake, leading to a long-term energy balance. Furthermore, it will be discussed how portion size, energy density and parental control interfere with children's ability to effectively regulate their energy intake.

INTERNAL CUES AS REGULATORS OF FOOD INTAKE

Regulation of food intake of children is determined by internal as well as external cues [5]. Internal cues are mainly hunger, thirst, satiety and satiation, which are regulated by a wide variety of peptides and hormones [6, 7]. External cues vary from portion size, to parenting styles. Research suggests that infants and children younger than 2 years of age have an innate ability to self regulate their energy intake [8]. Still, in industrialized countries, an increased number of children are obese [1], which suggests a long term energy imbalance. During childhood, children may lose the ability to regulate their food intake due to the presence of a variety of external cues present in the household and the wider environment they live in. It has, indeed, been hypothesized that young children (3-4 years of age) are better able to respond to their internal cues of satiety and hunger, than older aged children and adults [9]. The assumption is that older aged children and adults have had more opportunities to learn the association between a variety of external cues, food consumption and meal termination. Below we briefly review the evidence which is available to support such hypotheses.

One of the first researchers to suggest that infants and toddlers have an unlearned ability to self regulate their food intake comes from the research of Clara Davis in the 1920's and 1930's [10]. She performed a series of classic experiments in which she let 15 infants self regulate their food choice and intake. The experiment lasted for 4.5 years. Everyday children were presented with a variety of foods, of which they could freely choose and consume. At the end of the experiment all children were healthy and did not show signs of abnormal growth or development. These findings suggest that at an early age children are well able to regulate their own food intake. However, one important limitation needs to be taken into account. The foods offered were all rather "healthy". In fact Davis states in her article: "It should comprise of a wide range of foods of both animal and vegetable origin that would adequately provide all the food elements, amino acids, fats, carbohydrates, vitamins and minerals known to be necessary for human nutrition. The foods should be such as could generally be procured fresh in the market the year around. The list should contain only natural food materials and no incomplete foods or canned foods (…) sugars were not used nor were milk products, such as cream, butter or cheese." The extrapolation of Davis' findings with today's food environment where children do have access to high palatable, high energy dense foods should be used with caution [11]. Although some studies do suggest that breastfed infants infants are able to regulate their energy intake [12], it can not be concluded from David's studies that children older than 2 years of age can do the same.

CONTROLLED EXPERIMENTS

More recent investigations, which focused on children's ability to regulate their energy intake, can be split into *controlled experiments* and *observational studies*. One of the most cited studies which suggests that children are well able to regulate their energy intake during 24 hours was carried out by Birch and colleagues. In a controlled study they measured 2-to-5-year-olds' energy intake during breakfast, morning snack, lunch, afternoon snack, dinner and evening snack. Children were given access to two standardized menus of which they could eat as much as they wanted to. The researchers found that the variability in energy intake between children varied to a large extent between separate meals, but showed a low variability for total energy intake during the day. The authors concluded that children may have been compensating their meal intake according to the energy they consumed during other parts of the day [13]. Despite that, this research is often cited as evidence that children are able to regulate their food intake, the results also have been questioned. Several researchers claim that a lower variability in total energy consumption over 24 hours, compared to the high variability in energy consumption during a single meal can well be a statistical artifact [14-16]. Total energy intake exists of the summation of energy intake during separate meals, therefore total energy intake will most likely have a lower variability than the parts (meals) it is composed of. This statistical phenomenon has been demonstrated with artificial data sets, which were generated at random. Although in these data sets individual meal variations were not related to total daily energy consumption, the researchers demonstrated that for these data sets the variation of the individual meals was also far larger than the variation of the total daily energy consumption, comparable with the difference in variation found in the Birch's study [13]. The authors concluded that a difference between variability in energy intake during individual meals, and over 24 hours can largely be explained by this statistical artifact [15].

However, Birch's findings, as reported in the New England Journal of Medicine [13], do not stand on its own. Rather than investigating differences in variation on a *group level*, research also has focused on *individual's* ability to regulate energy intake. In these well controlled experiments, typically children are given a set amount of food to consume (i.e. pre load) after which they are given access to a meal 90 minutes after they consumed the pre-load. If children are able to regulate their food intake according to hunger and satiety (internal cues), they would eat less during the lunch when given a high energy pre-load compared to when a low energy pre-load was given. In other words, the total energy consumption from pre-load and lunch should remain fairly stable despite differences in the energy content of the pre-load. The energy content of the pre-load is usually manipulated by substituting high energy macro nutrients with low energy replacements (see [17] for a review).

Several studies investigated the hypothesis that children are able to self regulate their energy intake by using different pre-loads. For example, Cecil and colleagues gave children (6-9 yrs old) a high (1628kJ), low (783kJ) or a zero kJ preload. The provided preload needed to be consumed in full. After 90 minutes children were given access to a lunch and energy intake was measured. It was found that children did compensate their energy intake from the test meal in response to either the high or low energy preload. Young children (<7 years) showed a more accurate compensation in response to the different preloads than older aged children. This difference was most pronounced when children were given the high calorie preload. Young children consumed 22% less of the lunch after they consumed the high energy pre-load, compared to after they consumed the 0kJ preload. This difference was only 15% for older aged children. Furthermore, young children consumed 10% more energy at lunch after they were given a low energy preload, than after they were given a high energy preload. This difference in energy consumption was only 2% for older aged children. However, it is important to notice that these compensations were not fully accurate. This resulted in an average of 34% higher total energy intake (pre-load + test meal) when a high energy pre-load was consumed, compared to when a low energy preload was consumed [9]. The results do, however, suggest that younger aged children are better at regulating their energy intake than older aged children. Along the same line, studies with older aged children, failed to find evidence for self regulation of energy intake [18]. The results of Cecil's studies are in line with other experimental studies in which food consumption is highly controlled [17, 19, 20]. It is important to note that, in all these studies, although children showed the ability to adjust their energy intake in response to different preloads, only very few children showed a 100% compensation.

This incomplete compensation is likely to occur in response to high energy *preloads* as well as for *meals* in which high calorie macronutrients are replaced by low calorie substitutes. For example Leahy and colleagues found that when energy density of an entrée was decreased, children (2-to-5-year old) do compensate, but not fully, in terms of energy intake. In their study children only compensated for 16% of the energy deficit. It is important to note that the meals were equally liked, therefore, taste liking is not a confounding variable. This suggests that a decrease in energy density of a meal might result in a decrease in energy intake of that meal, because full energy compensation in response to low energy meal components does not take place. [21].

Large variations, in children's ability to regulate their energy intake do, however, exist. As mentioned earlier, older aged children (>7 years) are less able to accurately compensate for changes in the energy content of a preload, than younger aged children. Furthermore, it has been suggested that children with greater fat stores are less able to accurately compensate their calorie intake when a high calorie preload is given [20]. For example Jansen et al showed that overweight children are more responsive to cues which predict food intake (i.e. smell or eating a preload), than their lean counterparts. That is, overweight children consumed more after being exposed to food cues, than when they were not pre-exposed to these food cues. Such differences were not found for the normal weight children. The authors concluded that overweight children do not regulate their food intake as their normal weight peers do. Overweight children might be more susceptible to food cues, which are likely to trigger them to over eat [22].

Based on the available literature we can conclude that, in controlled experiments, children's ability to regulate their energy intake is reasonable, but far from perfect. A prolonged exposure to high energy dense foods may lead to a substantial increase in calorie consumption in the long term, because children's energy regulation is not able to fully adjust for increases in energy density of foods. Furthermore, large variations between children in their ability to accurately compensate do exist. Moreover, the external validity of controlled experiments which investigated children's ability to self-regulate their energy intake is poorly understood. The highly controlled situation in which these experiments take place may have little relevance for real life environments where external factors such as portion size and social context compete with children's ability to self-regulate their food intake.

OBSERVATIONAL STUDIES

Long term observational studies investigating children's ability to regulate energy intake are scarce. Shae and colleagues followed up 181 children for 3 years during which seven 24 hour recalls were conducted. Similarly to Birch's study [13], variation in calories consumed per meal were compared with the variation over 24 hours. Correspondingly to Birch's study, it was found that the variation per meal was significantly higher than the variation in 24 hours. Also, the results of this study, can however be explained by the same statistical artifact as mentioned previously [15].

In another observational study, researchers took 24h dietary recalls for 5 to 7 consecutive days of seventeen 4 –to-6-year old children [16]. Children were living in their normal environment and none of the foods, which were consumed, were manipulated or in any other way different to what children would normally eat. It was observed that children consumed less when the energy density of the meal was higher than average. However, the researchers also noticed that when the energy density of the meal was higher than average, the offered portion size decreased accordingly. When energy intake was adjusted for the serving size, no evidence of children's ability to compensate for high energy foods was observed. Another study with children in their natural environment also failed to replicate Birch's findings [13] and did not provide evidence that children are able to regulate their energy intake in a free living situation [23].

Conclusion

In conclusion, to our knowledge, there is little evidence that accurate calorie compensation takes place outside of lab controlled environments. This could possibly be due to the difference between a controlled lab environment and the presence of external cues which regulate children's food intake and are present in children's natural environment. Moreover, it is difficult to compare controlled experimental studies and observational studies. Controlled experiments give an answer to the question whether children *are able* to control their energy intake based on differences in energy content of food, whereas observational studies give an answer to the question whether children *are* indeed regulating their energy intake in their daily lives, when they are exposed to an abundance of foods which are high in calories, highly palatable. easily accessible, and which are given in a particular context. These external factors may well override children's ability to self regulate their energy intake.

External Cues as Regulators of Food Intake

External factors which either encourage children to eat, or stop eating are of large importance to children's control of energy intake [5]. First of all, in order for children to consume a particular food it needs to be available and accessible. Availability can be defined as the presence of a particular food in a particular environment. Accessibility concerns whether these foods can easily be eaten straight away without a substantial amount of effort [24]. Parents play a key role in the foods, which are available and accessible to children. This, however, does not mean that children are not able to influence parental decisions concerning food purchase [25-27].

Availability and Accessibility

According to the optimal foraging theory, individuals will thrive to optimize the benefit, which is a result of a certain behaviour for a minimal expenditure [28]. The net benefit will decrease when the amount of effort involved in consuming the product increases. Effort in eating may involve the price of the food relative to the available money, location of the food (ie. Do you need to travel long distances to buy or get a particular food?), preparation and the effort involved in eating the food. When food is readily available this may mean that a particular food is present in the household, or readily available in a fast food restaurant around the corner. The food becomes accessible when the food in the household is already prepared for consumption, the price of the readily available fast food is low and the fast food restaurant can be accessed by car, or is at a walking distance. Nowadays, high energy foods are more available than ever before. With the increase of fast food restaurants (especially in low income areas), convenience foods and low prices, high energy palatable foods are also highly accessible [29]. At the same time, in the past years, portion sizes of various food presented at home, in restaurants and fast food outlets have increased remarkably, with fast food outlets now serving the largest portions [30]. Taking the theory of optimal foraging into account, with the availability and accessibility of high energy food together, one could hypothesis an association between high energy consumption, or even the prevalence of obesity, and the availability and accessibility of high energy foods. In general, however, epidemiological studies failed to find such association [31, 32]. Only the variety of fast food restaurants seems to be positively significantly associated with fast food consumption [32].

Availability and Accessibility on Household Level

On a household level, however, significant associations between availability, accessibility and food consumption are found, but causality can not be concluded from these studies. For example, Pearson and colleagues found that the in-home availability of energy dense snack foods is associated with adolescence's change in consumption of these foods [33]. Other studies found that availability of soft drink in the household was strongly positively associated with soft drink consumption of adolescence [34]. By replacing nutritive sweeteners (i.e. sweet substances containing high levels of energy) with a non nutritive sweetener it has been suggested that energy intake can be reduced on the long term [35].

The association, on a household level, between availability, accessibility and consumption also holds up for healthy foods such as fruit, juice and vegetables. In a study with 4 to 6 graders it was found that availability of fruit, juice and vegetables, accounted for a significant 11% of the variance in consumption of these foods. Moreover, availability and accessibility accounted for 23% of the variance of consumption in children who did not even like the taste of fruit, juice and vegetables [24]. This suggests that availability and accessibility may play a key role in children's food consumption, but the causality of this association remains to be investigated. Alternatively the availability of snack foods is driven by children's request. In other words, children who consume large amounts of snack foods, may also requests these foods more which results in a higher availability of these foods in the household. The same could be true for healthy foods.

In terms of regulation of energy intake, from these epidemiological studies it cannot be concluded whether availability and accessibility can override internal hunger and satiety cues. It could well be that availability and accessibility of one food increases the consumption of that food, but decreases the consumption of other foods. We therefore need to have a look at experimental studies in which accessibility of a meal component is manipulated and total consumption of a meal is measured. One way to increase the availability and accessibility to food is by providing large portion sizes.

Effect of Increasing Portion Size on Energy Intake

Studies in adults demonstrated that portion size can influence meal consumption [36, 37]. In general, the more that is offered, the more that will be consumed. These findings have been replicated in children as young as 4 years of age. For example, Rolls and colleagues offered 3 to 5 year old children, in a cross over design over 3 weeks, either a portion that was smaller, equal or larger than the recommended serving size. Children older than 5 years of age, were significantly affected by the different portion sizes. In general, the larger the portion size, the more these children consumed. Three year olds seemed, however, to be unaffected by portion size [38]. Although the age difference has not been replicated elsewhere, the finding that children consume around 25% to 33% more when portion sizes double, has been confirmed by a number of studies [39, 40]. These percentages are similar to what has been found in adult populations (See [41] for review). The mechanisms by which increased portion sizes result in an increased consumption are not well understood in the case of children. It has been suggested that children are largely unaware when they are served a larger portion than usual (see [42] for a review). However, bite size portions have been shown to increase when larger portions are served during lunch [39]. This is in line with what has been shown with adults, who were being served double their normal portion size [43]. Furthermore, when an increase in portion size is combined with an increase in energy density, it has been demonstrated that children consume on average 76% more of the manipulated food and consumed on average 34% more energy from a meal of which the manipulated food was part of [44]. The results of these experiments could explain why real life observations of children failed to find evidence of children's ability to well regulate their energy intake. Furthermore, these studies are generally conducted with well liked foods. Whether an increase in portion size is able to increase the consumption of not so well liked foods remains to be investigated.

Long Term Energy Regulation

Although these studies do suggest that the manipulation of portion size and energy density significantly increases children's energy consumption within a meal, it still does not answer the question whether an increase in portion size (and energy density) would result in an increased energy balance over a day or longer. Studies with adults suggest that subjects who consumed up to 26% more in a single meal in response to an increased portion size, did not compensate for these additional calories in the short (2 days) [45], or long term (11 days) [46] . This suggests, that at least for an adult population, the increase in portion size will most likely result in an increased energy consumption in the long term. Studies with children concerning the long term energy effect of increased portion sizes are rare. To our knowledge, only one study sought to investigate this. Fisher and colleagues measured the 24h energy intake of 5-year-old children and their mothers after they were served different portion sizes of an entrée and snack food. All mothers and children were from low income, Hispanic and African American backgrounds. The manipulation of portion sizes took place throughout the day, resulting in 7 food items of which the portion size was doubled or kept at a normal serving. Similar to previous research, they observed a 23% increase in calorie consumption, from entrée and snacks when both were served in double the portion sizes. Across 24 hours children consumed on average 12% more energy when the large portion sizes where offered [47]. This suggests a significant role of portion size in children's regulation of energy intake. These findings have important implications for parents' everyday practice. Unintentionally, parents who serve their children large portions, encourage their children to over consume. This hypothesis is supported by Fishers' research which measured children's consumption when a large portion was provided and when children were given the opportunity to self regulate their serving size. It was demonstrated that when children selected their own portion size, less food was consumed, compared to when parents determined their children's portion sizes [40].

AVAILABILITY AND ACCESSIBILITY TO HEALTHY FOODS

Although the increase of portion sizes of unhealthy high energy dense foods can negatively impact on children's diets, a similar strategy with healthy foods might be able to advance their diet. The first line of evidence that this might be possible comes from epidemiological studies. Kratt and colleagues compared households with low, medium or high availability of fruit and vegetables on children's vegetable consumption. They found that children from households with a low availability of fruit and vegetables consumed significantly less fruit and vegetables compared to their peers from the remaining household [48]. Similarly, Pearson surveyed close to 2000 adolescents about their consumption, availability, and accessibility of fruit and vegetables in their family home. It was found that the availability of fruit and vegetables was positively associated with adolescence change in vegetable consumption, but not fruit consumption.

It is important to note, however, that although many studies group fruit and vegetables together [24, 48-50], it is well possible that the intake of these foods are regulated differently. For example, Reinaerts and colleagues concluded that based on epidemiological data, availability explained a significant proportion of the variance in fruit consumption, but not vegetable consumption. Accessibility for vegetables was, however, not measured. This is in line with an experimental study by Kral and colleagues. They presented children with different portion sizes of vegetables and fruits at the same eating occasion. They found that doubling the portion size of vegetables and fruit had little to no effect on children's consumption of vegetables, but increased fruit consumption by 43% [51]. In the latter study, however, it could well be that fruit was eaten instead of vegetables due to the higher taste liking for fruit. This is supported by Kral's finding that children who liked the taste of broccoli did increase their consumption of broccoli when this vegetable was served in a larger portion size [51]. Spill and colleagues gave children access to different portions sizes of carrots prior to dinner [52]. It was found that when children were served double the portion size of carrots (60 grams vs 30 grams), they, in general, consumed 47% more of the carrots, than when a single portion size was presented to them. It is important to note that in this study vegetables were served on their own rather than having competing foods children could choose from. Furthermore, carrots were particularly chosen for this study because of children's general liking for carrots. The influence of availability and accessibility on children's fruit and vegetable consumption is therefore likely facilitated by children taste preferences. Indeed, several epidemiological studies suggested that liking is strongly associated with children's fruit and vegetable consumption [53].

TASTE PREFERENCES AND CHILDREN'S FOOD CONSUMPTION

Many fruits contain sugars, which elicit a sweet taste upon consumption. Research repeatedly suggested that children have an inborn preference for sweet taste [54-57] and that children's food consumption can be increased by adding sweet tasting sugars to food [58-62]. Hypothetically liking for sweet tasting substances is driven by the need for energy, which the infant needs for growth and development [63, 64]. In nature, sweet tasting substances often signal energy contents. Furthermore, the first food infants usually encounter outside the womb is breast milk, which has a predominantly sweet taste [65]. Infants' innate preferences for sweet taste may facilitate an easy acceptance of breast milk. Some fruits may also have a sour taste, which is not necessarily disliked by children [66, 67]. Studies suggest that the liking for sour taste is positively associated with infants' and children's fruit consumption [68, 69]. This is in contrast with vegetables, which often have a bitter taste, that children do not like [56, 57, 70, 71]. The aversion for bitter taste may protect the human species from accidental poisoning. In nature, many toxic substances elicit a bitter taste [72].

BARRIERS FOR FRUIT AND VEGETABLE CONSUMPTION

Given that the taste of many fruits is not likely to be disliked by children, making fruits available to children may be an effective strategy to increase consumption, because taste is not an additional barrier. However, when vegetables are made available to children, taste can still be a major barrier for consumption. Furthermore, most fruits can be eaten straight away, or after a minor effort in preparation. It has been suggested that by simply slicing oranges in ready to eat pieces (decreasing the effort involved in eating) children's consumption of oranges increased [73]. In contrast, vegetables often need preparation in terms of cooking. Most children would, however, not be involved in the effort of preparing vegetables. However, parents may see it as a major effort and therefore are less likely to make vegetable accessible to children. Once vegetables are made accessible to children, taste might be the only barrier for consumption. It remains unknown whether an increase in accessibility to vegetables can decrease children's effort involved in eating vegetables and in such make the taste barrier less important. In adults it has been suggested that they can be tricked into eating something they would not particularly like, just by making it accessible and making use of an existing habit. For example, Wansink served 14-day old popcorn to adults who were watching a movie. They found that movie watchers who were provided with a large serving of popcorn consumed 33.6% more popcorn, than those who were served the medium serving size [37], even though the participants did not like the taste of the popcorn. In other words the taste barrier did not prevent participants from eating the popcorn while watching a movie. The habit of eating popcorn at the movies, the accessibility to a large amount, rather than consumers' taste liking of the popcorn, may have driven consumption. It remains to be investigated whether such strategy would work for children and their consumption of for example vegetables. In other words, can we increase children's consumption of vegetables by simply providing vegetables while children are watching tv or a movie.

Cullen found that the availability of and accessibility to fruit, juice and vegetables explained 23% of the variance of the consumption of these foods even though children did not like the taste of these foods [24]. Unfortunately, the authors did not report the exact contribution of vegetable accessibility on children's vegetable consumption. Furthermore, by making the consumption of vegetables more rewarding, the benefit of vegetable consumption might increase which in turn increases consumption [74-76]. Whether increasing the accessibility to vegetables, decreasing the amount of effort involved in eating vegetables and habit formation can increase children's vegetable consumption still remains to be tested in an experimental setting.

PARENTS AS EXTERNAL CUE FOR HUNGER AND SATIETY

Given that availability and accessibility of palatable foods is highly correlated with consumption as reviewed previously, the access to palatable foods might have to be restricted by parents. Parents can choose not to buy the highly palatable foods and in such way limit children's access to these foods. However, children's foods environment, especially when they grow older, expands beyond the household they are part of [26]. Highly palatable foods in grocery stores and the commercials and marketing activities for these foods are widely spread throughout the living environment of children. Food marketing can influence children's requests for these foods [77], children's choice of the advertised foods [78, 79] and children's consumption of these foods [80]. Parents may therefore have specific rules in place which limits children's access to highly palatable unhealthy foods (ie. only soda on Friday evening or weekends) [81, 82].

Several observational, as well as experimental studies suggest that food restriction can lead to children's increased desire and liking of the restricted food. This in turn can result in a high consumption of these foods when children are given free access to the previously restricted food. For example, we asked parents how much they restricted their children's access to sugary food [83]. We then measured children's liking for different concentrations of sucrose in an orange beverage. The results suggested that children of parents who gave their children very restricted access to sugary foods, preferred higher concentrations of sucrose, than those whose parents gave their child more freedom in the consumption of sugary foods. Causality can, however, not been drawn from this study. Studies by Birch do, however, suggest that children's liking and desire to consume particular foods increases in response to parental restriction [84, 85].

Fisher and Birch experimentally restricted children's access to medium liked foods by providing the target food in closed jars on a table amongst other similar foods, which were freely available during 2 sessions per week for a total of 5 weeks. The results of this study suggested that restriction resulted in an increase of children's positive comments about the restricted food, a higher frequency of selection of the restricted food, and a higher intake of the restricted food when children were given free access to the previously restricted food [84,

85]. Similar results were obtained by Jansen et al who experimentally restricted children's access to a particular colour of candy, whereas other colours of the same candy were freely available [86].

Similarly to the restriction of highly palatable unhealthy foods, parents often pressure children to consume healthy foods such as vegetables, or encourage children to eat more than they want by saying: "Clean your plate" [87], or by giving a reward for eating healthy foods (i.e. you can watch tv after you have eaten your vegetables). These parental practices might be received as "pressure to eat" by children [88]. It has been suggested that such strategies result in a decreased liking and desire to consume the foods which are eaten under pressure [88]. For example Birch and colleagues randomly assigned 45 pre-school children to one of four different instrumental eating conditions, which were different in the type of reward (praise or movie ticket) and the amount children were offered (baseline portion and baseline portion + an additional small amount) [89]. In addition two control groups were composed to investigate the effect of just the repeated exposure to the foods on children's liking. The foods children were offered existed of a milk beverage, which was neutrally liked by the child. Children were rewarded for consumption and liking was measured with a ranking procedure. In general preference for milk decreased when consumption was rewarded [89]. Other studies suggested that when a particular food is given as a reward for the consumption of another food (target food), preference for the target food decreases [88, 90]. However, reward may not always be perceived as pressure by the child. In situations where the parents tell the child to consume food A, otherwise the child will not be offered food B, it may likely to be perceived as pressure by the child. However, when other non-food rewards are given alongside the consumption of disliked foods, reward might increase consumption and may not have a negative effect on liking (the food is already low liked) as suggested by several studies [74, 76].

Although some, by no means "all", studies suggest that restriction and pressure lead to an increased and decreased liking and desire of the target food, respectively, it remains unknown how much children will consume of these foods when no rules are applied. In other words, are children able to self-regulate their consumption of candy, if nobody tells them that they are only allowed to eat a limited amount? Similarly, would children start eating vegetables themselves, if nobody told them they had to? We found that children whose parents applied rules, which aimed to restrict children's sugar consumption, consumed less sugary foods during the day, than children of parents who did not apply such rules [83]. Moreover, young children are mostly under the guardians of either teachers, parents or other caretakers. This limits children's opportunity to freely choose what they want and in which quantities. In other words, restriction may lead to an increased liking and desire, but as long as children are under the guardians of a caretaker who consistently applies the restriction rules, the consumption of the restricted foods may well be lower, than when no rules are applied.

However, it is important to realize that food restriction and pressure to eat may not only influence children's liking and desire for foods, but also affects children's ability to self regulate their energy intake. Both perceived pressure to eat, as well as perceived restriction to eat have been shown to be associated with 5 –year old girls' strong focus on external cues, rather than internal cues when eating (ie. hunger and satiety) [87]. That is, children are less likely to adjust their energy intake according to their feelings of hunger and satiety, when parents try to control their children's food intake, than when parents have more trust in children's own ability to regulate energy intake [91].

It has been suggested that girls' inability to respond to satiety signals as a result of parental food restricting when 5 years of age, can still be observed 2-4 years later. This suggests that parental restricting may have a long-term effect on the ability to effectively regulate energy intake, at least in girls [92]. Less data is available for boys. To our knowledge only one study investigated whether boys were similarly affected by food restriction as girls [91]. In this study they investigated close to 600 seven to twelve year old children and sought for correlations between children's external, restrained and emotional eating, and perceived parental pressure to eat. Although they did not observe an association between perceived parental pressure to eat and emotional and external eating for girls, they did observe such association for boys [91].

Besides explicit restriction or pressure, also casual comments such as:"are you done yet?" ,"just a couple of more bites, then you are finished" , may influence children's ability to self regulate their energy intake [93, 94]. Currently, to our knowledge, there are no studies available which investigated children's self-regulating mechanisms for vegetables. However, work with infants suggest that experience plays a key role in the regulation of vegetable intake [65, 95].

CONCLUSION

Children's ability to regulate their energy intake decreases with age. Similarly to adults, in a real life environment children's regulation of energy intake is disrupted by external cues such as portion sizes. Children are in general not well able to adjust their energy intake according to the energy density of food, which makes them prone to overconsumption in today's obeseogenic environment. Parental practices such as food restriction and pressure to eat, which aim to improve children's diet, are likely to be counterproductive as they are associated with children increased inability to self regulate their energy intake. Availability, accessibility and experience play a key role in children's consumption of both unhealthy energy dense food and healthy foods such as fruit and vegetables. More experimental research is needed into the causality of this association.

ACKNOWLEDGMENT

Reviewed by Dr Jullie Mennella, the Monell Chemical Senses Center, Philadelphia, US

REFERENCES

[1] Ebbeling, C.B., D.B. Pawlak, D.S. Ludwig, D.W. Haslam, and W.P. James, Childhood obesity: public-health crisis, common sense cure obesity. *Lancet*, 2002. 360(9331): p. 473-482.

[2] Fernandez, J.R., K. Casazza, J. Divers, and M. Lopez-Alarcon, Disruptions in energy balance: does nature overcome nurture? *Physiology & Behavior*, 2008. 94: p. 105-112.

[3] Melanson, K.J., M.S. Westerterp-Plantenga, L.A. Campfield, and W.H.M. Saris, *Short term regulation of food intake in humans, in Regulation of food intake and energy expenditure,* M.S. Westerterp-Plantenga, A.B. Steffens, and A. Tremblay, Editors. 1999, EDRA: Milano. p. 37-58.

[4] Swinburn, B., Obesity Prevention in Children and Adolescents Child and Adolescent *Psychiatric Clinics of North America*, 2009. 18(1): p. 209-223.

[5] Birch, L.L. and J.O. Fisher, Development of eating behaviors among children and adolescents. *Pediatrics*, 1998. 101(3 Pt 2): p. 539-549.

[6] Cumming, D. and J. Overduin, Gastrointestinal regulation of food intake. The *Journal of Clinical Investigation,* 2007. 117(1): p. 13-23.

[7] Druce, M. and S.R. Bloom, The regulation of appetite. *Archives of Disease in Childhood,* 2005. 91: p. 183-187.

[8] Fox, M.K., B. Devaney, K. Reidy, C. Razafindrakoto, and P. Ziegler, Relationship between portion size and energy intake among infants and toddlers: evidence of self regulation. *Journal of the American Dietetic Association,* 2006. 106: p. S77-S83.

[9] 9. Cecil, J.E., C.N.A. Palmer, W. Wrieden, I. Murrie, C. Bolton-Smith, P. Watt, D.J. Wallis, and M.M. Hetherington, Energy intakes of children after preloads: adjustment, not compensation. *American Journal of Clinical Nutrition,* 2005. 82: p. 302-308.

[10] Davis, C.M., Self selection of diet by newly weaned infants. *American Journal of Diseases of Children,* 1928. 36(4): p. 651-679.

[11] Story, M. and J.E. Brown, Do young children instinctively know what to eat. *New England Journal of Medicine,* 1987. 316(2): p. 103-105.

[12] Cohen, R.J., K.H. Brown, J. Canahuati, L.L. Rivera, and K.G. Dewey, Effects of age of introduction of complementary foods on infant breast milk intake, total energy intake, and growth: a randomized intervention study in Honduras. *The Lancet,* 1994. 344(July 30): p. 288-293.

[13] Birch, L.L., S.L. Johnson, G. Andresen, K.C. Peters, and M.C. Schulte, Variability of young children's energy intake. *New England Journal of Medicine*, 1991. 324: p. 232-235.

[14] Goldman, H.I., Self-regulation of energy intake in children, questioned. *Pediatrics,* 1993. 91: p. 1215.

[15] Hanley, J.A. and J.A. Hutcheon, Does children's energy intake at one meal influence their intake at subsequent meals? Or do we just think it does. *Paediatric and Perinatal epidemiology*, 2010. 24: p. 241-248.

[16] Mrdjenovic, G. and D.A. Levitsky, Children eat what they are served: the imprecise regulation of energy intake. *Appetite,* 2005. 44: p. 273-258.

[17] Birch, L.L. and J.O. Fisher, Food intake regulation in children. Fat and sugar substitutes and intake. *Annals of the New York Academy of Sciences,* 1997. 819: p. 194-220.

[18] Anderson, G.H.S., S. Saravis, R. Schacher, S. Zlotkin, and L.A. Leiter, Aspartame effect on lunch-time food intake, appetite and hedonic response in children. *Appetite*, 1989. 13: p. 93-103.

[19] Birch, L.L. and M. Deysher, Caloric compensation and sensory specific satiety: evidence for self regulation of food intake by young children. *Appetite*, 1986. 7: p. 323-331.

[20] Johnson, S.L. and L.L. Birch, Parents' and children's adiposity and eating style. *Pediatrics* 1994. 94(5): p. 653-661.

[21] Leahy, K.E., L.L. Birch, and B.J. Rills, Reducing the energy density of an entree decreases children's energy intake at lunch. *Journal of the American Dietetic Association*, 2008. 108: p. 41-48.

[22] Jansen, A., N. Theunissen, K. Slechten, C. Nederkoorn, B. Boon, S. Mulkens, and A. Roefs, Overweight children overeat after exposure to food cues. *Eating Behaviors*, 2003. 4: p. 197-209.

[23] Nielsen, S.B., C. Montgomery, L.A. Kelly, D.M. Jackson, and J.J. Reilly, Energy intake variability in free living young children. *Archives of Disease in Childhood*, 2010. 93: p. 971-973.

[24] Cullen, K.W., T. Baranowski, E. Owens, T. Marsh, L. Rittenberry, and C. de Moor, Availability, accessibility, and preferences for fruit, 100% fruit juice, and vegetables influence children's dietary behavior. *Health Education and Behavior* 2003. 30(5): p. 615-626.

[25] Flurry, L.A. and B. A.C., Children's influence in purchase decisions: a social power theory approach. *Journal of Business Research*, 2005. 58: p. 593-601.

[26] John, D.R., Consumer socialization of children: a retrospective look at twenty-five years of research. *Journal of Consumer Research*, 1999. 26(December 1999): p. 183-212.

[27] Berey, L.A. and R.W. Pollay, The influencing role of the child in family decision making. *Journal of Marketing Research*, 1968. 5(1): p. 70-72.

[28] Conner, M. and C.J. Armitage, *Food Choice, in The social psychology of food choice*, M. Conner and C.J. Armitage, Editors. 2002, Open University Press: Philadelphia. p. 12-42.

[29] Block, J.P., R.A. Scribner, and K.B. DeSalvo, Fast Food, Race/ethnicity, and income. A geographic analysis. *American Journal of Preventive Medicine*, 2004. 27(3): p. 211-217.

[30] Nielsen, S.J. and B.M. Popkin, Patterns and trends in food portion sizes, 1977-1998. *Journal of the American Medical Association*, 2010. 289(4): p. 450-453.

[31] Jeffery, R.W., J. Baxter, M. McGuire, and J. Linde, Are fast food restaurants an environmental risk factor for obesity. *International Journal of Behavioral Nutrition and Physical Activity*, 2006. 3(2).

[32] Thornton, L.E., R.J. Bentley, and A.M. Kavanagh, Fast food purchasing and access to fast food restaurants: a multilevel analysis of VicLANES. *International Journal of Behavioral Nutrition and Physical Activity*, 2009. 6(28).

[33] Pearson, N., K. Ball, and D. Crawford, Predictors of change in adolescents' consumption of fruit, vegetables and energy-dense snacks. *Britisch Journal of Nutrition*, 2010. 25: p. 1-9.

[34] Denney-Wilson, E., D. Crawford, T. Dobbins, L. Hardy, and A.D. Okely, Influences on consumption of soft drinks and fast foods in adolescents. *Asia Pacific Journal of Clinical Nutrition*, 2009. 18(3): p. 447-452.

[35] Mattes, R.D. and B.M. Popkin, Nonnutritive sweetener consumption in humans: effects on appetite and food intake and their putative mechanisms. *American Journal of Clincal Nutrition*, 2009. 89: p. 1-14.

[36] Wansink, B., J.E. Painter, and J. North, Bottomless bowls: why visual cues of portion size may influence intake. *Obesity Research*, 2005. 13(1): p. 93-100.

[37] Wansink, B. and J. Kim, Bad popcorn in big buckets: portion size can influence intake as much as taste. *Journal of Nutrition Education and Behavior* 2005. 37(5): p. 242.

[38] Rolls, B.J., D. Engell, and L.L. Birch, Serving portion size influences 5-year-old but not 3-year-old children's food intakes. *Journal of the American Dietetic Association,* 2000. 100(2): p. 232-234.

[39] Fisher, J.O., B.J. Rolls, and L.L. Birch, Children's bite size and intake of an entree are greater with large portions than with age-appropriate or self-selected portions. *American Journal of Clinical Nutrition,* 2003. 77(5): p. 1164-1170.

[40] Fisher, J.O., Effects of age on children's intake of large and self-selected food portions. *Obesity*, 2007. 15(2): p. 403-412.

[41] Steenhuis, I.H.M. and W.M. Vermeer, Portion size: review and framework for interventions. *International Journal of Behavioral Nutrition and Physical Activity,* 2009. 58(6).

[42] Fisher, J.A. and T.V.E. Kral, Super-size me: Portion size effects on young children's eating. *Physiology and Behavior*, 2008. 94: p. 39-47.

[43] Burger, K.S., J.O. Fisher, and S.L. Johnson, Mechanisms behind the portion size effect: visibility and bite size. *Obesity* 2010. a head of print.

[44] Fisher, J.O., Y. Liu, L.L. Birch, and B.J. Rolls, Effects of portion size and energy density on young children's intake at a meal. *American journal of Clinical Nutrition*, 2007. 86: p. 174-179.

[45] Rolls, B.J., L.S. Roe, and J.S. Meengs, Larger portion sizes lead to a sustained increase in energy intake over 2 days. *Journal of the American Dietetic Association*, 2006. 106: p. 543-549.

[46] Rolls, B.J., L.S. Roe, and J.S. Meengs, The effect of large portion sizes on energy intake is sustained for 11 days. *Obesity*, 2007. 15(6): p. 1535-1543.

[47] Fisher, J.O., A. Arreola, L.L. Birch, and B.J. Rolls, Portion size effects on daily energy intake in low-income Hispanic and African American children and their mothers. *American Journal of Clinical Nutrition*, 2007. 86: p. 1709-1716.

[48] Kratt, P., K. Reynolds, and R. Shewchuk, The role of availability as moderator of family fruit and vegetable consumption. *Health Education and Behavior,* 2000. 27(4): p. 471-481.

[49] Coulthard, H. and J. Blissett, Fruit and vegetable consumption in children and their mothers. Moderating effects of child sensory sensitivity. *Appetite*, 2009. 52(2): p. 410-415.

[50] Velde-te, S., J. Brug, M. Wind, C. Hildonen, M. Bjelland, C. Perez-Rodrigo, and K.-I. Klepp, Effects of a comprehensive fruit- and vegetable-promoting school-based intervention in three European countries: the Pro children study. *Britisch Journal of Nutrition*, 2008. 99: p. 893-903.

[51] Kral, T.V.E., A.C. Kabay, L.S. Roe, and B.J. Rolls, Effects of doubling the portion size of fruit and vegetable side dishes on children's intake at a meal. *Obesity*, 2010. 18: p. 521-527.

[52] Spill, M.K., L.L. Birch, L.S. Roe, and B.J. Rolls, Eating vegetables first: the use of portion size to increase vegetable intake in preschool children. *American Journal of Clinical Nutrition*, 2010. 91: p. 1237-1243.

[53] Brug, J., N. Tak, S. te Velde, E. Bere, and I. de Bourdeaudhuij, Taste preferences, liking and other factors related to fruit and vegetable intakes among schoolchildren: results from observational studies. *Britisch Journal of Nutrition,* 2008: p. S7-S14.

[54] Desor, J.A., O. Maller, and R.E. Turner, Taste in acceptance of sugars by human infants. *Journal of Comparative and Physiological Psychology*, 1973. 3: p. 496-501.

[55] Desor, J.A., O. Maller, R.E. Turner, and J.M. Weiffenbach, Preference for sweet in humans: infants, children and adults, in *Taste and development: the genesis of sweet preference.* 1977, US Government Printing Office: Washington, DC.

[56] Steiner, J.E. and J.M. Weiffenbach, Facial expressions of the neonate infant indication the hedonics of food-related chemical stimuli, in *Taste and development: the genesis of sweet preference.* 1977, U.S. Government Printing Office: Washington, DC. p. 173-188.

[57] Rossenstein, D. and H. Oster, Differential facial responses to four basic tastes in newborns. *Child Development*, 1988. 59: p. 1555-1568.

[58] Sullivan, S.A. and L.L. Birch, Pass the sugar, pass, the salt: experience dictates preference. *Developmental Psychology*, 1990. 26: p. 546-551.

[59] Filer, L.J., Studies of taste preference in infancy and childhood. *Pediatric Basics,* 1978. 12: p. 5-9.

[60] Bellisle, F., A.M. Dartois, C. Kleinknecht, and M. Broyer, Perceptions of and preferences for sweet taste in uremic children. *Journal of the American Dietetic Association,* 1990. 90(7): p. 951-954.

[61] Olson, C.M. and K.P. Gemmill, Association of sweet preference and food selection among four to five year old children. *Ecology of Food and Nutrition.*, 1981. 11: p. 145-150.

[62] Ritchey, N. and C. Olson, Relationship between family variables and children's preference for and consumption of sweet foods. *Ecology of Food and Nutrition.*, 1983. 13: p. 257-266.

[63] Beauchamp, G.K., B.J. Cowart, and J. Dobbing, *Development of sweet taste,* in *Sweetness.* 1987, Springer-Verlag: Berlin. p. 127-138.

[64] Coldwell, S.E., T.K. Oswald, and D.R. Reed, A marker of growth differs between adolesecents with high vs. low sugar preference. *Physiology & Behavior,* 2009. 96: p. 574-580.

[65] Mennella, J.A. and G.K. Beauchamp, Experience with a flavor in mother's milk modifies the infant's acceptance of flavored cereal. *Developmental Psychobiology,* 1999. 35(3): p. 197-203.

[66] Liem, D.G., S. Wolterink, A. Westerbeek, F.J. Kok, and C. De Graaf, Sour taste preferences of children relates to preference for novel and intense stimuli. *Chemical Senses,* 2004. 29(8): p. 713-720.

[67] Liem, D.G., *Sweet and sour taste preferences of children.* 2004, Wageningen, the Netherlands: Wageningen University.

[68] Liem, D.G., R.P. Bogers, P.C. Dagnelie, and C. De Graaf, Fruit consumption of young children is related to preference for sour taste. *Appetite,* 2006. 46(1): p. 93-96.

[69] Blossfeld I, C.A., Boland S, Baixauli R, Kiely M, Delahunty C., Relationships between acceptance of sour taste and fruit intakes in 18-month-old infants. *Britisch Journal of Nutrition,* 2007. 98(5): p. 1084-1091.

[70] Desor, J.A., O. Maller, and K. Andrews, Ingestive responses of human newborns to salty, sour, and bitter stimuli. *Journal of Comparative & Physiological Psychology*, 1975. 89(8): p. 966-970.

[71] Cowart, B.J., Development of taste perception in humans: sensitivity and preference throughout the life span. *Psychological Bulletin*, 1981. 90(1): p. 43-73.

[72] Drewnowski, A. and C. Gomez-Carneros, Bitter taste, phytonutrients, and the consumer: a review. *American Journal of Clinical Nutrition*, 2000. 72(6): p. 1424-1435.

[73] Swanson, M., A. Branscum, and P.J. Nakayima, Promoting consumption of fruit in elementary school cafeterias. The effects of slicing apples and oranges. *Appetite*, 2009. 53: p. 264-267.

[74] Lowe, C.F., P.J. Horne, K. Tapper, M. Bowdery, and C. Egerton, Effects of a peer modelling and rewards-based intervention to increase fruit and vegetable consumption in children. *European Journal of Clinical Nutrition*, 2004. 58(3): p. 510-522.

[75] Hendy, H., K. Williams, and T. Camise, "Kids choice" school lunch program increases children's fruit and vegetable acceptance. *Appetite*, 2005. 45: p. 250-263.

[76] Cooke, L.J., L.C. Chambers, E.V. Anez, H.A. Croker, D. Boniface, M.R. Yeomans, and J. Wardle, Eating for pleasure or profit: the effect of incentives on children's enjoyment of vegetables. *Psychological Science*, 2010. e-publucation ahead of print.

[77] Brody, H., Z. Stoneman, T.S. Lane, and A.K. Sanders, Television food commercials aimed at children, family grocery shopping, and mother-child interactions. *Family Relations*, 1981. 30: p. 435-439.

[78] Borzekowski, D.L. and T.N. Robinson, The 30-second effect: an experiment revealing the impact of television commercials on food preferences of preschooler. *Journal of the American Dietetic Association*, 2001. 101(1): p. 42-46.

[79] Robinson, T.N., D.L. Borzekowski, D.M. Matheson, and H.C. Kraemer, Effects of fast food branding on young children's taste preferences. *Archives of Pediatrics & Adolescent Medicine*, 2007.

[80] Halford, J.C., J. Gillespie, V. Brown, E.E. Pontin, and T.M. Dovey, Effect of television advertisements for foods on food consumption in children. *Appetite*, 2004. 42(2): p. 221.

[81] Seagren, J.S. and R.D. Terry, WIC female parents' behavior and attitudes towards their children's food intake- relationship to children's relative weight. *Society for Nutrition Education*, 1991. 23(5): p. 223-230.

[82] Bonorden, W.R., *Salt flavouring enhancing compositions, food products including such compositions and methods for preparing such products*. 2005, Campbell soup company.

[83] Liem, D.G., M. Mars, and C. De Graaf, Sweet preferences and sugar consumption of 4- and 5-year old children: role of parents. *Appetite*, 2003. 43: p. 235-245.

[84] Fisher, J.O. and L.L. Birch, Restricting access to foods and children's eating. *Appetite* 1999. 32(3): p. 405-419.

[85] Fisher, J.O. and L.L. Birch, Restricting access to palatable foods affects children's behavioral response, food selection, and intake. *American Journal of Clinical Nutrition*, 1999. 69(6): p. 1264-1272.

[86] Jansen, E., S. Mulkens, and A. Jansen, Do not eat the red food!: Prohibition of snacks leads to their relatively higher consumption in children. *Appetite*, 2007. 49(3): p. 572-577.

[87] Carper, J.L., F.J. Orlet, and L.L. Birch, Young girls' emerging dietary restraint and disinhibition are related to parental control in child feeding. *Appetite* 2000. 35(2): p. 121-129.

[88] Birch, L.L., D. Birch, D. Marlin, and L. Kramer, Effect of instrumental eating on children's food preferences. *Appetite*, 1982. 3: p. 125-134.

[89] Birch, L.L., D.W. Marlin, and J. Rotter, Eating as the "means" activity in a contingency: effects on young children's food preferences. *Child Development*, 1984. 55: p. 431-439.

[90] Newman, J. and A. Tayler, Effect of a means-end contingency on young children's food preferences. *Journal of Experimental Child Psychology,* 1992. 64: p. 200-216.

[91] van Strien, T. and F.G. Bazelier, Perceived parental control of food intake is related to external, restrained and emotional eating in 7-12-year-old boys and girls. *Appetite*, 2007. 49(3): p. 618-625.

[92] Birch, L.L., J.O. Fisher, and K.K. Davison, Learning to overeat: maternal use of restrictive feeding practices promotes girls' eating in the absence of hunger. *American Journal of Clinical Nutrition*, 2003. 78(2): p. 215-220.

[93] Ramsay, S.A., L.J. Branen, J. Fletcher, E. Price, S.L. Johnson, and M. Sigman-Grant, "Are you done?" child care provides' verbal communication at mealtimes that reinforce or hinder children's internal cues of hunger and satiation. *Journal of Nutrition Eduction and Behavior,* 2010. 42(4): p. 265-270.

[94] Orrell-Valente, J.K., L.G. Hill, W.A. Brechwald, K.A. Dodge, G.S. Pettit, and J.E. Bates, "Just three more bites": An observational analysis of parents' socialization of children's eating at mealtime. *Apptite*, 2007. 48: p. 37-45.

[95] Gerrish, C.J. and J.A. Mennella, Flavor variety enhances food acceptance in formula-fed infants. *American Journal of Clinical Nutrition*, 2001. 73(6): p. 1080-1085.

Chapter 10

PHYTOCHEMICALS FOR THE CONTROL OF HUMAN APPETITE AND BODY WEIGHT

S. A. Tucci[*], E. J. Boyland and J. C. Halford

Kissileff Laboratory for the Study of Human Ingestive Behaviour,
School of Psychology, University of Liverpool, Eleanor Rathbone Building,
Bedford Street South, Liverpool L69 7ZA, UK

ABSTRACT

The regulation of energy balance and body weight is under the influence of complex neural, metabolic and genetic interactions. Despite this, obesity is now a global epidemic associated with significant morbidity and mortality in adults and ill health in children. Thus the effective management of obesity has become an important clinical issue. To date there are very few approaches to weight management effective in the long term. This contrasts with disorders such as anorexia and bulimia nervosa which also appear in part to be phenomena of the modern environment and equally difficult to treat. This review will focus on the mechanisms of body weight regulation and the effect of plants or plant extracts (phytochemicals) on these mechanisms. As phytochemicals are often not single compounds but rather a mixture of different unrelated molecules, their mechanism of action usually targets several systems. In addition, since some cellular receptors tend to be widely distributed, sometimes a single molecule can have a widespread effect. This chapter will attempt to describe the main phytochemicals that have been suggested to affect the homeostatic mechanisms that regulate, and some non-homeostatic system that influence, body weight. The in vitro, pre-clinical and clinical data will be summarised and scientific evidence will be reviewed.

ABBREVIATIONS

2-AG	2-arachodonoyl glycerol
5-HT	Serotonin, 5-Hydroxytryptamine

---

[*] Corresponding author Email: sonia.tucci@liv.ac.uk; Tel: +44 (0) 151 7941121; Fax: + 44 (0) 151 7942945.

α-MSH	α- Melanocyte-stimulating hormone
Δ^9-THC	Δ^9-Tetrahydrocannabinol
A	Adrenaline
ARC	Arcuate nucleus
ATP	Adenosine-triphosphate
BMI	Body mass index
CART	Cocaine-and-amphetamine-regulated transcript
CCK	Cholecystokinin
CNS	Central nervous system
COMT	Catechol-o-methyl transferase
CPT	Carnitine palmitoyltransferase
CRH	Corticotropin releasing hormone
DA	Dopamine
DMN	Dorsomedial nucleus
EC	Epicatechin
ECG	Epicatechin gallate
EE	Energy expenditure
EGC	Epigallocatechin
EGCG	Epigallocatechin gallate
EI	Energy intake
FFA	Free fatty acids
GALP	Galanin-like peptide
GI	Gastrointestinal
GLP-1	Glucagon-like peptide-1
GCBE	Green coffee bean extract
GTE	Green tea extract
HCA	(−)- hydroxycitric acid
LH	Lateral hypothalamus
NA	Noradrenaline
NPY	Neuropeptide Y
PFC	Prefrontal cortex
PVN	Paraventricular nucleus
PYY	Peptide YY
TG	Triglycerides
SNS	Sympathetic nervous system
UCP-1	Uncoupling protein 1
VTA	Ventral tegmental area

INTRODUCTION

Ingestive behaviour in humans is influenced by a complex set of innate and cognate processes modulated by culture and the external environment [1]. From the physiological point of view, an appropriate supply of micro- and macronutrients is required for life. This has lead to the evolution of strong biological mechanisms that defend food supply just as they do for other biological needs [2]. Eating more food than necessary for daily energy expenditure (EE) in times of food plenty increased chances of survival during subsequent periods of famine. As a consequence, most vertebrates developed the ability to store a considerable amount of energy and some micronutrients for later use. However, this ability has now become one of the biggest health risks for many human populations [1]. The uninterrupted supply of cheap energy-dense foods together with an increasingly sedentary lifestyle has led to obesity in a large segment of the human population.

Weight gain and obesity are a result of positive energy balance due to a long-term mismatch between energy intake (EI) and EE. Obesity constitutes a major global health problem as it is a risk factor for several chronic disorders such as diabetes, hyperlipidemia, hypertension, cardiovascular disease, osteoarthritis and some forms of cancer [3] . The most widely advocated means of resolving the obesity epidemic are changes in lifestyle, dieting and exercise. Nevertheless, while losing weight in the short term is achievable, data suggest that maintaining reduced body weight over the long term has proven to be exceedingly difficult for most people [4, 5]. At least part of the reason behind the difficulty of maintaining a reduced body weight is the body's ability to activate adaptive mechanisms that act to minimize weight loss such as an increase in both the motivation to find food and the size of individual meals [6] which is accompanied by a decrease in metabolic rate [7] that lasts until energy stores are replenished. Therefore one rationale for pharmacotherapy and alternative approaches has been to sustain weight loss behaviour by dampening these compensatory mechanisms. Pharmacologic agents designed to suppress hunger have promoted weight loss, but were often accompanied by unacceptable side effects. For instance, amphetamine-based anorexigens have been effective in some patients, but in some also produced a variety of undesirable effects of mood and behavioural expression. These agents are also prone to abuse and may have the potential to produce chemical dependency [8].

Nonetheless, over the last 20 years, many drugs lacking amphetamine-like side effects have been successfully employed. Some of these agents were the beta-phenethylamine derivatives which had lower abuse potential and proved to be useful in some individuals. Nevertheless, side effects such as insomnia, anxiety and irritability precluded its widespread use [8]. The limited efficacy of beta-phenethylamine derivatives prompted research into a new class of agents, ones acting on serotonergic neurotransmission. Fenfluramine hydrochloride (Pondimin®) and then dexfenfluramine hydrochloride (Redux®, Adifax®) were widely effective, but were implicated in the development of cardiac valvulopathy [9] and subsequently withdrawn from the market. In 1997, sibutramine (Reductil®, Meridia®), a serotonin (5- hydroxytryptamine; 5 -HT)-and noradrenaline (NA)-reuptake inhibitor was introduced into the market. Sibutramine possesses effective weight loss and weight maintenance properties. However, its use has been associated with several psychiatric [10-14] and possible cardiovascular disorders related to transient increases in blood pressure and heart rate [15]. This may preclude its use in patients with particular psychiatric conditions (although the drug was originally developed as an anti-depressant [16]) and more importantly its effects on patients with cardiovascular conditions is still under investigation [17, 18]). Since such conditions are usually concomitant with obesity, potentially a proportion of obese patients may not be suitable for sibutramine therapy [19]. Orlistat (Xenical®), an intestinal lipase inhibitor, hinders the breakdown of fat in the intestines and as a consequence this undigested fat is not absorbed but excreted [20]. The presence of undigested fat in the bowels causes side effects (such as diarrhoea, abdominal pain, oily stools and faecal spotting) that limit use of orlistat [21]. Additionally, chronic gastrointestinal (GI) ailments like irritable bowel syndrome are clear contraindications for its use. These issues, along with the potential for abuse of this drug as a purgative, and possible deficiencies in fat soluble vitamins associated with use, have caused some concern. Nonetheless, a half dose of orlistat (Alli®, 60mg rather than 120 mg three times daily) has been approved in Australasia, USA and EU for over-the-counter use [21]. More recently, an approach that attempts to manipulate the mechanisms involved in the motivation to eat and the rewarding or hedonic properties of food is emerging. The drugs recently under investigation target the cannabinoid system which is thought to modulate food intake and energy balance.

MECHANISMS THAT REGULATE BODY WEIGHT

Signals of Energy Intake and Fat Storage

One of the major determinants of the survival of higher organisms including mammals is the ability to maintain a stable body weight. Body weight regulation mainly concerns adipose tissue since protein and carbohydrate stores in adults only vary a relatively small amount. Therefore, a chronic imbalance between EI and EE results in changes in adipose tissue mass [22]. Body weight, similarly to other physiological processes, is regulated by a feedback mechanism that integrates peripheral and central signals in order to generate an adequate response.

The afferent limb of the feedback mechanism of body weight regulation consists of substances that reflect the metabolic status of the organism. For instance, adipose tissue produces leptin. Leptin is the product of the *ob* gene [23] and correlates positively with the amount of adiposity [24]. Leptin levels are monitored by the hypothalamus, where the binding of leptin to its receptor alters the expression of several genes that encode for neuropeptides involved in modulating food intake and EE [25]. As with leptin, circulating levels of insulin are also proportional to adiposity [26]. Adiponectin is another protein produced by adipose tissue; similarly to leptin its secretion depends on fat store status but in contrast to leptin adiponectin plays a fundamental role in promoting lipolysis. Adiponectin plasma concentration is inversely correlated with adiposity and increases after food restriction [27]. Ghrelin is the first described GI hormone that stimulates food intake [28], it is released by the stomach and the intestine in the fasting state and situations of anticipated eating. It is suspected that the high levels of ghrelin generated by low calorie diets could be responsible for rebound weight gain [29, 30]. Cholecystokinin (CCK) is synthesised by endocrine cells in the duodenum and jejunum, and it was the first gut hormone shown to dose-dependently decrease food intake in several species, including humans [31-33]. CCK is one of the earliest short-term satiety signals. Similarly to CCK, peptide YY (PYY) and glucagon-like peptide 1 (GLP-1) also have satiating properties, being released by the ileum and colon in response to the presence of lipids and carbohydrates.

Central Control of Energy Balance

The detection and integration of the above mentioned orexigenic and anorexigenic signals (reviewed in [34]) occurs in the hypothalamus. Due to the absence of a blood-brain barrier, the arcuate nucleus (ARC) of the hypothalamus is considered to play a key integrative role between the initial afferent signals from the periphery and the central nervous system (CNS) responses. In addition to expressing receptors for the above mentioned peripheral signals [35, 36], ARC neurones also sense blood glucose levels [37]. The ARC has neuronal subpopulations that produce orexigenic (neuropeptide Y (NPY) and agouti-related peptide (AgRP)) as well as anorexigenic peptides (α-melanocyte-stimulating hormone (α-MSH), galanin-like peptide (GALP), and cocaine-and-amphetamine-regulated transcript (CART)). The ARC neurones project to "second-order" neurons implicated in the control of feeding such as the paraventricular nucleus of the hypothalamus (PVN), the dorsomedial hypothalamic nucleus (DMN), and the lateral hypothalamic area (LH) [38, 39]. When adiposity signals reach the ARC, anorexigenic peptides are released which activate a catabolic circuit. In contrast, when adiposity signal concentrations in the brain are low, orexigenic peptides are released activating an anabolic pathway [40].

Initially the LH was identified as a 'hunger centre' because lesions in this area produced temporary aphagia, adipsia, and reductions in body weight. Two sets of neurons that contain either orexin [41] or melanin concentrating hormone [42], both potent stimulators of food intake, have been identified in this area. Both types of neurons have a wide projection field to key cortical, limbic, and basal forebrain areas [43, 44]. The DMN receives inputs from cells in the ARC and from brainstem centres. Lesions restricted to the DMH typically result in hypophagia. The PVN integrates signals of different brain regions and triggers endocrine (through corticotropin-releasing hormone (CRH) and thyrotropin-releasing hormone), and autonomic responses.

Another system, the endocannabinoid system, has recently been implicated in the regulation of appetite. The role of this system in feeding regulation is supported by reports indicating that endocannabinoid systems are essential to suckling and growth in neonates [45], and are involved in feeding responses across the phylogenetic scale [46]. Brain endocannabinoid levels have been reported to be elevated in fasted rats [47], and administration of cannabinoid receptor agonists increase food intake [48, 49] while antagonists decrease it [50]. Overall, current data indicate that tonic endocannabinoid release may be crucial to the normal expression of feeding and possibly to the long-term regulation of body weight. In addition, the biosynthesis of the endocannabinoids anandamide and 2-arachodonoyl glycerol (2-AG) appears to be regulated by leptin [51]. Thus, leptin administration suppresses hypothalamic endocannabinoid levels in normal rats; while genetically obese, chronically hyperphagic rodents express elevated, leptin-reversible, hypothalamic anandamide or 2-AG levels [52].

In addition to receiving a fairly complex input on the individual's metabolic status, the hypothalamus integrates the motivation and emotion-related features of feeding behaviour (via direct interactions with medial prefrontal (PFC) and cingulate cortex, basal forebrain and medial septal nuclei) with more fundamental aspects of appetitive and aversive responses (via interaction with nucleus accumbens (NAc), amygdala, ventral tegmental area (VTA), substantia nigra and raphe [53-58]. After processing this information it sends its output mainly through three pathways: the endocrine system (pituitary gland), the sympathetic nervous system (SNS), and motor expression (promotion or inhibition of food intake) [59, 60]. These pathways constitute the efferent loop in the body weight control system. The endocrine system and SNS act mainly to control EE.

Systems Implicated in Energy Expenditure

EE is the second aspect of energy balance (the first being food intake). Total EE is the sum of resting EE, the thermic effect of food, and EE related to activity (for review, see [61, 62]). Resting EE or basal metabolic rate is the energy used for cell metabolism, to keep cells alive. The intrinsic inefficiency of these cellular events generates a certain amount of heat known as "obligatory thermogenesis". In humans, resting EE is relatively fixed, it primarily reflects body weight and composition, and is generally the largest component of total energy expenditure (65–75%) [63]. In addition, warm-blooded animals need to generate additional heat to reach the optimal core body temperature, also known as "adaptive thermogenesis." [64]. Since energy consumption during thermogenesis can involve oxidation of lipid fuel molecules, regulation of thermogenesis in response to metabolic signals can also contribute to energy balance and regulation of body adipose stores [65].

Food intake is associated with stimulation of EE, also known as diet-induced thermogenesis or the thermic effect of food. The magnitude of the thermic effect is 5 to 10% of the caloric content of ingested carbohydrates, 0 to 3% of that for lipids and 20 to 30% of that for proteins and is, in a situation of energy balance, approximately 10% of the daily energy intake [66]. This energy is consumed during intestinal absorption of nutrients, the initial steps of their metabolism in the body and their storage. In addition, when food is ingested, homeostatic mechanisms need to be activated in order to digest, absorb, distribute and store the nutrients as quickly as possible. The SNS plays a crucial role in this response, since it regulates postprandial blood flow distribution, blood pressure and thermogenic responses to a meal [67]. The SNS role in postprandial thermogenesis depends on the size and macronutrient composition of the meal and is most evident after high carbohydrate meals [68]. Obesity leads to increased levels of sympathetic activity, and overconsumption and high carbohydrate diets may lead to gradual downregulation of the β-adrenoceptor-mediated thermogenic and metabolic responses, which may be involved in the development of obesity [69-71].

In lean and obese adults weight loss significantly reduces EE beyond levels predicted solely on the basis of changes in weight and body composition [72]. However, there is little evidence of energy wastage in periods of overnutrition [73, 74]. Small increases in EE, if not accompanied by an equivalent increase in EI, would induce a slight negative energy balance and thereby influence body weight regulation in the long term. Thus, direct stimulation of EE may be used as a strategy to improve body weight loss and prevent (re)gain. It is well established that increasing EE at the same time as decreasing EI is more likely to result in significant weight loss and more importantly, weight loss maintenance.

PHYTOCHEMICALS AND WEIGHT CONTROL

When considering the mechanisms responsible for body weight maintenance it can be concluded that it could be achieved through manipulation of the following: EE (mainly thermogenesis), appetite suppression/satiety enhancement, and fat and glucose absorption blocking. The phytochemicals described below can alter either one single component but more frequently they exert their effect through a combination of modes of action.

Foods are an obvious source of phytochemicals and many may possess specific ingredients that alter appetite beyond the effects expected by normal nutrient loads. Additionally, many therapeutic herbs and nutrients have far fewer side effects and may provide an alternative treatment or could be used to enhance the effect of prescription medications. In this chapter, recent *in vitro*, animal and human studies on the effects of phytochemicals in body weight are examined and summarised. Although most phytochemicals that affect body weight regulation have a complex mechanism of action, for the purpose of this chapter they will be grouped according to their main effect (increase or decrease body weight) and the site of main mechanism of action (CNS, peripheral or both).

PHYTOCHEMICALS THAT DECREASE BODY WEIGHT MAINLY THROUGH A PERIPHERAL MECHANISM

Korean Pine Nut Oil

Nuts, in their various forms, are widely consumed across the globe, and have recently been linked with the positive health benefits of the Mediterranean diet [75]. Nut consumption is purported to have many health benefits, particularly some protective effects against cardiovascular disease [76, 77], and it has also been suggested that nuts have satiety enhancing ingredients as there is some epidemiological evidence linking nut consumption inversely with body weight [77]. These properties may relate to their general nutritional content such fibre and protein and/or specific oils. Oils are major constituents of nuts, constituting as much as 60% of the total weight in pine nuts.

Korean pine nut oil (Pinnothin®) is obtained by natural pressing of Korean pine nuts (*P. koraiensis*) and it contains triglycerides (TG) and more than 92% poly- and mono-unsaturated fatty acids (PUFAs and MUFAs) like pinolenic acid (C18:3), linoleic acid (C18:2) and oleic acid (C18:1) [78]. Korean Pine nut oil is claimed to be unique in that it contains approximately 15% pinolenic acid (C18:3). Previous studies on Korean pine nut oil have shown beneficial effects on lipoprotein metabolism and immune function [79, 80]. *In vitro*, Korean pine nut free fatty acids (FFA) have the ability to significantly increase the release of satiety hormones such as CCK from the murine neuroendocrine tumour cell line STC-1 [81]. *In vivo*, fat digestion leads to formation of monoglycerides and fatty acids. These products of fat digestion lead to an increase in CCK, GLP-1 and PYY secretion. However, only fatty acids with chain lengths ≥ C12 are capable of triggering the release of CCK and GLP-1 [82, 83]. Moreover, CCK delays gastric emptying and produces a subsequent increased feeling of satiety and a decreased appetite. In terms of inducing satiety hormone secretion, long chain fatty acids are more effective than medium chain fatty acids, and poly-unsaturated fatty acids are more effective than mono-unsaturated fatty acids [84, 85].

The fact that Korean pine nut FFA had the ability to significantly increase satiety hormones *in vitro* lead to the examination of this potential effect in human participants. Administration of pine nut FFA to overweight postmenopausal women produced a significant increase of CCK-8 and GLP-1 without altering ghrelin or PYY levels. In addition, Korean pine nut FFA also lowered the appetite sensation "prospective food intake" and "desire to eat", importantly, these effects lasted up to 4 hours [81, 86]. Another study showed that Korean pine nut FFA (2 grams) produced a significant 9% reduction in ad-libitum food intake thirty minutes after dosing compared with the placebo control. No differences between PinnoThin® and the placebo were seen at the evening meal, suggesting that there is no compensation for the lesser food intake during lunch [87]. Importantly, the studies performed so far report no adverse effect of the compound either during the study period or at post study debriefing. Whether Korean pine nut FFA produce beneficial effects on appetite and body weight beyond that of similar FFA remains to be demonstrated. Certainly, since there are other oil based satiety enhancing ingredients on the market, it could be possible to determine if these effects are due to distinct phytochemical components or are generic to these types of dietary lipids.

Palm Oil + Oat Oil Fractions

Olibra® is a fat emulsion formulated from palm oil (40%) and oat oil fractions (2.5%). Olibra® has a similar mechanism of action to that of Korean pine nut oil. This is an increased and prolonged release of PYY, CCK and GLP-1 [88, 89] that inhibits upper gut motility (to slow gastric emptying and intestinal transit) which generates an indirect satiety effect [90, 91].

Compared to other functional foods and phytochemicals, the evidence supporting the effects of this product on appetite is more comprehensive. Double-blind, placebo-controlled reports indicate that Olibra® administration to lean, overweight and obese individuals significantly decreased energy and macronutrient intake up to 36 h post-consumption [88, 92]. It also reduced hunger and desire to eat [93]. The chronic effects of Olibra® were investigated in a double-blind, placebo-controlled study where it was administered during a weight loss and weight maintenance scheme [89]. The results of this study suggest that Olibra® administration could help to maintain weight after weight loss programmes. Taken together these findings indicate that in addition to having acute effects on EI and hunger/satiety, Olibra® could be beneficial for weight maintenance.

Gallic Acid

Gallic acid is an organic acid found in gallnuts, sumac, witch hazel, tea leaves, oak bark, and other plants. Gallic acid, the major hydrolytic product of tannic acid, it is also found free [94]. In rodents, administration of both tannic and gallic acid reduces food intake [95-97]. Initially it was thought that the reduction in food intake was mediated through taste aversion, however, later it was demonstrated that intravenous and intraperitoneal infusion of gallic acid also reduced intake which indicates that the mechanism of action of this compound involves more than sensory or GI factors [94]. However, studies performed in humans have not replicated effects found in rodents [97].

It has been hypothesised that gallic acid competes with catecholamines for inactivation via the enzyme catechol-o-methyl transferase (COMT). This enzyme inactivates catecholamines such as NA and adrenaline (A) [98] whose administration into rats results in anorexia [99]. In addition, recent studies have shown that gallic acid inhibits squalene epoxidase (SE), an enzyme involved in cholesterol synthesis [100] and therefore alters lipid metabolism [101].

Garcinia Cambogia

G. cambogia (Commercially available as (−)- hydroxycitric acid (HCA) extract from *G. cambogia*: Super CitriMax® HCA-SXS (HCA-SX®)) is a tree indigenous to southeast Asia. The active component is in its small fruit, also known as Malabar tamarind. The dried and cured pericarp of the fruit of this species contains up to 30% by weight of HCA [102]. These pericarp rinds have been used for centuries in regional cooking practices and are reported to make meals more filling and satisfying [103, 104] without any reported harmful effects. Clinical studies with HCA have encountered some mild adverse events such as headache, and upper respiratory tract and GI symptoms [105].

Administration of HCA to rats and mice suppresses appetite and body fat accumulation [106-111]. These effects are also evident in animal models of genetic obesity such as Zucker rats [112], however the effects in these rats seem to be only achieved when toxic doses are given [113]. Studies performed in humans have provided conflicting results. Several randomized placebo-controlled, single-blinded cross-over trials have shown that administration of HCA (1.2-1.5 g/day) to overweight participants did not produce any significant decrease in body weight or appetite variables [105, 114]. On the other hand, a laboratory based study with a similar design reported that daily administration of a relatively low dose of HCA (900 mg/day) over 2 weeks, although only producing minor changes in body weight, reduced EI in and sustained satiety [115]. In an 8 week study Preuss et al [116] found that 2,800 mg/day of HCA produced a reduction of 5.4% and 5.2% in baseline body weight and BMI respectively compared to controls. In addition, food intake, total cholesterol, LDL, TG and serum leptin levels were significantly reduced, while HDL levels and excretion of urinary fat metabolites (a biomarker of fat oxidation) significantly increased.

HCA may promote weight reduction through suppressed de novo fatty acid synthesis, increased lipid oxidation and reduced food intake [117]. Enhanced satiety may also account for the reported suppression of energy consumption but this has yet to be demonstrated. One potential mechanism accounting for the satiety effect of HCA involves the inhibition of adenosine-triphosphate (ATP) -citrate lyase, the enzyme that converts excess glucose into fat [118, 119]. Furthermore, by inhibiting ATP-citrate lyase, HCA reduces the availability of acetyl-CoA, the building block for fat synthesis. As a result, carbohydrates and fatty acids that would have become fat are diverted to glycogen synthesis. This metabolic change may send a signal to the brain that results in reduced appetite, food intake, a decreased desire for sweets [107, 108]. A second possible mechanism for the anorectic effect of HCA is via acetyl CoA. By reducing acetyl CoA, malonyl CoA levels are reduced too, this decreases the negative feedback on carnitine acyltransferase[117] http://www. sciencedirect. com/science?_ob=ArticleURLand_udi=B6T0P-41XV7K8-Dand_user=6693785and_rdoc=1and_fmt=and_orig = searchand_sort=dandview=cand_ version=1and_urlVersion=0and_userid=6693785andmd5= 1a25b 03e0ae099a20de45bdc43b200b7 - bib21. This leads to increased lipid transport into the mitochondria and inefficient oxidation with resultant ketone body formation. Ketones are purported appetite suppressants, however, several groups have failed to observe an association between ketosis and reported hunger level [120, 121]. Several additional mechanisms of action of HCA have been proposed, one report showed that HCA administration decreased body weight by increasing EE [110], however, the mechanism responsible for this effect has not been elucidated. A recent study demonstrated that HCA alters the expression of genes associated with adipogenesis such as PPARγ2, SREBP1c, C/EBPα, and aP2 as well as other visceral obesity-related biomarkers [111].

The conclusion arising from studies in humans provides some support for the claim that HCA may be more effective at moderating weight gain [122] than at promoting weight loss, making the compound potentially more useful for weight maintenance after an initial loss. Again more clinical data are needed.

PHYTOCHEMICALS THAT BLOCK PANCREATIC LIPASE AND A-AMYLASE

Currently, malabsorptive surgery is one of the most effective treatments for obesity [123], therefore it is not surprising that non-surgical approaches have focused on drugs that inhibit the absorption of macronutrients. Acarbose, an inhibitor of carbohydrate absorption, has been shown to have modest efficacy in the treatment of diabetes, but does not cause weight loss [124]. Dietary fat is the most energy dense macronutrient, and most closely linked to overweight and obesity. Therefore, the blockage of fat absorption is a logical target for an anti-obesity drug. The phytochemicals described below act by blocking the breakdown and consequent absorption of dietary carbohydrates and/or lipids.

Salix Matsudana

S. matsudana (Chinese willow) (one ingredient of Rev Hardcore® and Methyl Ripped ®) is a species of willow native to north western China. Its leaves have been used for more than 3000 years in traditional Chinese medicine for the treatment of several ailments. It has recently been reported that the polyphenol extracts of S. matsudana have anti-obesity actions [125, 126]. This study showed that oral administration of polyphenol fractions to dietary-induced obese mice reduced adiposity and body weight. In vitro analysis revealed that S. matsudana extract enhanced NA-induced lipolysis and inhibited the enzyme α-amylase which is involved in the digestion and absorption of carbohydrates. In addition, the polyphenol fractions also had an effect on lipid absorption since its presence completely inhibited the intestinal absorption of palmitic acid which is a product of oil hydrolysis. These results conclude that the effects S. matsudana are mainly due to the inhibition of carbohydrate and lipid absorption, and the acceleration of fat mobilisation through enhancement of NA-induced lipolysis in adipocytes [125]. Although S. matsudana extracts have been shown to have anti-obesity actions in vitro and in rodents, research in humans, especially on the long term effects, is lacking.

Platycodi Radix

Platycodi radix is the root of *Platycodon grandiflorum* A. DC (*Campanulaceae*), commonly known as Doraji (Chinese drug, 'Jiegeng', and Japanese name, 'Kikyo'). It has been used as a traditional oriental medicine, as extracts have been reported to have wide-ranging health benefits [127]. In some Asian cultures Platycodi radix is used as a food and employed as a remedy for adult diseases including hypercholesterolemia and hyperlipidemia [128].

Platycodin saponins are the primary constituents of Platycodi Radix [129]. Similarly to ginseng, the anti-obesity and hypolipidemic properties of Platycodin saponins are due at least in part to an inhibition of pancreatic lipase [130, 131]. Nevertheless, a study by Zhao et al [132] found that in rats, the decrease in body weight correlated with decrease in caloric intake, an effect not obviously attributable to lipase inhibition. They ascribed this effect to the ability of Platycodin saponins to reduce gastric secretion [133], which in turn would cause a reduction in gastric digestion ability, generating food intake restriction. These results suggest that Platycodin saponins could be a potential therapeutic alternative in the treatment of obesity and hyperlipidemia [130, 131]. However, further data showing replication of these effects in humans are needed.

Kochia Scoparia

K. scoparia is a shrub whose fruits have been used in traditional Japanese and Chinese medicine, and also as food garnish in Japanese-style dishes [134]. There are several reports showing that in animals, the alcohol extract and saponins isolated from the fruit of *K. scoparia* inhibit blood glucose level increases through inhibition of glucose uptake in the small intestine [178-180], however, the exact mechanism responsible for this effect has not been elucidated. In addition, saponins from *K. scoparia* also inhibit pancreatic lipase. The oral administration of a saponin rich fraction significantly suppressed the increases in body and adipose tissue weights in dietary-induced obese mice [134]. However, human clinical data are lacking.

Aesculus Turbinata

A. turbinata is a medicinal plant widely distributed in northwestern China. Its dried ripe seeds have been used as a carminative, stomachic, and analgesic for the treatment of distension and pain in the chest and abdomen [135]. The saponins extracted from the seeds are called escins. Recently, escins have been reported to show inhibitory effects on both the elevation of blood glucose levels [136] and pancreatic lipase activity in mice [137, 138] but there are no data regarding these effects in humans.

Tea Saponins

Three kinds of tea: oolong, green, and black, are widely used as traditional healthy drinks all over the world. Among the three teas, green and oolong tea have been traditionally reported to have anti-obesity and hypolipidemic actions. Black tea also contains many active ingredients [139], however some of these may not survive processing. These teas contain several different active ingredients.

Oolong Tea

Catechins in oolong tea are reported to prevent dietary-induced obesity by inhibiting small-intestine micelle formation [140], limiting the absorption of sugars by inhibiting α-glucosidase activity [141]. In dietary-induced obese mice, oolong tea catechins suppressed increases in body weight, parametrial adipose tissue weights, and adipose cell size by delaying the intestinal absorption of dietary fat through the inhibition of pancreatic lipase activity [139]. In a double-blind, placebo-controlled study, twelve weeks daily administration of oolong tea (containing 690 mg of catechins) to normal and overweight males (with daily EI set at 90%) produced a significant reduction in body weight (1.5%), body mass index (BMI) (1.5%), waist circumference (2.0%), and body fat mass (3.7%), compared to the placebo group [142]. These results suggest that oolong tea catechin consumption might be useful as an adjuvant during weight loss programmes.

Green Tea

In Asia, green tea is a widely consumed beverage and for centuries has been thought to possess significant health promoting effects [143]. The long term consumption of green tea and its extract (GTE) (commercially available as pills, patches, gums, mints, extracts, and ice creams) have been associated with weight loss mainly through a thermogenic mechanism [144]. It is particularly the catechins from the flavanols fraction of green tea which have received a lot of attention. Green tea is derived from drying and steaming the fresh tea leaves and thus no oxidation occurs, resulting in high levels of catechins. In contrast, black tea undergoes a full fermentation stage before drying and steaming [145] which lowers levels of catechins. The main active ingredients in GTE: the catechins epigallocatechin gallate (EGCG; Teavigo®), epigallocatechin (EGC), epicatechin gallate (ECG), and epicatechin (EC) are responsible for many of the beneficial effects of green tea [146, 147].

In vitro data suggest that the anti-obesity effects of green tea are at least partially mediated via inhibition of adipocyte differentiation and proliferation [148-150]. There is also evidence that green tea could reduce glucose and fat absorption by inhibiting GI enzymes involved in nutrient digestion [151, 152] . In addition, EGCG directly inhibits COMT, an enzyme that degrades NA, thus prolonging the action of sympathetically released NA [153][153][153][153][153][153][153][153][153][153][153][153][153][153, 154]. GTE is also rich in caffeine which is a potent amplifier of thermogenesis when given in conjunction with other SNS agonists such as ephedrine, nicotine, catechins or capsaicin from chillies [155-159].

Studies have shown that green tea reduces adipose tissue weight in rodent models of obesity. These effects appear to be mediated via increased EE and decreased glucose uptake by skeletal muscle and adipose tissue [160-162]. In humans the majority of studies that investigated the effects of GTE administration showed a significant decrease in body weight and body fat when compared to baseline. Body weight changes (corrected for changes in placebo group) ranged from 0.6 to −1.25 kg, whereas the change in body fat ranged from 0.5 to −1.8 kg [163-168]. However, it is important to highlight that in some of these studies participants were also subjected to moderate energy restriction (90% of individual energy requirements) [142, 169] or exercise [168]. In an open, uncontrolled study (not blinded and lacking a control group) administration of GTE to overweight participants produced a 4.6% decrease in body weight compared to baseline [170]. Nevertheless the majority of these studies were not strictly controlled for EI and physical activity. However, when food intake was monitored, there was no significant difference in EI between groups. Therefore it has been suggested that thermogenesis and fat oxidation are the main mechanisms responsible for weight loss [171-173]. Catechins from GTE have been associated with an increase in SNS activity, thermogenesis and fat oxidation in humans [142, 171].

A number of *in vitro*, pre-clinical and clinical studies were, and are currently, being performed to investigate the anti-obesity effects of green tea. As of today, a body of evidence has accumulated, which scientifically supports the traditional notion that green tea reduces body weight by "eliminating fat". The results from preclinical and clinical studies strongly suggest that GTE, rich in catechins and caffeine, is an effective potentiator of sympathetically mediated thermogenesis and could be used as an adjuvant in the management of obesity [174]. Certainly the effects of GTE on weight control are worthy of further clinical investigation.

Green Coffee Bean

Green coffee bean extract (GCBE) (Quest Green Coffee ®, Svetol®) contains 10% caffeine and 27% chlorogenic acid as the principal constituents. However, the roasting process of coffee drastically reduces the level of chlorogenic acid and its related compounds [175]. Chlorogenic acid is a polyphenolic compound with antioxidative activity which has been reported to have a hypotensive effect [176] and to selectively inhibit hepatic glucose-6-phosphatase [177], which is a rate-limiting enzyme involved in gluconeogenesis. Administration of GCBE or chlorogenic acid to mice has a suppressive effect on weight gain and visceral fat accumulation [178]. Moreover, chlorogenic acid also reduces the level of hepatic TG. Interestingly, this effect is more potent than that of GCBE.

Carnitine palmitoyltransferase (CPT) is a rate-limiting enzyme that catalyses the transportation of metabolised and fatty acid to liver mitochondria for β-oxidation. GCBE administration enhances CPT activity [178]. However, CPT activity does not seem to be affected when caffeine and chlorogenic acid are administered alone. In humans, a comparative, randomized, double-blind study showed that the administration of instant coffee enriched with chlorogenic acid induced a reduction in body fat and body mass at least in part due to a reduction in the absorption of glucose [179]. In addition, inhibition of the activity of glucose-6-phosphatase would limit the release of glucose into the general circulation [180] and, therefore lower insulin levels. This would ultimately lead to an increase in the consumption of fat reserves, due to the reduced availability of glucose as an energy source [179]. Nonetheless, the efficacy of these products in those already regularly exposed to caffeine remains to be demonstrated. Both coffee drinking and obesity appear co-existing in most developed societies.

Citrus Aurantium

C. aurantium (Citrus Aurantium extract ®, Bitter Orange extract®), also known as bitter orange, sour orange, or Seville orange has been used for thousands of years in ancient Chinese medicine. *C. aurantium* contains alkaloids such as *p*-Octopamine and synephrines which exert adrenergic agonist activity [181] and are present in supplements designed to aid weight loss [182].

Due to their adrenergic agonist properties *C. aurantium* alkaloids are used clinically as decongestants, vasopressors during surgical procedures, for acute treatment of priapism and in ophthalmological exams for pupil dilation [183]. In terms of their effects on body weight, synephrines could potentially increase energy expenditure and decrease food intake [184]. In addition, there is some evidence that adrenergic agonists, including *C. aurantium* synephrines, decrease gastric motility [185].

In vitro studies have shown that synephrines promote lipolysis in adipocytes [186]. In rodents, synephrines administration reduces body weight [185, 187], 188] and increases lipoprotein lipase activity [188]. Nevertheless, similarly to other sympathetic agonists, *C. aurantium* fruit extracts seem to have cardiotoxic effects [189].

In humans a few trials have examined the effects of C. aurantium synephrines alone, or in combination with other ingredients, on body weight and/or body composition. Overall, these studies reported a loss of 2.4–3.4 kg among participants using SAs, while placebo groups lost 0.94–2.05 kg [183]. Although these results might suggest some beneficial effects from synephrines supplementation, they cannot be considered conclusive at this point because they do not separate the effects of *C. aurantium* or SAs from those of other ingredients, particularly ephedrine. In addition these trials were of short duration and sample sizes were frequently inadequate. Therefore it can be concluded that since the available data on *C. aurantium* weight loss properties are limited, and its toxic effects relevant, it would be difficult to formulate *C. aurantium* related public health recommendations with confidence.

PHYTOCHEMICALS THAT DECREASE BODY WEIGHT THROUGH A COMBINATION OF CENTRAL AND PERIPHERAL MECHANISMS

Gingseng

Ginseng based supplements (Nature's Resource Ginseng®, Pharmanex® Energy Formula, Puritan's Pride®, Korean Ginseng®, Vitamin World®, Puritan's Pride®, and American Ginseng®) are some of the most popular and highly regarded supplements on the market today.

Ginsenosides have been regarded as the principal components responsible for the pharmacological activities of both Panax ginseng (including red ginseng) and American ginseng (*P. quinquefolium*) [190]. Saponins are extracts of the stem, leaves and roots of both Panax ginseng and American ginseng. They contain several active ginsenosides [191]. *In vivo* studies have shown that saponins from *P. quinquefolium* inhibit pancreatic lipase activity [192]. Studies in rodents have shown that the saponin and purified ginsenosides of ginseng have an anti-obesity effect in dietary and genetically obese rodents [163-166]. The majority of reports agree that the main effect of ginsenosides is the inhibition of pancreatic lipase, however there are other suggested mechanisms which may work independently or concurrently, such as increasing EE, improving sensitivity to insulin and changing blood insulin levels [165, 167, 168] and very interestingly, a central effect in the hypothalamus. A study by Etou et al [193] showed that intracerebroventricular infusion of the ginsenoid Rb-1 potently decreased food intake dose-dependently. The analysis of meal patterns revealed that the suppressive effect was due to decreasing meal size. The anorectic effects of central Rb-1 seem to be site-specific since its administration into the VMH reduced food intake, whereas in the lateral hypothalamus it did not alter intake. The specificity of Rb-1 in reducing meal size suggests a particular action on within-meal controls of food consumption [194]. Very recently, it has been demonstrated that the administration of the ginseng saponins protopanaxadiol and protopanaxatriol to dietary-induced obese rats decreased body weight, total food intake, adiposity, serum total cholesterol and leptin to levels equal to or below the normal diet animals [195]. When investigating the mechanisms responsible for these effects the authors found that the animals that received the saponins had lower level of hypothalamic NPY and higher levels of CCK. These results suggest that the anti-obesity actions of saponins target central and peripheral mechanisms. Whilst these potential mechanisms of action are entirely plausible, the efficacy of ginsenosides in weight management is, as far as we are aware, undemonstrated.

Caffeine

Caffeine (Caffeine Pro®) is the most widely consumed behaviourally active substance in the world [196]. Almost all caffeine consumed comes from dietary sources (beverages and food), most of it from coffee and tea [196]. The central effects of caffeine at habitually consumed doses are due to its effects on the widely distributed adenosine A1, A2A and A2B receptors [186, 187]. Adenosine is known to modulate the action of neurotransmitters, including dopamine (DA) in the NAc [197, 198] and PFC [199]. Some studies demonstrate that a functional DA/adenosine interaction in the NAc is necessary to induce the reinforcing effects of rewards [200], and that adenosine is involved in sweet taste perception [201, 202].

Experiments performed in rodents have shown that that long-term consumption of caffeine decreases body weight, body fat mass, adipocyte number and palatable food consumption [155, 203-205]. By blocking adenosine receptors, caffeine could blunt the dopaminergic tone in the NAc and thus decrease the perception of the rewarding effects of palatable food ultimately leading to a decrease in consumption of palatable food. In addition, the effect of caffeine on intake of palatable food could also be the consequence of an increased cholinergic transmission in the NAc. Cholinergic transmission is also related to feeding behaviour as it is a signal of satiation [206, 207], and acute and chronic administration of caffeine increase the release of acetylcholine in the NAc [208]. Moreover, caffeine disrupts operant responding in rats trained to press levers for food rewards, however, tolerance develops to this effect [209]. Apart from its effect on adenosine receptors, it is known that caffeine alters serotonergic and noradrenergic neurotransmission [196]. It has been reported that in addition to decreasing fat deposits, caffeine administration to dietary obese mice increases 5-HT content in several brain structures including the hypothalamus, hippocampus and striatum [210]. This is an interesting finding since 5-HT increases correlate with decreases in appetite [211].

Although long-term intervention studies in humans showed no effect of caffeine consumption on body weight [212-215], acute administration in controlled experiments appears to have a small reducing effect on caloric intake [174, 216-218]. Also, reintroduction of caffeine after a period of abstinence in regular coffee consumers was found to reduce daily EI by decreasing the number of meals [219]. Increased caffeine intake has been reported to produce slightly smaller weight gains in men and women when compared to controls [220]. A possible explanation for the lack of a long-term effect of caffeine is the development of a tolerance to its effects [212].

In addition to its central actions, caffeine has also been reported to reduce body weight through a thermogenic action. However, the thermogenic effect of caffeine seems to be more relevant in normal weight individuals [221-223]. Similarly, caffeine-induced lipolysis seems to be more prominent in non obese subjects [224]. It has been suggested that caffeine inhibits the phosphodiesterase-induced degradation of intracellular cyclic AMP (cAMP) [225]. Furthermore, it has been reported that caffeine stimulates substrate cycles like the Cori cycle (conversion of glycogen and glucose to lactate) and the FFA-triglyceride cycle [226-228]. Caffeine administration to humans increases urinary catecholamine excretion, this effect is mainly on A rather than NA excretion, suggesting that it acts primarily via adrenomedullary stimulation and not through peripheral sympathetic discharge [229]. To conclude, caffeine seems to act through central and peripheral mechanisms which would, over the long term, help with achieving weight loss. However, because of the issue of tolerance, the potential benefits of such an approach to weight control in societies of individuals already exposed to high levels of caffeine may be somewhat limited.

Nicotine

Nicotine is an alkaloid naturally occurring in tobacco leaves [230] and is their major addictive component. Among several effects, nicotine reduces appetite and alters feeding patterns typically resulting in reduced body weight [231]. The results of many epidemiologic studies agree on a strong inverse relationship between cigarette smoking and body weight, with smokers weighing significantly less than non-smokers of the same age and sex [232, 233]. In addition, smoking cessation is usually accompanied by hyperphagia and weight gain which is more prominent in women [234-237]. Similarly to caffeine, nicotine exerts its effect through central and metabolic actions.

Peripherally, nicotine could lead to weight loss by both increasing metabolic rate and decreasing metabolic efficiency. Smoking a single cigarette has been shown to induce a 3% rise in EE within 30 minutes [238]. Although studies of nicotine-induced changes in overall metabolic rate are more variable [239, 240], nicotine administration has been shown to alter metabolic processing *in vivo* (humans and animals) and in both hepatocytes and adipocytes [240-242]. *In vitro* studies have shown that nicotine decreases lipolysis by inhibiting lipoprotein lipase activity, decreasing triglyceride uptake and hence lessening net storage in adipose tissue [240]. Activation of nicotinic receptors in both white and brown adipose tissue induces the expression of uncoupling protein 1 (UCP1) [242]. As UCP1 shifts the balance of energy metabolism from the generation of ATP to the generation of heat, this represents a shift in metabolic efficiency compatible with the average lower bodyweight of smokers [235].

Besides its metabolic properties, nicotine also alters intake and appetite by modulating the central pathways that regulate the various aspects of food intake. Studies performed in rodents have shown that the reduction in food intake observed after nicotine administration is associated with contemporary changes in hypothalamic neurotransmitters involved in appetite regulation [243, 244] (for an extensive review see [233]). For instance, acute and chronic exposure to nicotine decreases hypothalamic NPY levels [219, 245]. Chronic administration of nicotine down regulates orexin binding sites [246]. Moreover, nicotine enhances dopaminergic and serotonergic activity in the LH [233, 247] which may promote satiety, and the increased food intake associated with smoking cessation has been hypothesized to be due to a desensitisation of these neurons [248]. Nicotine also increases DA release in the NAc [249] and VTA [250], which are related to reward. However, an attempt to confirm an acute anorectic effect of nicotine mediated by DA or by systemic administration of antagonists prior to nicotine has yielded negative results [251].

In humans, numerous clinical and epidemiological studies indicate that body weight and BMI are lower in cigarette smokers than in non-smokers [252-255]. Body leanness is particularly associated with the duration, rather than the intensity of smoking [232]. Studies of feeding behaviour reveal that although in both smokers and non-smokers nicotine does not change hunger sensations [231], its administration decreases meal size, without substantial changes in meal number [256, 257]. The effects of chronic nicotine administration on appetite suppression, decreased food intake, and leanness are not confined to humans [256, 258, 259]. In rodents, chronic nicotine administration has also been found to cause weight loss or decrements in the rate of weight gain [234, 258-264], an effect which has been found by some studies to be due, in part, to decreased food intake [260, 264, 265]. Due to its abuse potential, nicotine preparations are almost exclusively used to delay post cessation weight gain [266-268]. Moreover, given health and addiction issues surrounding smoking, it is unlikely that non-prescription nicotine based weight control products could enter the market without considerable demonstration of efficacy and absence of psychological side effects both during treatment and at cessation.

Khat

Chewing leaves of the khat plant (*Catha edulis*) is a prevalent social custom in the Republic of Yemen and parts of East Africa [269]. The appetite suppressant effects of khat chewing have been reported for several centuries. As cited by Le Bras and Fretillere [270], Naguib Ad-Din, in 1237 prescribed in his "Livre de médicaments composés" the use of khat by warriors and messengers to relieve tiredness and hunger. Several other more recent reports also mention the anorexigenic effects of *C. edulis* [271, 272]. The predominant active ingredients of *C. edulis* are cathinone (1-a-aminopropiophenone) and cathine (D-norpseudoephedrine). These compounds share similarities with amphetamine, with up to 90% being absorbed during chewing, predominantly via the oral mucosa [273].

Amphetamine-like compounds affect appetite centrally, by acting in the hypothalamus. Cathinone and cathine need, like amphetamine, recently synthesized brain cathecolamines to be active [274]. In rats, systemic administration of cathinone and cathine decreases food intake [272, 275]. However, as with amphetamine, tolerance to the anorectic effects of these amines develops after 7 days [272]. Apart from direct effects in the hypothalamus, cathinone also delays gastric emptying. In a placebo-controlled study performed in healthy volunteers, khat chewing prolonged gastric emptying significantly when compared to lettuce chewing. This effect is attributed to the enhanced sympathomimetic action of cathinone [276]. This, together with central effects, explains the correlation between cathinone levels and hunger and fullness scores. However, both effects are likely to be secondary to the central sympathomimetic effect and do not appear to be associated with changes in the levels of peripheral peptides such as ghrelin and PYY [269].

Hoodia Gordonii

H. gordonii (commercially available as pills, patches, and liquid: Hoodia pure®, Hoodia MAX®, Pure Hoodia®, RapidSlim SX®, Hooderma®, Hoodia-HG57®), a member of the large milkweed family, is a desert-originating, succulent, slow growing plant which is widely distributed through the arid areas of South Africa and Namibia [277]. Anecdotal reports and interviews of native and non-native South Africans, reported that the ingestion of Hoodia sap apparently decreased both the feelings and sensations (e.g., 'pangs') of hunger that occurred during long treks in the dry bush [278]115. The pharmacological properties of the sap of the *Hoodia* species (including subspecies *H.* or *H. lugardi*), were examined in detail as part of a project carried out by the National Food Research Institute, CSIR, Pretoria, South Africa in 1963 which investigated more than a thousand species of indigenous plants that were used as food [279]. Preliminary experiments that evaluated the thirst quenching properties of *Hoodia* extracts in mice also found that the extract had an appetite-suppressant activity. This led to further research and the identification of the active compound which is a tri-rhabinoside, 14-OH, 12-tigloyl pregnane steroidal glycoside [280, 281]. Currently, there are more than twenty international patent applications/ registrations on *H. gordonii* relating to the appetite suppressant, anti-diabetic activity and the treatment of gastric acid secretion [279]. The available literature offers limited reports on the biological effects of *H. gordonii* and its active compounds [279]. Initial feeding experiments in rats showed that both the crude extract and the pregnane glycoside, administered over an eight day period, decreased food consumption and body mass when compared to animals receiving placebo [281]. This reduction in body weight has been replicated in a second study in rats [282]. Studies performed in diabetic obese Zucker rats showed that the dried extracts of the plant sap exerted anorectic activity and reversal of diabetes which were maintained for the duration of dosing (up to 8 weeks). Interestingly, the decrease in food intake and subsequent weight loss seemed to be independent of the nutrient content of the diet and also occurred in animals that exposed to a highly palatable diet (Phytopharm and Pfizer, unpublished). In addition, Phytopharm, who in 1997 were granted the license for the patent for the active component of the Hoodia "P57" extract, have recently disclosed phase 1 studies in healthy overweight humans where significant reductions in calorie intake and body weight were achieved [283].

To determine whether P57 exerts its effect through a central mechanism, MacLean and Luo [284] administered the compound directly into the brain ventricles and found a 50-60% decrease in food intake over 24 h. The same study found that P57 increased the ATP content in hypothalamic cells. Increased hypothalamic ATP correlates with decreased appetite, while diet restriction produces a decrease in ATP in the hypothalamus. This assertion is supported by the finding that hypothalamic ATP was reduced after four days of moderate food deprivation, and central administration of P57 was able to reverse this effect [284]. This finding suggests that one mechanism of action of P57 is through a central mechanism. However this by no means rules out the possibility that P57 could also act through a peripheral mechanism, for example on vagal afferent nerves on gastric emptying, or on potentially anorectic peripheral hormones, such as CCK[285]. P57 has been in the market for some time. First developed in partnership with Pfizer for a drug application, and then with Unilever as a food ingredient, the product is currently with an industrial partner. This suggests that it has been difficult to successfully develop P57 as a weight controlling product, which brings into question the potential of hoodia for this type of product per se.

Caralluma Fimbriata

Similarly to *H. gordonii*, *C. fimbriata* (Slimaluma®), is also well known as a famine food, an appetite suppressant, a portable food for hunting and a thirst quencher among tribal populations. *C. fimbriata* is an edible succulent cactus that belongs to the family Asclepiadaceae and is cooked as a vegetable, used in preserves like chutneys and pickles, or eaten raw. There are no adverse event reports on the Indian subcontinent over the centuries of use [286]. It is widely found in India, Africa, the Canary Islands, Arabia, southern Europe, Ceylon, and Afghanistan [287].

The key ingredients in *C. fimbriata* are pregnane glycosides, flavone glycosides, megastigmane glycosides, bitter principles, saponins and various other flavonoids [288]. The appetite suppressing action of *C. fimbriata* could be mainly attributed to the pregnane glycosides. These compounds seem to have peripheral and central effects. In the adipose tissue, pregnane glycosides exert their effect at least in part by blocking both ATP-citrate lyase, an extra- mitochondrial enzyme involved in the initial steps of *de novo* lipogenesis [289], and malonyl Coenzyme A [290] leading to a reduction in lipogenesis. In the central structures regulating appetite, pregnane glycosides and its related molecules seem to share a similar mechanism of that of *H. gordonii* where they act by amplifying the signaling of the energy sensing function in the basal hypothalamus [284, 291].

A placebo-controlled randomized trial performed in overweight humans showed that administration of *C. fimbriata* extracts over a period of two months lead to a reduction in self-reported measures of appetite, body weight and waist circumference when compared to a control group [291]. Interestingly *C. fimbriata* selectively reduced the intake of refined sugars, sweets, cholesterol and saturated fats, without altering fruit, vegetable or fish intake. This could provide an additional mechanism of reduction in body weight since the consumption of foods such as whole grains, fruit and vegetables has been found to be directly associated with reduction in hunger and increased satiety levels, which could lead to lowered voluntary EI [292].

Coleus Forskohlii

C. forskohlii (ForsLean®) is a plant native to India that belongs to the mint family and has been used traditionally as a herbal medicine to treat various disorders of the cardiovascular, respiratory, GI, and CN systems [293]. Chemically, it is a plant rich in alkaloids, which are considered likely to have influence on the biological systems [294]. One of the main active compounds in *C. forskohlii* is forskolin, a diterpene that acts directly on adenylate cyclase [295]. Adenylate cyclase is an enzyme that activates cyclic adenosine monophosphate (cAMP). In turn cAMP promotes lipolysis, increases the body's basal metabolic rate, and increases utilisation of body fat [296].

A placebo-controlled randomized trial performed in free-living overweight women showed that although *C. forskohlii* supplementation did not promote weight loss, it helped mitigate weight gain with apparently no clinically significant side effects [297]. These data would suggest further clinical study of *C. forskohlii* may be worthwhile.

PHYTOCHEMICALS THAT INCREASE APPETITE AND BODY WEIGHT

Cannabis Sativa

Although the use of cannabis (*C. sativa*) for medicinal and other purposes dates back at least four thousand years, understanding of the underlying pharmacology dates back only forty years. Rapid progress in this understanding has only been made since the discovery of the receptors that bind to exogenous as well as the recently discovered endogenous cannabinoids. Cannabis contains more than sixty bioactive 'cannabinoid' compounds [298]. Of these, Δ^9-tetrahydrocannabinol (Δ^9-THC) (Marinol®, Dronabinol®, Sativex®) is widely regarded to be primarily responsible for many of the well-known physiological and psychoactive properties of the plant, and has been the focus of many recent pharmacological and therapeutic developments. Unlike the majority of plant derived drugs, Δ^9-THC is an aromatic hydrocarbon rather than an alkaloid [299].

Cannabinoids are known for their rewarding effects and for their ability to stimulate increases in food intake (i.e. the marijuana 'munchies') [48]. It is now reasonable to assume that cannabis hyperphagia is largely attributable to Δ^9-THC actions at brain CB1 cannabinoid receptors, and reflects a biologically significant role of endocannabinoids in appetite processes. However, despite recent advances in cannabinoid pharmacology and the aforementioned promotion of CB1 antagonists in an anti-obesity role, the past decade has seen surprisingly little progress in our understanding of the mechanisms whereby exogenous or endogenous cannabinoids promote eating.

Typically, healthy volunteers (often experienced marijuana users) show substantial increases in caloric intake, most frequently derived from snack foods after acute and chronic dosing (typically in the form of cannabis cigarettes, and less frequently oral Δ^9-THC administration) [48, 300-305]. Δ^9-THC seems to predominantly enhance the orosensory qualities of food, particularly sweet, palatable items [306, 307]. However, it has recently been demonstrated that Δ^9-THC can have broad, dose-related effects on appetite that are not restricted to specific flavours or food types (Townson and Kirkham, unpublished observations). It is probable, but untested, that these actions are CB1 receptor-mediated, since the broader psychological actions of cannabis in people are reversed by the selective CB1 antagonist rimonabant (Acomplia®) [308]. Additionally, a small number of clinical trials have assessed the possible benefits of cannabinoids in the treatment of wasting and appetite loss in cancer cachexia and AIDS. Treatment with Δ^9-THC improved appetite ratings, increased food intake, and attenuated weight loss or induced weight gain [309-312]. In animals, systemic and central administration of Δ^9-THC and endogenous cannabinoids such as anandamide and 2-AG has been shown to stimulate feeding [313-319]. Importantly, this effect has been shown to be mediated by CB1 receptors, being reversed by rimonabant but not the CB2 selective antagonist SR144258 [320]. The hyperphagic effect of Δ^9-THC in rats is also remarkably potent, causing animals to overconsume even when replete. Interestingly, low doses of Δ^8-THC (another phytocannabinoid), have been reported to have significantly greater hyperphagic potency than Δ^9-THC [321]. Such data indicate the importance of exploring the behavioural actions of other phytocannabinoids.

Regarding the relation between reward and appetite effects, a promising hypothesis is that cannabinoids increase appetite and food intake at least in part by enhancing the hedonic impact or palatability of food [322-324]. Systemic and central administration of Δ^9-THC potently increased intake of sweet foods more than less palatable foods [325], and enhanced voluntary licking bouts at a sucrose spout in a manner consistent with palatability enhancement [326]. Moreover, systemic administration of Δ^9-THC in rats is reported to cause eventual increase in affective orofacial 'liking' reactions elicited by the taste of sucrose, suggesting enhancement of taste palatability [323].

The brain substrates of cannabinoid hedonic effects are so far unknown, but hypotheses suggest that endogenous cannabinoid neurotransmission in limbic brain structures such as the NAc mediates the hedonic impact of natural rewards like sweetness [327]. The NAc is an especially likely candidate for cannabinoid mediation of hedonic impact because it is known to contribute to the generation, via other neurotransmitters, of hedonic affect ('liking') and appetitive motivation ('wanting') for food and drug rewards [328].

Sutherlandia (Lessertia Frutescens)

Sutherlandia *(L. frutescens)* is commonly given in the belief that this herb will treat some of the symptoms associated with HIV/AIDS, such as nausea and lack of appetite, amongst others [329]. A recent randomized, double-blind, placebo-controlled trial of *Sutherlandia* leaf powder in healthy adults showed that 800 mg/d during 3 months increased appetite ratings [330]. The constraints of the investigation related to limited sample size, precluding firm conclusions from being drawn about these preliminary data or any speculation related to mechanisms of action.

CONCLUSION

Table 1. Mechanisms of action of various phytochemicals

Product	Mechanism of action	Ref
Korean pine nut FFA and TG	↑ CCK and GLP-1.	[81, 86, 87]
Palm and oat oil (Olibra®)	↑ PYY, CCK and GLP-1.	[88]
Gallic acid	Competes with cathecolamines for inactivation via COMT. Inhibits SE and decreases lipid absorption.	[94, 101]
G. cambogia	Inhibits ATP-citrate lyase. Alters the expression of adipogenesis related genes.	[110, 111, 118, 119]
Product	Mechanism of action	Ref
S. matsudana (polyphenol extract)	↑ NA induced lipolysis. Inhibits α-amylase activity and palmitic acid absorption.	[125]
Platycodi radix saponins	Inhibit pancreatic lipase. ↓ gastric secretion.	[130-132]
K scoparia saponins and alcohol extract	Inhibit pancreatic lipase.	[134]
A. turbinata escins	Inhibit pancreatic lipase.	[136, 138]
Oolong tea catechins	Inhibit pancreatic lipase.	[139]
Green tea catechins	Inhibit phospho-ERK1, phospho-ERK2, Cdk2, PPARc2, and C/EBP, GI enzymes, COMT, α-amylase and sucrose.	[149, 151-153, 331, 332]
GCBE and chlorogenic acid	Enhances CPT activity. ↓ Glucose absorption.	[178, 179]
C. aurantium synephrines	Adrenergic agonist activity, ↑ EE and ↓ gut motility.	[183]
Ginseng saponins	Inhibit pancreatic lipase. ↑CCK. ↓ NPY in the hypothalamus.	[192, 195]
Caffeine	CNS: Blocks adenosine receptors, ↓ DA transmission in NAc. ↑ DA in PFC. ↑ cholinergic transmission. Alters 5-HT transmission. Peripheral: ↑ thermogenesis.	[156, 184, 225-229]
Nicotine	CNS: ↑ DA release in LHA, NAc and VTA. ↑ 5-HT release. Modulates orexin neurotransmission Peripheral: inhibits lipoprotein lipase. Induces the expression of UCP-1.	[233, 240, 242, 246, 247, 249, 250]
Khat cathinone and cathine	↑ sympathetic activity. Delay gastric emptying.	[272]
Hoodia gordonii extract	↑ ATP content in hypothalamic cells.	[284]
C. fimbriata	CNS: ↑ ATP content in hypothalamic cells. Peripheral: Inhibits ATP-citrate lyase and malonyl CoA.	[284, 289-291]
C. forskohlii	Stimulates adenyl cyclase. ↑ cAMP.	[296]
THC	Modulates opioid and DA neurotransmission in CNS rewarding areas.	[322-324]

Overall, no single phytochemical can be considered to a proven weight control product. Whilst, some of the phytochemicals reviewed above show potentially promising effects for weight control, for the majority of cases more data are needed to define safety, the optimal dose required, the mechanism of action and the actual magnitude of effects that can be expected during use in practice. Moreover, many of these substances may also produce substantial and potentially averse side effects.

Moreover, for the majority of compounds described here, there are tantalizing but still inconsistent or incomplete data relating to the mechanism of action and benefits for weight control. In some cases (e.g. *A. turbinata*, sutherlandia), it is not yet even established, even in the most basic terms, what aspects of energy balance (intake, uptake, or expenditure) are actually affected. Some of these phytochemicals probably do not directly affect body weight or weight loss, but could benefit body composition during weight maintenance or (re)gain periods. Other ingredients present significant obstacles to use in foods, because of issues such as safety (caffeine, nicotine, Δ^9-THC, *C. aurantium*). On the other hand, some proposed ingredients (e.g. green tea) could be particularly attractive because they have a long history of safe consumption, and also may bring other added health benefits beyond weight control. For bulk fats such as plant derived oils, the levels that would need to be used may be quite high as a replacement for traditional food oils. This may limit the food formats where they would be of most value, and the putative 'functional' benefit for weight control needs to be balanced against the significant amounts of energy delivered by such ingredients at effective doses.

Additionally, it is important to note here that although some phytochemicals that can be acquired over the counter have been scientifically tested, others have shown no proven efficacy (i.e. *S. matsudana*, caffeine, ginseng).

Table 2. *In vitro* effects of phytochemicals and their doses

Product	Dose	Effect	Ref
Korean pine nut FFA	50 μM	↑ CCK-8 release.	[81]
G. cambogia HCA SX	10 μM-1 mM	↑ 5-HT release in isolated rat brain cortex. Lowers abdominal fat leptin expression.	[333, 334]
S. matstudana (polyphenol extract)	250–5000 g/mL	↑ NA induced lypolisis. Inhibits α-amylase activity. Inhibits of palmitic acid absorption.	[125]
	0.5 and 1.0 g/L	Inhibits pancreatic lipase.	[130, 132]
K. scoparia alcohol extract and saponins	0.25 mg/ml	Inhibit pancreatic lipase.	[134]
A. turbinata escins	20-100 μM	Inhibit pancreatic lipase.	[136]
Oolong tea catechins	05-2 g/L	Inhibit pancreatic lipase.	[139]
Green tea catechins	5 -30 μM	Inhibit adipocytes differentiation Inhibit α-amylase and sucrase.	[148-150, 152]
C. aurantium synephrines	0.1 μM	↑ lipolysis	[186]
H. gordonii	5000 nM	↑ ATP content in hypothalamic cells.	[284]

Table 3. *In vivo* effects of Phytochemicals, their routes of administration and doses

Product	Dose	Effect	Ref
Korean pine nut FFA and TG	Humans: 2-3g/day VO	↑ CCK and GLP-1 ↓ Desire to eat and prospective food intake.	[81, 86, 87, 89]
Palm and oat oil (Olibra®)	Humans: 5-15 g/day VO	↓ Food intake. ↓ Hunger and desire to eat.	[88, 92, 93]
Gallic acid	Rats: 360 mg IV, 400 mg intragastric. 1-5% of diet. 2% IP infusion. Humans: 2.4 g/day VO	↓ Food intake. No effect.	[94, 97] [97]
G. cambogia (HCA)	Rodents: 0, 0.2, 2.0 and 5.0% of feed intake, 52.6 mmol OH-CIT/kg in diet.	↓ EI, body weight, visceral fat, leptin levels and adipocyte size. ↑ EE.	[109-111, 333, 334]
	Humans 900, 2800 mg/day VO	↓ EI and body weight. Sustained satiety.	[115, 116]
S. matstudana (polyphenol extract)	Mice: 5% polyphenol fraction in diet	↓ Adiposity and body weight.	[125]
Platycodi radix saponins	Dietary obese rodents: 35-70 mg/kg VO	↓ Body weight and caloric intake.	[130, 132]
K. scoparia	Rodents: 1-3% in diet	↓ Body weight increase induced by high fat diet.	[134]
A. turbinata escins	Dietary obese mice: 1 mg/kg VO Mice: 100 mg/kg VO	↓ Body weight increase -induced by high fat diet. Attenuates increase in glucose levels.	[136, 138]
Oolong tea catechins	Rodents: 0.5% in diet. 690 mg of catechins	↓ Body weight increase -induced by high fat diet. ↓ Adipocyte size ↓ body weight, BMI and adiposity.	[139, 142]
Green tea catechins	Rats: 20 gr/kg in drinking water. EGCG: 75-85 mg/kg i.p. Humans: 130-600 mg/day alone or in combination with caffeine.	↓ Adiposity. ↓ Body weight and adiposity.	[160-164, 335, 336]
Green coffee bean extract (GCBE) and chlorogenic acid	Mice: GCBE (0.5-1% in diet or 200-400 mg/kg VO), Chlorogenic acid: (0.15-0.3% in diet or 60-120mg/kg VO) Humans: 140 mg/d VO	↓ Body weight and visceral fat. ↓ Hepatic TG levels. ↓ Glucose absorption. ↓ BMI and adiposity.	[178, 179]
C. aurantium synephrine	Rodents: 10mg/kg IP Humans: 32-300 mg/d VO	↓ Lipoprotein lipase activity. ↓ Body weight	[187, 188, 337]
Ginseng saponins	Rodents: 1-3% of diet, 50- 250mg/kg IP 0.05, 0.10 and 0.20 μ mol ICV	↓ Food intake, body weight and adiposity.	[192, 193, 195, 338]
Caffeine	Rats: 1g/L drinking water Humans: 50-100 mg VO	↓ Palatable food intake, ↓ adiposity. Slight anorectic effect.	[205, 210]
Product	Dose	Effect	Ref
Nicotine	Rats: μM in LHA, NAc by microdialysis. 0.5-12 mg/kg SC or IP Humans: smoking chewing gum and patches	↓ Food intake and body weight ↓ Food intake and body weight.	[231, 240, 247, 249, 262, 339, 340]
Khat cathinone and cathine	Rats: 4-10 mg/kg rats IP	↓ Food intake	[272, 275]
H. gordonii extract	Rats: 0.4–40 nmol ICV Humans: 500-750 mg/day VO	↓ Food intake and body weight. ↓ Food intake and body weight	[284]
C. fimbriata extract	Humans 1 g/day VO	↓ Hunger levels, food intake, body weight and waist circumference	[291]
C. forskohlii	Overweight women: 250 mg/day VO	Prevents weight gain	[297]
Δ⁹-THC	Rodents: 0.5-4 mg/kg VO, SC, IP. 2.5, 10 and 25 μg ICV Humans: smoking cigarettes with 1.8-3.1% THC, 20- 210 mg/day VO	↑ Food intake and body weight ↑ Food intake and body weight	[48, 300-305, 314, 315, 317, 319-321, 341, 342]
Sutherlandia	800 mg/d for 3 months	↑ Appetite ratings	[330]

Table 4. Effects on food intake and / or body weight of various phytochemicals and their recommended uses

Product	Acute effect	Chronic effect	Recommended use	Ref
Korean pine nut	↓ 9% ad libitum food intake		Supports long term weight loss.	[87]
Palm and oat oil (Olibra®)	↓ Energy (25%) and macronutrient intake up to 36 h post-consumption	Helps to maintain weight after weight loss programmes.	Helps weight maintenance after weight loss programmes.	[89]
Gallic acid		No dose-related weight loss or reduction in food intake.	Not conclusive	[97]
G. cambogia (HCA)		5.4% and 5.2% in baseline body weight and BMI. ↓ 24 h EI by 15-30%	Helps weight maintenance after weight loss programmes.	[115, 116]
S. matsudana			No human studies.	
Platycodi radix			No human studies.	
K. scoparia			No human studies.	
turbinata			No human studies	
Oolong tea saponins		↓ body weight (1.5%), BMI (1.5%), waist circumference (2.0%), body fat mass (3.7%)	As an adjuvant in weight loss programmes.	[142]
Green tea		↓ body weight 0.6 –1.25 kg, ↓ body fat 0.5–1.8 kg	As an adjuvant in the management of obesity.	[163-167]
CGBE (chlorogenic acid)		↓ 5.7 kg when compared to placebo	As an adjuvant in the management of obesity.	[179]
C. aurantium synephrine	↑ Heart rate and blood pressure	↓.4–3.4 kg compared to 0.94–2.05 kg in placebo	Use limited by side effects.	[185, 189]
Ginseng saponins			No human studies	
Caffeine	↓ 3% EI compared to placebo	No effect	Not conclusive	[174, 213, 343]
Nicotine		Less weight gain (0.47 kg vs 1.02 kg) in smoking cessation programmes	Delay post cessation weight gain.	[268]
Khat			No human studies.	
H. gordonii		↓ EI to 1000 kcal/d	Not conclusive.	[279, 283]
fimbriata		↓ Hunger levels. Non significant trend towards ↓EI, BMI and body weight.	Helps to suppress appetite during weight loss programmes.	[291]
forskohlii			No human studies	
Δ^9-THC	↑ Appetite, enhances hedonic qualities of food	Attenuates weight loss or induces weight gain	Could helps in the management of appetite and weight in cachexia/cancer/AIDS.	[309-312]
Sutherlandia		↑ appetite ratings	Could help in the management of appetite and weight in cachexia/cancer/AIDS.	[330]

Improved understanding and evidence on each of the reviewed and other proposed weight control ingredients will guide further research, as well as the selection of ingredients and product formats that can deliver the most attractive and effective benefits to consumers.

Ultimately, only randomised, double blinded, placebo-controlled clinical trials of phytochemicals in humans can demonstrate their true potential. With regard to appetite and food intake this will involve proving phytochemical based products significantlu reduce daily caloric intake but adjusting appetite rather than by causing behavioural disruption or inducing malaise. For all ingredient purported to be useful in weight control, significant placebo subtracted weight loss needs be demonstrated at least in the medium term i.e. up to 24 weeks of use.

REFERENCES

[1] Prentice, AM. Early influences on human energy regulation: thrifty genotypes and thrifty phenotypes. *Physiol. Behav.* 2005 86: 640-645.

[2] Berthoud, HR; Morrison, C. The brain, appetite, and obesity. *Annu. Rev. Psychol.* 2008 59: 55-92.

[3] Bray, GA. Medical consequences of obesity. *J. Clin. Endocrinol. Metab.* 2004 89: 2583-2589.

[4] Wadden, TA. Treatment of obesity by moderate and severe caloric restriction. Results of clinical research trials. *Ann. Intern. Med.* 1993 119: 688-693.

[5] Rosenbaum, M; Leibel, RL. The physiology of body weight regulation: relevance to the etiology of obesity in children. *Pediatrics.* 1998 101: 525-539.

[6] Dulloo, AG; Jacquet, J; Girardier, L. Poststarvation hyperphagia and body fat overshooting in humans: a role for feedback signals from lean and fat tissues. *Am. J. Clin. Nutr.* 1997 65: 717-723.

[7] Dulloo, AG; Jacquet, J. Adaptive reduction in basal metabolic rate in response to food deprivation in humans: a role for feedback signals from fat stores. *Am. J. Clin. Nutr.* 1998 68: 599-606.

[8] Silverstone, T. Appetite suppressants: a review. *Drugs.* 1992 43: 820-836.

[9] Khan, MA; Herzog, CA; St. Peter, JV; Hartley, GG; Madlon-Kay, R; Dick, CD; Asinger, RW; Vessey, JT. The prevalence of cardiac valvular insufficiency assessed by transthoracic echocardiography in obese patients treated with appetite-suppressant drugs. *N. Engl. J. Med.* 1998 339: 713-718.

[10] Dogangun, B; Bolat, N; Rustamov, I; Kayaalp, L. Sibutramine-induced psychotic episode in an adolescent. *J. Psychosom. Res.* 2008 65: 505-506.

[11] Taflinski, T; Chojnacka, J. Sibutramine-associated psychotic episode. *Am. J. Psychiatry.* 2000 157: 2057-2058.

[12] Benazzi, F. Organic hypomania secondary to sibutramine-citalopram interaction. *J. Clin. Psychiatry.* 2002 63: 165.

[13] Binkley, K; Knowles, SR. Sibutramine and panic attacks. *Am. J. Psychiatry.* 2002 159: 1793-1794.

[14] Lee, J; Teoh, T; Lee, TS. Catatonia and psychosis associated with sibutramine: a case report and pathophysiologic correlation. *J. Psychosom. Res.* 2008 64: 107-109.

[15] King, DJ; Devaney, N. Clinical pharmacology of sibutramine hydrochloride (BTS 54 524), a new antidepressant, in healthy volunteers. *Br. J. Pharmacol.* 1988 26: 607-611.

[16] Weintraub, M; Rubio, A; Golik, A; Byrne, L; Scheinbaum, ML. Sibutramine in weight control: a dose-ranging, efficacy study. *Clin. Pharmacol. Ther.* 1991 50: 330-337.

[17] Sharma, AM; Caterson, ID; Coutinho, W; Finer, N; Van Gaal, L; Maggioni, AP; Torp-Pedersen, C; Bacher, HP; Shepherd, GM; James, WP. Blood pressure changes associated with sibutramine and weight management - an analysis from the 6-week lead-in period of the sibutramine cardiovascular outcomes trial (SCOUT). *Diabetes Obes. Metab.* 2008.

[18] Maggioni, AP; Caterson, I; Coutinho, W; Finer, N; Gaal, LV; Sharma, AM; Torp-Pedersen, C; Bacher, P; Shepherd, G; Sun, R; James, P. Tolerability of sibutramine during a 6-week treatment period in high-risk patients with cardiovascular disease and/or diabetes: a preliminary analysis of the Sibutramine Cardiovascular Outcomes (SCOUT) Trial. *J. Cardiovasc. Pharmacol.* 2008 52: 393-402.

[19] Cummings, S; Parham, ES; Strain, GW. Position of the American Dietetic Association: Weight management. *J. Am. Diet. Assoc.* 2002 102: 1145-1155.

[20] Halford, JCG. Pharmacotherapy for obesity. *Appetite.* 2006: 6-10.

[21] Filippatos, TD; Derdemezis, CS; Gazi, IF; Nakou, ES; Mikhailidis, DP; Elisaf, MS. Orlistat-associated adverse effects and drug interactions: a critical review. *Drug Saf.* 2008 31: 53-65.

[22] Jequier, E; Tappy, L. Regulation of body weight in humans. *Physiol. Rev.* 1999 79: 451-480.

[23] Zhang, Y; Proenca, R; Maffei, M; Barone, M; Leopold, L; Friedman, JM. Positional cloning of the mouse obese gene and its human homologue. *Nature.* 1994 372: 425-432.

[24] Schwartz, M; Peskind, E; Raskind, M; Boyko, E; Porte, DJ. Cerebrospinal fluid leptin levels: relationship to plasma levels and to adiposity in humans. *Nat. Med.* 1996 2: 589-593.

[25] Woods, S; Seeley, C; Porte, RJJ; Schwartz, M. Signals that regulate food intake and energy homeostasis. *Science.* 1998 280: 1478-1383.

[26] Bagdade, JD; Bierman, E; Porte, D. The significance of basal insulin levels in the evaluation of the insulin response to glucose in diabetic and nondiabetic subjects. *J. Clin. Invest.* 1967 46: 1549-1557.

[27] Reinehr, T; Roth, C; Menke, T; Andler, W. Adiponectin before and after weight loss in obese children. *J. Clin. Endocrinol. Metab.* 2004 89: 3790-3794.

[28] Kojima, M; Hosoda, H; Date, Y; Nakazato, M; Matsuo, H; Kangawa, K. Ghrelin is a growth-hormone-releasing acylated peptide from stomach. *Nature.* 1999 402: 656-660.

[29] Wynne, K; Stanley, S; McGowan, B; Bloom, S. Appetite control. *J. Endocrinol.* 2005 184: 291-318.

[30] Morton, GJ; Cummings, DE; Baskin, DG; Barsh, GS; Schwartz, MW. Central nervous system control of food intake and body weight. *Nature.* 2006 443: 289-295.

[31] Gibbs, J; Young, RC; Smith, GP. Cholecystokinin decreases food intake in rats. *J. Comp. Physiol. Psychol.* 1973 84: 488-495.

[32] Kissileff, HR; Pi-Sunyer, FX; Thornton, J; Smith, GP. C-terminal octapeptide of cholecystokinin decreases food intake in man. *Am. J. Clin. Nutr.* 1981 34: 154-160.

[33] Lieverse, RJ; Jansen, JBMJ; Masclee, AAM; Lamers, CBHW. Role of cholecystokinin in the regulation of satiation and satiety in humans. *Ann. N.Y. Acad. Sci.* 1994 713: 268-272.

[34] Kalra, S; Dube, M; Pu, S; Xu, B; TL, H; Kalra, P. Interacting appetite-regulating pathways in the hypothalamic regulation of body weight. *Endocr. Rev.* 1999 20: 68-100.

[35] Cowley, MA; Smart, JL; Rubinstein, M; Cerdan, MG; Diano, S; Horvath, TL; Cone, RD; Low, MJ. Leptin activates anorexigenic POMC neurons through a neural network in the arcuate nucleus. *Nature.* 2001 411: 480-484.

[36] Elmquist, JK; Elias, CF; Saper, CB. From lesions to leptin: hypothalamic control of food intake and body weight. *Neuron.* 1999 22: 221-232.

[37] Spanswick, D; Smith, MA; Mirshamsi, S; Routh, VH; Ashford, ML. Insulin activates ATP-sensitive K channels in hypothalamic neurons of lean, but not obese rats. *Nat. Neurosci.* 2000 3: 757-758.

[38] Elias, CF; Saper, CB; Maratos-Flier, E; Tritos, NA; Lee, C; Kelly, J; Tatro, JB; Hoffman, GE; Ollmann, MM; Barsh, GS; Sakurai, T; Yanagisawa, M; Elmquist, JK. Chemically defined projections linking the mediobasal hypothalamus and the lateral hypothalamic area. *J. Comp. Neurol.* 1998 402: 442-459.

[39] Elias, CF; Aschkenasi, C; Lee, C; Kelly, J; Ahima, RS; Bjorbaek, C; Flier, JS; Saper, CB; Elmquist, JK. Leptin differentially regulates NPY and POMC neurons projecting to the lateral hypothalamic area. *Neuron.* 1999 23: 775-786.

[40] Valassi, E; Scacchi, M; Cavagnini, F. Neuroendocrine control of food intake. *Nutr. Metab. Cardiovasc. Dis.* 2008 18: 158-168.

[41] Sakurai, T; Amemiya, A; Ishii, M; Matsuzaki, I; Chemelli, R; Tanaka, H; Williams, S; Richarson, J; Kozlowski, G; Wilson, S; Arch, J; Buckingham, R; Haynes, A; Carr, S; Annan, R; McNulty, D; Liu, W; Terrett, J; Elshourbagy, N; Bergsma, D; Yanagisawa, M. Orexins and orexin receptors: a family of hypothalamic neuropeptides and G protein-coupled receptors that regulate feeding behavior. *Cell.* 1998 92: 573-585.

[42] Qu, D; Ludwig, DS; Gammeltoft, S; Piper, M; Pelleymounter, MA; Cullen, MJ; Mathes, WF; Przypek, R; Kanarek, R; Maratos-Flier, E. A role for melanin-concentrating hormone in the central regulation of feeding behaviour. *Nature.* 1996 380: 243-247.

[43] Abizaid, A; Gao, Q; Horvath, TL. Thoughts for food: brain mechanisms and peripheral energy balance. *Neuron.* 2006 51: 691-702.

[44] Breivogel, CS; Childers, SR. The functional neuroanatomy of brain cannabinoid receptors. *Neurobiol. Dis.* 1998 5: 417-431.

[45] Fride, E; Ginzburg, Y; Breuer, A; Bisogno, T; Di Marzo, V; Mechoulam, R. Critical role of the endogenous cannabinoid system in mouse pup suckling and growth. *Eur. J. Pharmacol.* 2001 419: 207-214.

[46] De Petrocellis, L; Melck, D; Bisogno, T; Milone, A; Di Marzo, V. Finding of the endocannabinoid signalling system in Hydra, a very primitive organism: possible role in the feeding response. *Neuroscience.* 1999 92: 377-387.

[47] Kirkham, TC; Williams, CM; Fezza, F; Di Marzo, V. Endocannabinoid levels in rat limbic forebrain and hypothalamus in relation to fasting, feeding and satiation: stimulation of eating by 2-arachidonoyl glycerol. *Br. J. Pharmacol.* 2002 136: 550-557.

[48] Greenberg, I; Kuehnle, J; Mendelson, JH; Bernstein, JG. Effects of marihuana use on body weight and caloric intake in humans. *Psychopharmacology. (Berl)*, 1976 49: 79-84.

[49] Abel, EL. Cannabis: effects on hunger and thirst. *Behavioral Biology.* 1975 15: 255-281.

[50] Colombo, G; Agabio, R; Diaz, G; Lobina, C; Reali, R; Gessa, GL. Appetite suppression and weight loss after the cannabinoid antagonist SR 141716. *Life Sci.* 1998 63: PL113-7.

[51] Friedman, JM; Halaas, JL. Leptin and the regulation of body weight in mammals. *Nature.* 1998 395: 763-770.

[52] Di Marzo, V; Goparaju, SK; Wang, L; Liu, J; Batkai, S; Jarai, Z; Fezza, F; Miura, G; Palmiter, RD; Sugiura, T; Kunos, G. Leptin-regulated endocannabinoids are involved in maintaining food intake. *Nature.* 2001 410: 822-825.

[53] Bittencourt, JC; Elias, CF. Melanin-concentrating hormone and neuropeptide EI projections from the lateral hypothalamic area and zona incerta to the medial septal nucleus and spinal cord: a study using multiple neuronal tracers. *Brain Res.* 1998 805: 1-19.

[54] Broberger, C; De Lecea, L; Sutcliffe, JG; Hokfelt, T. Hypocretin/orexin- and melanin-concentrating hormone-expressing cells form distinct populations in the rodent lateral hypothalamus: relationship to the neuropeptide Y and agouti gene-related protein systems. *J. Comp. Neurol.* 1998 402: 460-474.

[55] Peyron, C; Tighe, DK; van den Pol, AN; de Lecea, L; Heller, HC; Sutcliffe, JG; Kilduff, TS. Neurons containing hypocretin (orexin) project to multiple neuronal systems. *J. Neurosci.* 1998 18: 9996-10015.

[56] Stratford, T; Kelley, A. Evidence of a functional relationship between the nucleus accumbens shell and lateral hypothalamus subserving the control of feeding behavior. *J. Neurosci.* 1999 19: 11040-11048.

[57] Pajolla, GP; Crippa, GE; Correa, SA; Moreira, KB; Tavares, RF; Correa, FM. The lateral hypothalamus is involved in the pathway mediating the hypotensive response to cingulate cortex-cholinergic stimulation. *Cell Mol. Neurobiol.* 2001 21: 341-356.

[58] Fadel, J; Deutch, AY. Anatomical substrates of orexindopamine interactions: lateral hypothalamic projections to the ventral tegmental area. *Neuroscience.* 2002 111: 379-387.

[59] Berthoud, HR. Multiple neural systems controlling food intake and body weight. *Neurosci. Biobehav. Rev.* 2002 26: 393-428.

[60] Broberger, C. Brain regulation of food intake and appetite: molecules and networks. *J. Intern. Med.* 2005 258: 301-327.

[61] Danforth, EJ; Burger, A. The role of thyroid hormones in the control of energy expenditure. *Clin. Endocrinol. Metab.* 1984 13: 581-595.

[62] Silva, JE. The multiple contributions of thyroid hormone to heat production. *J. Clin. Invest.* 2001 108: 35-37.

[63] Paddon-Jones, D; Westman, E; Mattes, RD; Wolfe, RR; Astrup, A; Westerterp-Plantenga, M. Protein, weight management, and satiety. *Am. J. Clin. Nutr.* 2008 87: 1558S-1561S.

[64] Kim, B. Thyroid hormone as a determinant of energy expenditure and the basal metabolic rate. *Thyroid.* 2008 18: 141-144.

[65] Morrison, SF; Nakamura, K; Madden, CJ. Central control of thermogenesis in mammals. *Exp. Physiol.* 2008 93: 773-797.

[66] Tappy, L. Thermic effect of food and sympathetic nervous system activity in humans. *Reprod. Nutr. Dev.* 1996 36: 391-397.

[67] van Baak, MA. Meal-induced activation of the sympathetic nervous system and its cardiovascular and thermogenic effects in man. *Physiol. Behav.* 2008 94: 178-186.

[68] Welle, S; Lilavivat, U; Campbell, RG. Thermic effect of feeding in man: increased plasma norepinephrine levels following glucose but not protein or fat consumption. *Metabolism.* 1981 30: 953-958.

[69] van Baak, MA. The peripheral sympathetic nervous system in human obesity. *Obes. Rev.* 2001 2: 3-14.

[70] Blaak, EE; van Baak, MA; Kester, AD; Saris, WH. Beta-adrenergically mediated thermogenic and heart rate responses: effect of obesity and weight loss. *Metabolism.* 1995 44: 520-524.

[71] Seals, DR; Bell, C. Chronic sympathetic activation: consequence and cause of age-associated obesity? *Diabetes.* 2004 53: 276-284.

[72] Rosenbaum, M; Hirsch, J; Gallagher, DA; Leibel, RL. Long-term persistence of adaptive thermogenesis in subjects who have maintained a reduced body weight. *Am. J. Clin. Nutr.* 2008 88: 906-912.

[73] Jebb, SA. Metabolic response to slimming, In: Cottrell, R, editor. *Weight Control: The Current Perspective.* London: Chapman and Hall; 1995.

[74] Ravussin, E; Schutz, Y; Acheson, KJ; Dusmet, M; Bourquin, L; Jequier, E. Short-term, mixed-diet overfeeding in man: no evidence for "luxuskonsumption". *Am. J. Physiol.* 1985 249: E470-477.

[75] Salas-Salvado, J; Fernandez-Ballart, J; Ros, E; Martinez-Gonzalez, MA; Fito, M; Estruch, R; Corella, D; Fiol, M; Gomez-Gracia, E; Aros, F; Flores, G; Lapetra, J; Lamuela-Raventos, R; Ruiz-Gutierrez, V; Bullo, M; Basora, J; Covas, MI. Effect of a Mediterranean diet supplemented with nuts on metabolic syndrome status: one-year results of the PREDIMED randomized trial. *Arch. Intern. Med.* 2008 168: 2449-2458.

[76] Fraser, GE; Sabate, J; Beeson, WL; Strahan, TM. A possible protective effect of nut consumption on risk of coronary heart disease. *The Adventist Health Study Arch. Intern. Med.* 1992 1524: 1416-1424.

[77] Hu, FB; Stampfer, MJ; Manson, JE; Rimm, EB; Colditz, GA; Rosner, BA; Speizer, FE; Hennekens, CH; Willett, WC. Frequent nut consumption and risk of coronary heart disease in women: prospective cohort study. *BMJ.* 1998 317: 1341-1345.

[78] Alper, CM; Mattes, RD. Effects of chronic peanut consumption on energy balance and hedonics. *Int. J. Obes. Relat. Metab. Disord.* 2000 26: 1129-1137.

[79] Lee, JW; Lee, KW; Lee, SW; Kim, IH; Rhee, C. Selective increase in pinolenic acid (all-cis-5,9,12-18:3) in Korean pine nut oil by crystallization and its effect on LDL-receptor activity. *Lipids.* 2004 39: 383-387.

[80] Asset, G; Staels, B; Wolff, RL; Baugé, E; Madj, Z; Fruchart, JC; Dallongeville, J. Effects of Pinus pinaster and Pinus koraiensis seed oil supplementation on lipoprotein metabolism in the rat. *Lipids.* 1999 34: 39-44.

[81] Pasman, WJ; Heimerikx, J; Rubingh, CM; van den Berg, R; O'Shea, M; Gambelli, L; Hendriks, HF; Einerhand, AW; Scott, C; Keizer, HG; Mennen, LI. The effect of Korean pine nut oil on in vitro CCK release, on appetite sensations and on gut hormones in post-menopausal overweight women. *Lipids Health Dis.* 2008 7: 10.

[82] Matzinger, D; Degen, L; Drewe, J; Meuli, J; Duebendorfer, R; Ruckstuhl, N; D'Amato, M; Rovati, L; Beglinger, C. The role of long chain fatty acids in regulating food intake and cholecystokinin release in humans. *Gut.* 2000 46: 688-693.

[83] Feltrin, KL; Little, TJ; Meyer, JH; Horowitz, M; Smout, AJ; Wishart, J; Pilichiewicz, AN; Rades, T; Chapman, IM; Feinle-Bisset, C. Effects of intraduodenal fatty acids on appetite, antropyloroduodenal motility, and plasma CCK and GLP-1 in humans vary with their chain length. *Am. J. Physiol. Regul. Integr. Comp. Physiol.* 2004 287: R524-R533.

[84] McLaughlin, J; Grazia Luca, M; Jones, MN; D'Amato, M; Dockray, G; Thompson, DG. Fatty acid chain length determines cholecystokinin secretion and effect on human gastric motility. *Gastroenterology.* 1999 116: 46-53.

[85] Lawton, CL; Delargy, HJ; Brockman, J; Smith, FC; E, BJ. The degree of saturation of fatty acids influences post-ingestive satiety. *Br. J. Nutr.* 2000 83: 473-482.

[86] Scott, C; Pasman, W; Hiemerikx, J; Rubingh, C; Van Den Berg, R; O'Shea, M; Gambelli, L; Hendricks, H; Mennen, L; Einerhand, A. Pinnothin™ suppresses appetite in overweight women. *Appetite.* 2007 49: 330.

[87] Hughes, GM; Boyland, EJ; Williams, NJ; Mennen, L; Scott, C; Kirkham, TC; Harrold, JA; Keizer, HG; Halford, JC. The effect of Korean pine nut oil (PinnoThin) on food intake, feeding behaviour and appetite: a double-blind placebo-controlled trial. *Lipids Health Dis.* 2008 7: 6.

[88] Burns, AA; Livingstone, MB; Welch, RW; Dunne, A; Rowland, IR. Dose-response effects of a novel fat emulsion (Olibra) on energy and macronutrient intakes up to 36 h post-consumption. *Eur. J. Clin. Nutr.* 2002 56: 368-377.

[89] Diepvens, K; Soenen, S; Steijns, J; Arnold, M; Westerterp-Plantenga, M. Long-term effects of consumption of a novel fat emulsion in relation to body-weight management. *Int. J. Obes. (Lond)*, 2007 31: 942-949.

[90] Welch, I; Saunders, K; Read, NW. Effect of ileal and intravenous infusions of fat emulsions on feeding and satiety in human volunteers. *Gastroenterology.* 1985 89: 1293-1297.

[91] Welch, IM; Sepple, CP; Read, NW. Comparisons of the effects on satiety and eating behaviour of infusion of lipid into the different regions of the small intestine. *Gut.* 1988 29: 306-311.

[92] Burns, AA; Livingstone, MB; Welch, RW; Dunne, A; Robson, PJ; Lindmark, L; Reid, CA; Mullaney, U; Rowland, IR. Short-term effects of yoghurt containing a novel fat emulsion on energy and macronutrient intakes in non-obese subjects. *Int. J. Obes. Relat. Metab. Disord.* 2000 24: 1419-1425.

[93] Diepvens, K; Steijns, J; Zuurendonk, P; Westerterp-Plantenga, MS. Short-term effects of a novel fat emulsion on appetite and food intake. *Physiol. Behav.* 2008 95: 114-117.

[94] Glick, Z. Modes of action of gallic acid in suppressing food intake of rats. *J. Nutr.* 1981 111: 1910-1916.

[95] Joslyn, MA; Glick, Z. Comparative effects of gallotannic acid and related phenolics on the growth of rats. *J. Nutr.* 1969 98: 119-126.

[96] Mueller, WS. The significance of tannic substances and theobromine in chocolate milk. *J. Dairy Sci.* 1942 25: 221-230.

[97] Roberts, AT; Martin, CK; Liu, Z; Amen, RJ; Woltering, EA; Rood, JC; Caruso, MK; Yu, Y; Xie, H; Greenway, FL. The safety and efficacy of a dietary herbal supplement and gallic acid for weight loss. *J. Med. Food.* 2007 10: 184-188.

[98] Axelrod, J; Senoh, S; Witkop, B. O-methylation of catecholamines in vivo. *J. Biol. Chem.* 1958 233: 697-701.

[99] Russek, M; Mogenson, G; Stevenson, JA. Calorigenic hyperglycemia and anorexigenic effects of adrenaline and noradrenaline. *Physiol. Behavior.* 1967 2: 429-433.

[100] Abe, I; Prestwich, GD. *Comprehensive Natural Products Chemistry.* Oxford, Pergamon; 1999.

[101] Jang, A; Srinivasan, P; Lee, NY; Song, HP; Lee, JW; Lee, M; Jo, C. Comparison of hypolipidemic activity of synthetic gallic acid-linoleic acid ester with mixture of gallic acid and linoleic acid, gallic acid, and linoleic acid on high-fat diet induced obesity in C57BL/6 Cr Slc mice. *Chem. Biol. Interact.* 2008 174: 109-117.

[102] Lewis, YS; Neelakantan, S. (−)-Hydroxycitric acid - the principal acid in the fruits of Garcinia cambogia. *Desr. Psytochem.* 1965 4: 619-625.

[103] Clouatre, D; Rosenbaum, ME. *The Diet and Health Benefits of HCA.* New Canaan, Connecticut, Keats Publishing; 1994.

[104] Sergio, W. A natural food, the Malabar Tamarind, may be effective in the treatment of obesity. *Med. Hypotheses.* 1988 27: 39-40.

[105] Heymsfield, SB; Allison, D; Vasselli, JR; Pietrobelli, A; Greenfield, D; Nuñez, C. Garcinia cambogia (hydroxycitric acid) as a potential antiobesity agent: a randomized controlled trial. *JAMA.* 1998 280: 1596-1600.

[106] Sullivan, AC; Hamilton, JG; Miller, ON; Wheatley, VR. Inhibition of lipogenesis in rat liver by (−)-hydroxycitrate. *Arch. Biochem. Biophys.* 1972 150: 183-190.

[107] Sullivan, AC; Triscari, J; Hamilton, JG; Miller, ON. Effect of (-)-hydroxycitrate upon the accumulation of lipid in the rat. II. appetite. *Lipids.* 1974 9: 129-134.

[108] Sullivan, AC; Triscari, J; Hamilton, JG; Miller, ON; Wheatley, VR. Effect of (-)-hydroxycitrate upon the accumulation of lipid in the rat. I. lipogenesis. *Lipids.* 1974 9: 121-128.

[109] Rao, RN; Sakaria, KK. Lipid-lowering and antiobesity effect of (−)-hydroxycitric acid. *Nutr. Res.* 1988 8: 209-212.

[110] Vasselli, JR; Shane, E; Boozer, CN; Heymsfield, SB. Garcinia cambogia extract inhibits body weight gain via increased Energy Expenditure (EE) in rats. *FASEB J.* 1998 12: A505.

[111] Kim, KY; Lee, HN; Kim, YJ; Park, T. Garcinia cambogia extract ameliorates visceral adiposity in C57BL/6J mice fed on a high-fat diet. *Biosci. Biotechnol. Biochem.* 2008 72: 1772-1780.

[112] Asghar, M; Monjok, E; Kouamou, G; Ohia, SE; Bagchi, D; Lokhandwala, MF. Super CitriMax (HCA-SX) attenuates increases in oxidative stress, inflammation, insulin resistance, and body weight in developing obese Zucker rats. *Mol. Cell Biochem.* 2007 304: 93-99.

[113] Saito, M; Ueno, M; Ogino, S; Kubo, K; Nagata, J; Takeuchi, M. High dose of Garcinia cambogia is effective in suppressing fat accumulation in developing male Zucker obese rats, but highly toxic to the testis. *Food Chem. Toxicol.* 2005 43: 411-419.

[114] Mattes, RD; Bormann, L. Effects of (-)-hydroxycitric acid on appetitive variables. *Physiol. Behav.* 2000 71: 87-94.

[115] Westerterp-Plantenga, MS; Kovacs, EM. The effect of (-)-hydroxycitrate on energy intake and satiety in overweight humans. *Int. J. Obes. Relat. Metab. Disord.* 2002 26: 870-872.

[116] Preuss, HG; Rao, CV; Garis, R; Bramble, J; Ohia, SE; Bagchi, M; Bagchi, D. An overview of the safety and efficacy of a novel, natural(-)-hydroxycitric acid extract (HCA-SX) for weight management. *J. Med.* 2004 35: 33-48.

[117] McCarty, M; Majeed, M. The pharmacology of Citrin, In: Majeed, M, et al., editor. *Citrin®. A revolutionary, herbal approach to weight management*. Burlingame, CA: New Editions Publishing; 1994;p. 34-52.

[118] Sullivan, AC; Singh, M; Srere, PA; Glusker, JP. Reactivity and inhibitor potential of hydroxycitrate isomers with citrate synthase, citrate lyase, and ATP citrate lyase. *J. Biol. Chem.* 1977 252: 7583-7590.

[119] Watson, JA; Fang, M; Lowenstein, JM. Tricarballylate and hydroxycitrate: substrate and inhibitor of ATP: citrate oxaloacetate lyase. *Arch. Biochem. Biophys.* 1969 135: 209-217.

[120] Baird, I; Parsons, R; Howard, AN. Clinical and metabolic studies of chemically defined diets in the management of obesity. *Metabolism.* 1974 23: 654-657.

[121] Silverston, J; Stark, JE; Buckle, R. Hunger during total starvation. *Lancet.* 1966 1: 343-344.

[122] Greenwood, MR; Cleary, MP; Gruen, R; Blase, D; Stern, JS; Triscari, J; Sullivan, AC. Effect of (-)-hydroxycitrate on development of obesity in the Zucker obese rat. *Am. J. Physiol.* 1981 240: E72-E78.

[123] Korenkov, M; Sauerland, S; Junginger, T. Surgery for obesity. *Curr. Opin. Gastroenterol.* 2005 21: 679-683.

[124] Chiasson, JL; Josse, RG; Gomis, R; Hanefeld, M; Karasik, A; Laakso, M. Acarbose for prevention of type 2 diabetes mellitus: the STOP-NIDDM randomised trial. *Lancet.* 2002 359: 2072-2077.

[125] Han, LK; Sumiyoshi, M; Zhang, J; Liu, MX; Zhang, XF; Zheng, YN; Okuda, H; Kimura, Y. Anti-obesity action of Salix matsudana leaves (Part 1). Anti-obesity action by polyphenols of Salix matsudana in high fat-diet treated rodent animals. *Phytother. Res.* 2003 17: 1188-1194.

[126] Han, LK; Sumiyoshi, M; Zheng, YN; Okuda, H; Kimura, Y. Anti-obesity action of Salix matsudana leaves (Part 2). Isolation of anti-obesity effectors from polyphenol fractions of Salix matsudana. *Phytother. Res.* 2003 17: 1195-1198.

[127] Lee, EB. Pharmacological studies on Platycodon grandiflorum A. DC. IV. A comparison of experimental pharmacological effects of crude platycodin with clinical indications of platycodi radix *Yakugaku Zasshi.* 1973 93: 1188-1194.

[128] Kim, KS; Ezaki, O; Ikemoto, S; Itakura, H. Effects of Platycodon grandiflorum feeding on serum and liver lipid concentrations in rats with diet-induced hyperlipidemia. *J. Nutr. Sci. Vitaminol. (Tokyo)*, 1995 41: 485-491.

[129] Hiroahi, I; Kauzuo, T; Yohko, Y. Saponins from the roots of Platycodon grandiflorum. Part 1: structure of prosapogenins. *J. Chem. Soc. Perkin. Trans.* 1981: 1928−1933.

[130] Han, L; Zheng, Y; Xu, B; Okuda, H; Kimura, Y. Saponins from Platycodi radix ameliorate high fat diet-induced obesity in mice. *J. Nutr.* 2002 132: 2241-2245.

[131] Han, LK; Xu, BJ; Kimura, Y; Zheng, Y; Okuda, H. Platycodi radix affects lipid metabolism in mice with high fat diet-induced obesity. *J. Nutr.* 2000 130: 2760-2764.

[132] Zhao, HL; Sim, JS; Ha, YW; Kang, SS; Kim, YS. Antiobese and hypolipidemic effects of platycodin saponins in diet-induced obese rats: evidences for lipase inhibition and calorie intake restriction. *Int. J. Obes. (Lond)*, 2005 29: 983-990.
[133] Lee, EB. Pharmacological activities of crude platycodin. *J. Pharmaceut. Soc. Korea.* 1975 19: 164-176.
[134] Han, L; Nose, R; Li, W; Gong, X; Zheng, Y; Yoshikawa, M; Koike, K; Nikaido, T; Okuda, H; Kimura, Y. Reduction of fat storage in mice fed a high-fat diet long term by treatment with saponins prepared from Kochia scoparia fruit. *Phytother. Res.* 2006 20: 877-882.
[135] Qian, XZ. *Colored Illustrations of Chinese Herbs: Part II.* Beijing, People's Health Press; 1996.
[136] Kimura, H; Ogawa, S; Jisaka, M; Kimura, Y; Katsube, T; Yokota, K. Identification of novel saponins from edible seeds of Japanese horse chestnut (Aesculus turbinata Blume) after treatment with wooden ashes and their nutraceutical activity. *J. Pharm. Biomed. Anal.* 2006 41: 1657-1665.
[137] Kimura, H; Ogawa, S; Katsube, T; Jisaka, M; Yokota, K. Antiobese effects of novel saponins from edible seeds of Japanese horse chestnut (Aesculus turbinata BLUME) after treatment with wood ashes. *J. Agric Food Chem.* 2008 56: 4783-4788.
[138] Hu, JN; Zhu, XM; Han, LK; Saito, M; Sun, Y; Yoshikawa, M; Kimura, Y; Zheng, YN. Anti-obesity effects of escins extracted from the seeds of Aesculus turbinata BLUME (Hippocastanaceae). *Chem. Pharm. Bull. (Tokyo)*, 2008 56: 12-16.
[139] Han, LK; Kimura, Y; Kawashima, M; Takaku, T; Taniyama, T; Hayashi, T; Zheng, YN; Okuda, H. Anti-obesity effects in rodents of dietary teasaponin, a lipase inhibitor. *Int. J. Obes.* 2001 25: 1459-1464.
[140] Muramatsu, K; Fukuyo, M; Hara, Y. Effect of green tea catechins on plasma cholesterol level in cholesterol-fed rats. *J. Nutr. Sci. Vitaminol. (Tokyo)*, 1986 32: 613-622.
[141] Ikeda, I; Imasato, Y; Sasaki, E; Nakayama, M; Nagao, H; Takeo, T; Yayabe, F; Sugano, M. Tea catechins decrease micellar solubility and intestinal absorption of cholesterol in rats. *Biochim. Biophys. Acta.* 1992 1127: 141-146.
[142] Nagao, T; Komine, Y; Soga, S; Meguro, S; Hase, T; Tanaka, Y; Tokimitsu, I. Ingestion of a tea rich in catechins leads to a reduction in body fat and malondialdehyde-modified LDL in men. *Am. J. Clin. Nutr.* 2005 81: 122-129.
[143] Balentine, DA; Wiseman, SA; Bouwens, LC. The chemistry of tea flavonoids. *Crit. Rev. Food Sci. Nutr.* 1997 37: 693-704.
[144] Wolfram, S; Wang, Y; Thielecke, F. Anti-obesity effects of green tea: from bedside to bench. *Mol. Nutr. Food Res.* 2006 50: 176-187.
[145] Thielecke, F; Boschmann, M. The potential role of green tea catechins in the prevention of the metabolic syndrome - A review. *Phytochemistry.* 2009 Epub ahead of printing.
[146] Sano, M; Tabata, M; Suzuki, M; Degawa, M; Miyase, T; Maeda-Yamamoto, M. Simultaneous determination of twelve tea catechins by high-performance liquid chromatography with electrochemical detection. *Analyst.* 2001 126: 816-820.
[147] Mandel, SA; Amit, T; Weinreb, O; Reznichenko, L; Youdim, MB. Simultaneous manipulation of multiple brain targets by green tea catechins: a potential neuroprotective strategy for Alzheimer and Parkinson diseases. *CNS Neurosci. Ther.* 2008 14: 352-365.

[148] Wolfram, S; Raederstorff, D; Wang, Y; Teixeira, SR; Elste, V; Weber, P. TEAVIGO (epigallocatechin gallate) supplementation prevents obesity in rodents by reducing adipose tissue mass. *Ann. Nutr. Metab.* 2005 49: 54-63.

[149] Furuyashiki, T; Nagayasu, H; Aoki, Y; Bessho, H; Hashimoto, T; Kanazawa, K; Ashida, H. Tea catechin suppresses adipocyte differentiation accompanied by down-regulation of PPARgamma2 and C/EBPalpha in 3T3-L1 cells. *Biosci. Biotechnol. Biochem.* 2004 68: 2353-2359.

[150] Hung, PF; Wu, BT; Chen, HC; Chen, YH; Chen, CL; Wu, MH; Liu, HC; Lee, MJ; Kao, YH. Antimitogenic effect of green tea (-)-epigallocatechin gallate on 3T3-L1 preadipocytes depends on the ERK and Cdk2 pathways. *Am. J. Physiol. Cell Physiol.* 2005 288: C1094-1108.

[151] Shimizu, M; Kobayashi, Y; Suzuki, M; Satsu, H; Miyamoto, Y. Regulation of intestinal glucose transport by tea catechins. *Biofactors.* 2000 13: 61-65.

[152] Matsumoto, N; Ishigaki, F; Ishigaki, A; Iwashina, H; Hara, Y. Reduction of blood glucose levels by tea catechin. *Biosci. Biotechnol. Biochem.* 1993 57: 525-527.

[153] Dulloo, AG; Seydoux, J; Girardier, L; Chantre, P; Vandermander, J. Green tea and thermogenesis: interactions between catechin-polyphenols, caffeine and sympathetic activity. *Int. J. Obes. Relat. Metab. Disord.* 2000 24: 252-258.

[154] Borchardt, RT; Huber, JA. Catechol O-methyltransferase. 5. Structure-activity relationships for inhibition by flavonoids. *J. Med. Chem.* 1975 18: 120-122.

[155] Zheng, G; Sayama, K; Okubo, T; Juneja, LR; Oguni, I. Anti-obesity effects of three major components of green tea, catechins, caffeine and theanine, in mice. *In Vivo.* 2004 18: 55-62.

[156] Dulloo, AG; Seydoux, J; Girardier, L. Paraxanthine (metabolite of caffeine) mimics caffeine's interaction with sympathetic control of thermogenesis. *Am. J. Physiol.* 1994 267: E801-E804.

[157] Yoshioka, M; Doucet, E; Drapeau, V; Dionne, I; Tremblay, A. Combined effects of red pepper and caffeine consumption on 24 h energy balance in subjects given free access to foods. *Br. J. Nutr.* 2001 85: 203-211.

[158] Dulloo, AG. Herbal simulation of ephedrine and caffeine in treatment of obesity. *Int. J. Obes. Relat. Metab. Disord.* 2002 26: 590-592.

[159] Jessen, AB; Toubro, S; A, A. Effect of chewing gum containing nicotine and caffeine on energy expenditure and substrate utilization in men. *Am. J. Clin. Nutr.* 2003.

[160] Choo, JJ. Green tea reduces body fat accretion caused by high-fat diet in rats through beta-adrenoceptor activation of thermogenesis in brown adipose tissue. *J. Nutr. Biochem.* 2003 14: 671-676.

[161] Hasegawa, N; Yamda, N; Mori, M. Powdered green tea has antilipogenic effect on Zucker rats fed a high-fat diet. *Phytother. Res.* 2003 17: 477-480.

[162] Ashida, H; Furuyashiki, T; Nagayasu, H; Bessho, H; Sakakibara, H; Hashimoto, T; Kanazawa, K. Anti-obesity actions of green tea: possible involvements in modulation of the glucose uptake system and suppression of the adipogenesis-related transcription factors. *Biofactors.* 2004 22: 135-140.

[163] Hase, T; Komine, Y; Meguro, S; Takeda, Y; Takahashi, H; Matusi, Y. Anti-obesity effects of tea catechins in humans. *J. Oleo Sci.* 2001 50: 599-605.

[164] Tsuchida, T; Itakura, H; Nakamura, H. Reduction of body fat in humans by long-term ingestion of catechins. *Prog. Med.* 2002 22: 2189-2203.

[165] Kovacs, EM; Mela, DJ. Metabolically active functional food ingredients for weight control. *Obes. Rev.* 2006 7: 59-78.

[166] Auvichayapat, P; Prapochanung, M; Tunkamnerdthai, O; Sripanidkulchai, BO; Auvichayapat, N; Thinkhamrop, B; Kunhasura, S; Wongpratoom, S; Sinawat, S; Hongprapas, P. Effectiveness of green tea on weight reduction in obese Thais: A randomized, controlled trial. *Physiol. Behav.* 2008 93: 486-491.

[167] Nagao, T; Hase, T; Tokimitsu, I. A green tea extract high in catechins reduces body fat and cardiovascular risks in humans. *Obesity. (Silver Spring)*, 2007 15: 1473-1483.

[168] Maki, KC; Reeves, MS; Farmer, M; Yasunaga, K; Matsuo, N; Katsuragi, Y; Komikado, M; Tokimitsu, I; Wilder, D; Jones, F; Blumberg, JB; Cartwright, Y. Green tea catechin consumption enhances exercise-induced abdominal fat loss in overweight and obese adults. *J. Nutr.* 2009 139: 264-270.

[169] Diepvens, K; Kovacs, EM; Vogels, N; Westerterp-Plantenga, MS. Metabolic effects of green tea and of phases of weight loss. *Physiol. Behav.* 2006 87: 185-191.

[170] Chantre, P; Lairon, D. Recent findings of green tea extract AR25 (Exolise) and its activity for the treatment of obesity. *Phytomedicine.* 2002 9: 3-8.

[171] Dulloo, AG; Duret, C; Rohrer, D; Girardier, L; Mensi, N; Fathi, M; Chantre, P; Vandermander, J. Efficacy of a green tea extract rich in catechin polyphenols and caffeine in increasing 24-h energy expenditure and fat oxidation in humans. *Am. J. Clin. Nutr.* 1999 70: 1040-1045.

[172] Rumpler, W; Seale, J; Clevidence, B; Judd, J; Wiley, E; Yamamoto, S; Komatsu, T; Sawaki, T; Ishikura, Y; Hosoda, K. Oolong tea increases metabolic rate and fat oxidation in men. *J. Nutr.* 2001 131: 2848-2852.

[173] Rudelle, S; Ferruzzi, MG; Cristiani, I; Moulin, J; Mace, K; Acheson, KJ; Tappy, L. Effect of a thermogenic beverage on 24-hour energy metabolism in humans. *Obesity. (Silver Spring)*, 2007 15: 349-355.

[174] Belza, A; Toubro, S; A, A. The effect of caffeine, green tea and tyrosine on thermogenesis and energy intake. *Eur. J. Clin. Nutr.* 2007 Epub ahead of print.

[175] del Castillo, MD; Ames, JM; Gordon, MH. Effect of roasting on the antioxidant activity of coffee brews. *J. Agric Food Chem.* 2002 50: 3698-3703.

[176] Suzuki, A; Kagawa, D; Ochiai, R; Tokimitsu, I; Saito, I. Green coffee bean extract and its metabolites have a hypotensive effect in spontaneously hypertensive rats. *Hypertens. Res.* 2002 25: 99-107.

[177] Arion, WJ; Canfield, WK; Ramos, FC; Schindler, PW; Burger, HJ; Hemmerle, H; Schubert, G; Below, P; Herling, AW. Chlorogenic acid and hydroxynitrobenzaldehyde: new inhibitors of hepatic glucose 6-phosphatase. *Arch. Biochem. Biophys.* 1997 339: 315-322.

[178] Shimoda, H; Seki, E; Aitani, M. Inhibitory effect of green coffee bean extract on fat accumulation and body weight gain in mice. *BMC Complement Altern. Med.* 2006 6: 9.

[179] Thom, E. The effect of chlorogenic acid enriched coffee on glucose absorption in healthy volunteers and its effect on body mass when used long-term in overweight and obese people. *J. Int. Med. Res.* 2007 35: 900-908.

[180] Herling, AW; Burger, HJ; Schwab, D; Hemmerle, H; Below, P; Schubert, G. Pharmacodynamic profile of a novel inhibitor of the hepatic glucose-6-phosphatase system. *Am. J. Physiol.* 1998 274: G1087-1093.

[181] Pellati, F; Benvenuti, S; Melegari, M; Firenzuoli, F. Determination of adrenergic agonists from extracts and herbal products of Citrus aurantium L. var. amara by LC. *J. Pharm. Biomed. Anal.* 2002 29: 1113-1119.

[182] Preuss, HG; DiFerdinando, D; Bagchi, M; Bagchi, D. Citrus aurantium as a thermogenic, weight-reduction replacement for ephedra: an overview. *J. Med.* 2002 33: 247-264.

[183] Haaz, S; Fontaine, KR; Cutter, G; Limdi, N; Perumean-Chaney, S; Allison, DB. Citrus aurantium and synephrine alkaloids in the treatment of overweight and obesity: an update. *Obes. Rev.* 2006 7: 79-88.

[184] Astrup, A. Thermogenic drugs as a strategy for treatment of obesity. *Endocrine.* 2000 13: 207-212.

[185] National Toxicology Program. NTP toxicology and carcinogenesis studies of ephedrine sulfate (CAS, 134-72-5) in F344/N rats and B6C3F1 mice (Feed Studies). *Natl. Toxicol. Program Tech. Rep. Series.* 1986 307: 1-186.

[186] Mooney, RA; McDonald, JM. Effect of phenylephrine on lipolysis in rat adipocytes: no evidence for an alpha-adrenergic mechanism. *Int. J. Biochem* 1984 16: 55-59.

[187] Yeh, SY. Comparative anorectic effects of metaraminol and phenylephrine in rats. *Physiol. Behav.* 1999 68: 227-234.

[188] Desfaits, AC; Lafond, J; Savard, R. The effects of a selective alpha-1 adrenergic blockade on the activity of adipose tissue lipoprotein lipase in female hamsters. *Life Sci.* 1995 57: 705-713.

[189] Calapai, G; Firenzuoli, F; Saitta, A; Squadrito, F; Arlotta, M; Costantino, G; Inferrera, G. Antiobesity and cardiovascular toxic effects of Citrus aurantium extracts in the rat: a preliminary report. *Fitoterapia.* 1999 70: 586-592.

[190] Attele, AS; Wu, JA; Yuan, CS. Ginseng pharmacology: multiple constituents and multiple actions. *Biochem. Pharmacol.* 1999 58: 1685-1693.

[191] Yuan, CS; Wu, JA; Osinski, J. Ginsenoside variability in American ginseng samples. *Am. J. Clin. Nutr.* 2002 75: 600-601.

[192] Liu, W; Zheng, Y; Han, L; Wang, H; Saito, M; Ling, M; Kimura, Y; Feng, Y. Saponins (Ginsenosides) from stems and leaves of Panax quinquefolium prevented high-fat diet-induced obesity in mice. *Phytomedicine.* 2008 15: 1140-1145.

[193] Etou, H; Sakata, T; Fujimoto, K; Terada, K; Yoshimatsu, H; Ookuma, K; Hayashi, T; Arichi, S. Ginsenoside-Rb1 as a suppressor in central modulation of feeding in the rat. *Nippon Yakurigaku Zasshi.* 1988 91: 9-15.

[194] Cooper, SJ; Al-Naser, HA; Clifton, PG. The anorectic effect of the selective dopamine D1-receptor agonist A-77636 determined by meal pattern analysis in free-feeding rats. *Eur. J. Pharmacol.* 2006 532: 253-257.

[195] Kim, JH; Kang, SA; Han, SM; Shim, I. Comparison of the antiobesity effects of the protopanaxadiol- and protopanaxatriol-type saponins of red ginseng. *Phytother. Res.* 2009 23: 78-85.

[196] Fredholm, BB; Bättig, K; Holmén, J; Nehlig, A; Zvartau, EE. Actions of caffeine in the brain with special reference to factors that contribute to its widespread use. *Pharmacol. Rev.* 1999 51: 83-133.

[197] Quarta, D; Borycz, J; Solinas, M; Patkar, K; Hockemeyer, J; Ciruela, F; Lluis, C; Franco, R; Woods, AS; Goldberg, SR; Ferré, S. Adenosine receptor-mediated modulation of dopamine release in the nucleus accumbens depends on glutamate

neurotransmission and N-methyl-D-aspartate receptor stimulation. *J. Neurochem.* 2004 91: 873-880.

[198] Krugel, U; Schraft, T; Regenthal, R; Illes, P; Kittner, H. Purinergic modulation of extracellular glutamate levels in the nucleus accumbens in vivo. *Int. J. Dev. Neurosci.* 2004 22: 565-570.

[199] De Luca, MA; Bassareo, V; Bauer, A; Di Chiara, G. Caffeine and accumbens shell dopamine. *J. Neurochem.* 2007 103: 157-163.

[200] Arolfo, MP; Yao, L; Gordon, AS; Diamond, I; Janak, PH. Ethanol operant self-administration in rats is regulated by adenosine A2 receptors. *Alcohol. Clin. Exp. Res.* 2004 28: 1308-1316.

[201] Schiffman, SS; Diaz, C; Beeker, TG. Caffeine intensifies taste of certain sweeteners: role of adenosine receptor. *Pharmacol. Biochem. Behav.* 1986 24: 429-432.

[202] Schiffman, SS; Gill, JM; Diaz, C. Methyl xanthines enhance taste: evidence for modulation of taste by adenosine receptor. *Pharmacol. Biochem. Behav.* 1985 22: 195-203.

[203] Cheung, WT; Lee, CM; Ng, TB. Potentiation of the anti-lipolytic effect of 2-chloroadenosine after chronic caffeine treatment. *Pharmacology.* 1988 36: 331-339.

[204] Muroyama, K; Murosaki, S; Yamamoto, Y; Odaka, H; Chung, HC; Miyoshi, M. Anti-obesity effects of a mixture of thiamin, arginine, caffeine, and citric acid in non-insulin dependent diabetic KK mice. *J. Nutr. Sci. Vitaminol. (Tokyo),* 2003 49: 56-63.

[205] Pettenuzzo, L; Noschang, C; von Pozzer Toigo, E; Fachin, A; Vendite, D; Dalmaz, C. Effects of chronic administration of caffeine and stress on feeding behavior of rats. *Physiol. Behav.* 2008 95: 295-301.

[206] Kelley, AE; Baldo, BA; Pratt, WE; Will, MJ. Corticostriatal-hypothalamic circuitry and food motivation: Integration of energy, action and reward. *Physiol. Behav.* 2005 86: 773-795.

[207] Meister, B. Neurotransmitters in key neurons of the hypothalamus that regulate feeding behavior and body weight. *Physiol. Behav.* 2007 92: 263-271.

[208] Acquas, E; Tanda, G; Di Chiara, G. Differential effects of caffeine on dopamine and acetylcholine transmission in brain areas of drug-naive and caffeine-pretreated rats. *Neuropsychopharmacology.* 2002 27: 182-193.

[209] Carney, JM. Effects of caffeine, theophylline and theobromine on scheduled controlled responding in rats. *Br. J. Pharmacol.* 1982 75: 451-454.

[210] Chen, MD; Lin, WH; Song, YM; Lin, PY; Ho, LT. Effect of caffeine on the levels of brain serotonin and catecholamine in the genetically obese mice. *Zhonghua Yi Xue Za Zhi. (Taipei),* 1994 53: 257-261.

[211] Halford, JC; Blundell, JE. Pharmacology of appetite suppression. *Prog. Drug Res.* 2000 54: 25-58.

[212] Diepvens, K; Westerterp, KR; Westerterp-Plantenga, MS. Obesity and thermogenesis related to the consumption of caffeine, ephedrine, capsaicin, and green tea. *Am. J. Physiol. Regul. Integr. Comp. Physiol.* 2007 292: R77-R85.

[213] Astrup, A; Breum, L; Toubro, S; Hein, P; Quaade, F. The effect and safety of an ephedrine/caffeine compound compared to ephedrine, caffeine and placebo in obese subjects on an energy restricted diet. A double blind trial. *Int. J. Obes. Relat. Metab. Disord.* 1992 16: 269-277.

[214] Pasman, WJ; Westerterp-Plantenga, MS; Saris, WH. The effectiveness of long-term supplementation of carbohydrate, chromium, fibre and caffeine on weight maintenance. *Int. J. Obes. Relat. Metab. Disord.* 1997 21: 1143-1151.

[215] Westerterp-Plantenga, MS; Lejeune, MP; Kovacs, EM. Body weight loss and weight maintenance in relation to habitual caffeine intake and green tea supplementation. *Obes. Res.* 2005 13: 1195-1204.

[216] Tremblay, A; Masson, E; Leduc, S; A, H; Despres, JP. Caffeine reduces spontaneous energy intake in men but not in women. *Nutr. Res.* 1988 8: 553-558.

[217] Racotta, S; Leblanc, J; Richard, D. The effect of caffeine on food intake in rats: involvement of corticotropin-releasing factor and the sympatho-adrenal system. *Pharmacol. Biochem. Behav.* 1994 48: 887-892.

[218] Comer, SD; Haney, M; W, FR; Fischman, MW. Effects of caffeine withdrawal on humans living in a residential laboratory. *Exp. Clin. Psychopharmacol.* 1997 5: 399-403.

[219] Jessen, A; Buemann, B; Toubro, S; Skovgaard, IM; Astrup, A. The appetite-suppressant effect of nicotine is enhanced by caffeine. *Diab. Ob. Metab.* 2005 7: 327-333.

[220] Lopez-Garcia, E; van Dam, RM; Rajpathak, S; Willett, WC; Manson, JE; Hu, FB. Changes in caffeine intake and long-term weight change in men and women. *Am. J. Clin. Nutr.* 2006 83: 674-680.

[221] Jung, RT; Shetty, PS; James, WP; Barrand, MA; Callingham, BA. Caffeine: its effect on catecholamines and metabolism in lean and obese humans. *Clin. Sci. (Lond)*, 1981 60: 527-535.

[222] Hollands, MA; Arch, JR; Cawthorne, MA. A simple apparatus for comparative measurements of energy expenditure in human subjects: the thermic effect of caffeine. *Am. J. Clin. Nutr.* 1981 34: 2291-2294.

[223] Graham, TE. Caffeine and exercise: metabolism, endurance and performance. *Sports Med.* 2001 31: 785-807.

[224] Acheson, KJ; Zahorska-Markiewicz, B; Pittet, P; Anantharaman, K; Jequier, E. Caffeine and coffee: their influence on metabolic rate and substrate utilization in normal weight and obese individuals. *Am. J. Clin. Nutr.* 1980 33: 989-997.

[225] Dulloo, AG. Ephedrine, xanthines and prostaglandin-inhibitors: actions and interactions in the stimulation of thermogenesis. *Int. J. Obes. Relat. Metab. Disord.* 1993 17 S35-S40.

[226] Astrup, A; Toubro, S. Thermogenic, metabolic, and cardiovascular responses to ephedrine and caffeine in man. *Int. J. Obes. Relat. Metab. Disord.* 1993 17 S41-S43.

[227] Astrup, A; Toubro, S; Cannon, S; Hein, P; Breum, L; Madsen, J. Caffeine: a double-blind, placebo-controlled study of its thermogenic, metabolic, and cardiovascular effects in healthy volunteers. *Am. J. Clin. Nutr.* 1990 51: 759-767.

[228] Yoshida, T; Sakane, N; Umekawa, T; Kondo, M. Relationship between basal metabolic rate, thermogenic response to caffeine, and body weight loss following combined low calorie and exercise treatment in obese women. *Int. J. Obes. Relat. Metab. Disord.* 1994 18: 345-350.

[229] Haller, CA; Jacob, Pr; Benowitz, N. Enhanced stimulant and metabolic effects of combined ephedrine and caffeine. *Clin. Pharmacol. Ther.* 2004 75: 259-273.

[230] Taylor, P. Ganglionic stimulating and blocking agents, In: Oillman, AG, et al., editor. *The Pharmacological Basis of Therapeutics*. New York: McMiilan; 1985.

[231] Perkins, KA; Epstein, LH; Stiller, RL; Fernstrom, MH; Sexton, JE; Jacob, RG; Solberg, R. Acute effects of nicotine on hunger and caloric intake in smokers and nonsmokers. *Psychopharmacology.* 1991 103: 103-109.

[232] Albanes, D; Jones, DY; Micozzi, MS; Mattson, ME. Associations between smoking and body weight in the U.S. population: analysis of NHANES II. *Am. J. Public Health.* 1987 77: 439-444.

[233] Jo, YH; Talmage, DA; Role, LW. Nicotinic receptor-mediated effects on appetite and food intake. *J. Neurobiol.* 2002 53: 618-632.

[234] Grunberg, NE; Bowen, DJ; Winders, SE. Effects of nicotine on body weight and food consumption in female rats. *Psychopharmacology. (Berl)*, 1986 90: 101-105.

[235] Klesges, RC; Meyers, AW; Klesges, LM; La Vasque, ME. Smoking, body weight, and their effects on smoking behavior: a comprehensive review of the literature. *Psychol. Bull.* 1989 106: 204-230.

[236] Pomerleau, CS. Issues for women who wish to stop smoking, In: Seidman, DF and Covey, LS, editor. *Helping the hard-core smoker.* London: Lawrence Erlbaum; 1999;p. 73-91.

[237] Pomerleau, CS; Pomerleau, OF; Namenek, RJ; Mehringer, AM. Short-term weight gain in abstaining women smokers. *J. Subst. Abuse Treat.* 2000 18: 339-342.

[238] Dallosso, HM; James, WP. The role of smoking in the regulation of energy balance. *Int. J. Obes.* 1984 8: 365-375.

[239] Stamford, BA; Matter, S; Fell, RD; Papanek, P. Effects of smoking cessation on weight gain, metabolic rate, caloric consumption, and blood lipids. *Am. J. Clin. Nutr.* 1986 43: 486-494.

[240] Sztalryd, C; Hamilton, J; Horowitz, BA; Johnson, P; Kraemer, FB. Alterations of lipolysis and lipoprotein lipase in chronically nicotine-treated rats. *Am. J. Physiol.* 1996 270: E215-E223.

[241] Ashakumary, L; Vijayammal, PL. Effect of nicotine on lipoprotein metabolism in rats. *Lipids.* 1997 32: 311-315.

[242] Arai, K; Kim, K; Kaneko, K; Iketani, M; Otagiri, A; Yamauchi, N; Shibasaki, T. Nicotine infusion alters leptin and uncoupling protein 1 mRNA expression in adipose tissues of rats. *Am. J. Physiol. Endocrinol. Metab.* 2001 280: E867-E876.

[243] Sanigorski, A; Fahey, R; Cameron-Smith, D; Collier, GR. Nicotine treatment decreases food intake and body weight via a leptin-independent pathway in Psammomys obesus. *Diabetes Obes. Metab.* 2002 4: 346-350.

[244] Winders, SE; Grunberg, NE. Effects of nicotine on body weight, food consumption and body composition in male rats. *Life Sci.* 1990 46: 1523-1530.

[245] Chen, H; Hansen, MJ; Jones, JE; Vlahos, R; Bozinovski, S; Anderson, GP; Morris, MJ. Regulation of hypothalamic NPY by diet and smoking. *Peptides.* 2007 28: 384-389.

[246] Kane, JK; Parker, SL; Li, MD. Hypothalamic orexin-A binding sites are downregulated by chronic nicotine treatment in the rat. *Neurosci. Lett.* 2001 298: 1-4.

[247] Yang, ZJ; Blaha, V; Meguid, MM; Oler, A; Miyata, G. Infusion of nicotine into the LHA enhances dopamine and 5-HT release and suppresses food intake. *Pharmacol. Biochem. Behav.* 1999 64: 155-159.

[248] Miyata, G; Meguid, MM; Fetissov, SO; Torelli, GF; Kim, HJ. Nicotine's effect on hypothalamic neurotransmitters and appetite regulation. *Surgery.* 1999 126: 255-263.

[249] Mifsud, JC; Hernandez, L; Hoebel, BG. Nicotine infused into the nucleus accumbens increases synaptic dopamine as measured by in vivo microdialysis. *Brain Res.* 1989 478: 365-367.

[250] Nisell, M; Nomikos, GG; Svensson, TH. Infusion of nicotine in the ventral tegmental area or the nucleus accumbens of the rat differentially affects accumbal dopamine release. *Pharmacol. Toxicol.* 1994 75: 348-352.

[251] Zarrindast, MR; Oveisi, MR. Effects of monoamine receptor antagonists on nicotine-induced hypophagia in the rat. *Eur. J. Pharmacol.* 1997 321: 157-162.

[252] Williamson, DF; Madans, J; Anda, RF; Kleinman, JC; Giovino, GA; Byers, T. Smoking cessation and severity of weight gain in a national cohort. *N. Engl. J. Med.* 1991 324: 739-745.

[253] Shimokata, H; Muller, DC; Andres, R. Studies in the distribution of body fat. III. Effects of cigarette smoking. *JAMA.* 1989 261: 1169-1173.

[254] Flegal, KM; Troiano, RP; Pamuk, ER; Kuczmarski, RJ; Campbell, SM. The influence of smoking cessation on the prevalence of overweight in the United States. *N. Engl. J. Med.* 1995 333: 1165-1170.

[255] Huot, I; Paradis, G; Ledoux, M. Quebec Heart Health Demonstration Project Research Group. Factors associated with overweight and obesity in Quebec adults. *Int. J. Obes. Relat. Metab. Disord.* 2004 28: 766-774.

[256] Blaha, V; Yang, ZJ; Meguid, M; Chai, JK; Zadak, Z. Systemic nicotine administration suppresses food intake via reduced meal sizes in both male and female rats. *Acta Med.* 1998 41: 167-173.

[257] Miyata, G; Meguid, MM; Varma, M; Fetissov, SO; Kim, HJ. Nicotine alters the usual reciprocity between meal size and meal number in female rat. *Physiol. Behav.* 2001 74: 169-176.

[258] Bray, GA. Reciprocal relation of food intake and sympathetic activity: experimental observations and clinical implications. *Int. J. Obes. Relat. Metab. Disord.* 2000 24: S8-S17.

[259] Zhang, L; Meguid, MM; Miyata, G; Varma, M; Fetissov, SO. Role of hypothalamic monoamines in nicotine-induced anorexia in menopausal rats. *Surgery.* 2001 130: 133-142.

[260] McNair, E; Bryson, R. Effects of nicotine on weight change and food consumption in rats. *Pharmacol. Biochem. Behav.* 1983 18: 341-344.

[261] Grunberg, NE; Bowen, DJ; Morse, DE. Effects of nicotine on body weight and food consumption in rats. *Psychopharmacology. (Berl)*, 1984 83: 93-98.

[262] Schechter, MD; Cook, PG. Nicotine-induced weight loss in rats without an effect on appetite. *Eur. J. Pharmacol.* 1976 38: 63-69.

[263] Morgan, MM; Ellison, G. Different effects of chronic nicotine treatment regimens on body weight and tolerance in the rat. *Psychopharmacology. (Berl)*, 1987 91: 236-238.

[264] Wager-Srdar, SA; Levine, AS; Morley, JE; Hoidal, JR; Niewoehner, DE. Effects of cigarette smoke and nicotine on feeding and energy. *Physiol. Behav.* 1984 32: 389-395.

[265] Grunberg, NE; Bowen, DJ; Maycock, VA; Nespor, SM. The importance of sweet taste and caloric content in the effects of nicotine on specific food consumption. *Psychopharmacology. (Berl)*, 1985 87: 198-203.

[266] Filozof, C; Fernandez Pinilla, MC; Fernandez-Cruz, A. Smoking cessation and weight gain. *Obes. Rev.* 2004 5: 95-103.

[267] Gross, J; Stitzer, ML; Maldonado, J. Nicotine replacement: effects of postcessation weight gain. *J. Consult. Clin. Psychol.* 1989 57: 87-92.

[268] Allen, SS; Hatsukami, D; Brintnell, DM; Bade, T. Effect of nicotine replacement therapy on post-cessation weight gain and nutrient intake: a randomized controlled trial of postmenopausal female smokers. *Addict. Behav.* 2005 30: 1273-1280.

[269] Murray, CD; Le Roux, CW; Emmanuel, AV; Halket , JM; Przyborowska, AM; Kamm, MA; Murray-Lyon, IM. The effect of Khat (Catha edulis) as an appetite suppressant is independent of ghrelin and PYY secretion. *Appetite.* 2008 51: 747-750.

[270] Le Bras, M; Fretillere, Y. Les aspects mrdicaux de la consommation habituelle du Cath. *Mdd trop.* 1965 25: 720-731.

[271] Halbach, H. Medical aspects of the chewing of khat leaves. *Bull. Wld Hlth Org.* 1972 47: 21-29.

[272] Zelger, JL; Carlini, EA. Anorexigenic effects of two amines obtained from Catha edulis Forsk. (Khat) in rats. *Pharmacol. Biochem. Behav.* 1980 12: 701-705.

[273] Toennes, SW; Harder, S; Schramm, M; Niess, C; Kauert, GF. Pharmacokinetics of cathinone, cathine and norephedrine after the chewing of khat leaves. *Br. J. Clin. Pharmacol.* 2003 56: 125-130.

[274] Zelger, JL; Schorno, HX; Carlini, EA. Behavioural effects of cathinone, an amine obtained from Catha edulis Forsk.: comparisons with amphetamine, norpseudoephedrine, apomorphine and nomifensine. *Bull. Narc.* 1980 32: 67-81.

[275] Eisenberg, MS; Maher, TJ; Silverman, HI. A comparison of the effects of phenylpropanolamine, d-amphetamine and d-norpseudoephedrine on open-field locomotion and food intake in the rat. *Appetite.* 1987 9: 31-37.

[276] Heymann, TD; Bhupulan, A; Zureikat, NE; Bomanji, J; Drinkwater, C; Giles, P; Murray-Lyon, IM. Khat chewing delays gastric emptying of a semi-solid meal. *Aliment Pharmacol. Ther.* 1995 9: 81-83.

[277] Van Beek, TA; Verpoorte, R; Svendsen, AB; Leeuwenberg, AJ; Bisset, NG. Tabernaemontana L. (Apocynaceae): a review of its taxonomy, phytochemistry, ethnobotany and pharmacology. *J. Ethnopharmacol.* 1984 10: 1-156.

[278] Bruyns, P. A revision of hoodia and lavrania (Asclepidaceae-Stapeliaeae Botanische Jahrbucher:fuer). *Syst. Pflanzenges Pflanzengeogr.* 1993 115: 145-270.

[279] van Heerden, FR. Hoodia gordonii: A natural appetite suppressant. *J. Ethnopharmacol.* 2008 119 434-437.

[280] Van Heerden, FR; Horak, RM; Learmonth, RA; Maharaj, V; Whittal, RD, *Pharmaceutical compositions having appetite-suppressant activity.* 1998.

[281] Van Heerden, FR; Horak, RM; Maharaj, VJ; Vleggaar, R; Senabe, JV; Gunning, PJ. An appetite suppressant from Hoodia species. *Phytochemistry.* 2007 68: 2545-2553.

[282] Tulp, OL; Harbi, NA; Mihalov, J; DerMarderosian, A. Effect of Hoodia plant on food intake and body weight in lean and obese LA/Ntul//-cp rats. *FASEB J*, 2001 15: A404.

[283] Phytopharm open offer and placing prospectus 080228. 2008: 1-129.

[284] MacLean, DB; Luo, LG. Increased ATP content/production in the hypothalamus may be a signal for energy-sensing of satiety: studies of the anorectic mechanism of a plant steroidal glycoside. *Brain Res.* 2004 1020: 1-11.

[285] MacLean, DB. Abrogation of peripheral cholecystokinin-satiety in the capsaicin treated rat. *Regul. Pept.* 1985 11: 321-333.

[286] Laddha, KS, *Medicinal Natural Products Research Laboratory*, University of Mumbai: Mumbai, India.

[287] *Wealth of India. A Dictionary of Indian Raw Materials and Industrial Products*. 1992. p. 266-267.

[288] Bader, A; Braca, A; De Tommasi, Na; Morelli, I. Further constituents from Caralluma negevensis. *Phytochemistry*. 2003 62: 1277-1281.

[289] Preuss, HG; Bagchi, D; Bagchi, M; Rao, CV; Dey, DK; Satyanarayana, S. Effects of a natural extract of (-)-hydroxycitric acid (HCA-SX) and a combination of HCA-SX plus niacin-bound chromium and Gymnema sylvestre extract on weight loss. *Diabetes Obes Metab*, 2004 6: 171-180.

[290] Preuss, HG, *Report on the Safety of Caralluma Fimbriata and its Extract*. 2004: Washington, D C.

[291] Kuriyan, R; Raj, T; Srinivas, SK; Vaz, M; Rajendran, R; Kurpad, AV. Effect of Caralluma fimbriata extract on appetite, food intake and anthropometry in adult Indian men and women. *Appetite*. 2007 48: 338-344.

[292] Roberts, SB; Heyman, MB. Dietary composition and obesity: do we need to look beyond dietary fat? *J. Nutr.* 2000 130: 267S.

[293] Agarwal, KC; Parks, REJ. Forskolin: a potential antimetastatic agent. *Int. J. Cancer.* 1983 32: 801-804.

[294] Caprioli, J; Sears, M. Forskolin lowers intraocular pressure in rabbits, monkeys, and man. *Lancet.* 1983 1: 958-960.

[295] Burns, TW; Langley, PE; Terry, BE; Bylund, DB; Forte, LRJ. Comparative effects of forskolin and isoproterenol on the cyclic AMP content of human adipocytes. *Life Sci.* 1987 40: 145-154.

[296] Litosch, I; Hudson, TH; Mills, I; Li, SY; Fain, JN. Forskolin as an activator of cyclic AMP accumulation and lipolysis in rat adipocytes. *Mol. Pharmacol.* 1982 22: 109-115.

[297] Henderson, S; Magu, B; Rasmussen, C; Lancaster, S; Kerksick, C; Smith, P; Melton, C; Cowan, P; Greenwood, M; Earnest, C; Almada, A; Milnor, P; Magrans, T; Bowden, R; Ounpraseuth, S; Thomas, A; Kreider, RB. Effects of coleus forskohlii supplementation on body composition and hematological profiles in mildly overweight women. *J. Int. Soc. Sports Nutr.* 2005 2: 54-62.

[298] Gaoni, Y; Mechoulam, R. Isolation, structure and partial synthesis of an active constituent of hashish. *J. Am. Chem. Soc.* 1964 86: 1646.

[299] Woelkart, K; Salo-Ahen, OM; Bauer, R. CB receptor ligands from plants. *Curr. Top. Med. Chem.* 2008 8: 173-186.

[300] Foltin, RW; Brady, JV; Fischman, MW. Behavioral analysis of marijuana effects on food intake in humans. *Pharmacol. Biochem. Behav.* 1986 25: 577-582.

[301] Foltin, RW; Fischman, MW; Byrne, MF. Effects of smoked marijuana on food intake and body weight of humans living in a residential laboratory. *Appetite*. 1988 11: 1-14.

[302] Haney, M; Rabkin, J; Gunderson, E; Foltin, RW. Dronabinol and marijuana in HIV+ marijuana smokers: acute effects on caloric intake and mood. *Psychopharmacology. (Berl)*, 2005 181: 170-178.

[303] Hart, CL; Ward, AS; Haney, M; Comer, SD; Foltin, RW; Fischman, MW. Comparison of smoked marijuana and oral D9-tetrahydrocannbinol in humans. *Psychopharmacology. (Berl)*, 2002 164: 407-415.

[304] Haney, M; Ward, AS; Comer, SD; Foltin, RW; Fischman, MW. Abstinence symptoms following oral THC administration to humans. *Psychopharmacology. (Berl)*, 1999 141: 385-394.

[305] Haney, M; Gunderson, EW; Rabkin, J; Hart, CL; Vosburg, SK; Comer, SD; Foltin, RW. Dronabinol and marijuana in HIV-positive marijuana smokers. Caloric intake, mood, and sleep. *J. Acquir. Immune Defic. Syndr.* 2007 45: 545-554.

[306] Abel, EL. Effects of marijuana on the solution of anagrams, memory and appetite. *Nature.* 1971 231: 260-261.

[307] Hollister, LE. Hunger and appetite after single doses of marihuana, alcohol, and dextroamphetamine. *Clin. Pharmacol. Ther.* 1971 12: 44-49.

[308] Huestis, MA; Gorelick, DA; Heishman, SJ; Preston, KL; Nelson, RA; Moolchan, ET; Frank, RA. Blockade of effects of smoked marijuana by the CB1 selective cannabinoid receptor antagonist SR141716. *Arch. Gen. Psychiatry.* 2001 58: 322-328.

[309] Regelson, W; Butler, JR; Schultz, J. Delta-9-tetrahydrocannabinol as an effective antidepressant and appetitestimulating agent in advanced cancer patients, In: Braude, M and Szara, S, editor. *The Pharmacology of Marijuana.* New York:: Raven Press; 1976;p. 763-776.

[310] Beal, JE; Olson, R; Laubenstein, L; Morales, JO; Bellman, P; Yangco, B; Lefkowitz, L; Plasse, TF; Shepard, KV. Dronabinol as a treatment for anorexia associated with weight loss in patients with AIDS. *J. Pain Symptom. Manage.* 1995 10: 89-97.

[311] Plasse, TF; Gorter, RW; Krasnow, SH; Lane, M; Shepard, KV; Wadleigh, RG. Recent clinical experience with dronabinol. *Pharmacol. Biochem. Behav.* 1991 40: 695-700.

[312] Struwe, M; Kaempfer, S; Geiger, C; Pavia, A; Plasse, T; Shepard, K; Ries, K; Evans, T. Effect of dronabinol on nutritional status in HIV infection. *Ann. Pharmacother.* 1993 27: 827-831.

[313] Kirkham, TC; Rogers, EK; Tucci, S, *Eating stimulated by intra-PVN infusion of the endocannabinoid 2-AG is reversed by opioid receptor blockade,* in *Society for Neuroscience 35th Annual Meeting.* 2005: Washington USA. p. 533.15.

[314] Williams, CM; Kirkham, TC. Reversal of delta 9-THC hyperphagia by SR141716 and naloxone but not dexfenfluramine. *Pharmacol. Biochem. Behav.* 2002 7: 333-340.

[315] Brown, JE; Kassouny, M; Cross, JK. Kinetic studies of food intake and sucrose solution preference by rats treated with low doses of delta9-tetrahydrocannabinol. *Behav. Biol.* 1977 20: 104-110.

[316] Anderson-Baker, WC; McLaughlin, CL; Baile, CA. Oral and hypothalamic injections of barbiturates, benzodiazepines and cannabinoids and food intake in rats. *Pharmacol. Biochem. Behav.* 1979 11: 487-491.

[317] Williams, CM; Rogers, PJ; Kirkham, TC. Hyperphagia in pre-fed rats following oral delta9-THC. *Physiol. Behav.* 1998 65: 343-346.

[318] Williams, CM; Kirkham, TC. Anandamide induces overeating: mediation by central cannabinoid (CB1) receptors. *Psychopharmacology.* 1999 143: 315-317.

[319] Williams, CM; Kirkham, TC. Reversal of cannabinoid hyperphagia by naloxone but not dexfenfluramine. *Appetite.* 2000 35: 317.

[320] Williams, CM; Kirkham, TC. Observational analysis of feeding induced by Delta9-THC and anandamide. *Physiol. Behav.* 2002 76: 241-250.

[321] Avraham, Y; Ben-Shushan, D; Brener, A; Zolotarev, O; Okon, O; Fink, N; Katz, V; Berry, EM. Very low dose of tetrahydrocannabinol (THC) improves food consumption

and cognitive function in an animal model of anorexia nervosa. *Pharmacol. Biochem. Behav.* 2004 77: 657-684.

[322] Cooper, S. Endocannabinoids and food consumption: comparisons with benzodiazepine and opioid palatability-dependent appetite. *Eur. J. Pharmacol.* 2004 500: 37-49.

[323] Jarrett, MM; Limebeer, CL; Parker, LA. Effect of delta9-tetrahydrocannabinol on sucrose palatability as measured by the taste reactivity test. *Physiol. Behav.* 2005 86: 475-479.

[324] Kirkham, TC. Endocannabinoids in the regulation of appetite and body weight. *Behav. Pharmacol.* 2005 16: 297-313.

[325] Koch, JE; Matthews, SM. Delta9-tetrahydrocannabinol stimulates palatable food intake in Lewis rats: effects of peripheral and central administration. *Nutr. Neurosci.* 2001 4: 179-187.

[326] Higgs, S; Williams, C; Kirkham, T. Cannabinoid influences on palatability: microstructural analysis of sucrose drinking after delta(9)-tetrahydrocannabinol, anandamide, 2-arachidonoyl glycerol and SR141716. *Psychopharmacology.* 2003 165: 370-377.

[327] Mahler, SV; Smith, KS; Berridge, KC. Endocannabinoid hedonic hotspot for sensory pleasure: anandamide in nucleus accumbens shell enhances 'liking' of a sweet reward. *Neuropsychopharmacology.* 2007 32: 2267-2278.

[328] Berridge, KC; Robinson, TE. Parsing reward. *Trends Neurosci.* 2003 26: 507-513.

[329] van Wyk, BE; Albrecht, C. A review of the taxonomy, ethnobotany, chemistry and pharmacology of Sutherlandia frutescens (Fabaceae). *J. Ethnopharmacol.* 2008 119: 620-629.

[330] Johnson, Q; Syce, J; Nell, H; Rudeen, K; Folk, WR. A randomized, double-blind, placebo-controlled trial of Lessertia frutescens in healthy adults. *PLoS Clin. Trials.* 2007 2: e16.

[331] Schwarz, EJ; Reginato, MJ; Shao, D; Krakow, SL; Lazar, MA. Retinoic acid blocks adipogenesis by inhibiting C/EBPbeta-mediated transcription. *Mol. Cell. Biol.* 1997 17: 1552-1561.

[332] Elberg, G; Gimble, JM; Tsai, SY. Modulation of the murine peroxisome proliferator-activated receptor gamma 2 promoter activity by CCAAT/enhancer-binding proteins. *J. Biol. Chem.* 2000 275: 27815-27822.

[333] Roy, S; Rink, C; Khanna, S; Phillips, C; Bagchi, D; Bagchi, M; Sen, CK. Body weight and abdominal fat gene expression profile in response to a novel hydroxycitric acid-based dietary supplement. *Gene Expr.* 2004 11: 251-262.

[334] Shara, M; Ohia, SE; Yasmin, T; Zardetto-Smith, A; Kincaid, A; Bagchi, M; Chatterjee, A; Bagchi, D; Stohs, SJ. Dose- and time-dependent effects of a novel (-)-hydroxycitric acid extract on body weight, hepatic and testicular lipid peroxidation, DNA fragmentation and histopathological data over a period of 90 days. *Mol. Cell Biochem.* 2003 254: 339-346.

[335] Kao, YH; Hiipakka, RA; Liao, S. Modulation of endocrine systems and food intake by green tea epigallocatechin gallate. *Endocrinology.* 2000 141: 980-987.

[336] Kovacs, EM; Lejeune, MP; Nijs, I; Westerterp-Plantenga, MS. Effects of green tea on weight maintenance after body-weight loss. *Br. J. Nutr.* 2004 91: 431-437.

[337] Calapai, G; Crupi, A; Firenzuoli, F; Costantino, G; Inferrera, G; Campo, GM; Caputi, AP. Effects of Hypericum perforatum on levels of 5-hydroxytryptamine, noradrenaline

and dopamine in the cortex, diencephalon and brainstem of the rat. *J. Pharm. Pharmacol.* 1999 51: 723-8.
[338] Xie, JT; Wang, CZ; Ni, M; Wu, JA; Mehendale, SR; Aung, HH; Foo, A; Yuan, CS. American ginseng berry juice intake reduces blood glucose and body weight in ob/ob mice. *J. Food Sci.* 2007 72: S590-S594.
[339] Moffatt, RJ; Owens, SG. Cessation from cigarette smoking: changes in body weight, body composition, resting metabolism, and energy consumption. *Metabolism.* 1991 40: 465-470.
[340] Perkins, KA; Epstein, LH; Marks, BL; Stiller, RL; Jacob, RG. The effect of nicotine on energy expenditure during light physical activity. *N. Engl. J. Med.* 1989 320: 898-903.
[341] Koch, JE. Delta(9)-THC stimulates food intake in Lewis rats: effects on chow, high-fat and sweet high-fat diets. *Pharmacol. Biochem. Behav.* 2001 68: 539-543.
[342] Koch, JE; Matthews, SM. Delta9-tetrahydrocannabinol stimulates palatable food intake in Lewis rats: effects of peripheral and central administration. *Nutr. Neurosci.* 2001 4: 179-187.
[343] Greenberg, JA; Boozer, CN; Geliebter, A. Coffee, diabetes, and weight control. *Am. J. Clin. Nutr.* 2006 84: 682-693.

In: Appetite: Regulation, Role in Disease and Control
Editor: Steven R. Mitchell, pp. 217-264

ISBN 978-1-61209-842-5
© 2011 Nova Science Publishers, Inc.

Chapter 11

GHRELIN: A PEPTIDE INVOLVED IN THE CONTROL OF APPETITE

*Carine De Vriese, Jason Perret and Christine Delporte**
Laboratory of Biological Chemistry and Nutrition,
Université Libre de Bruxelles, Brussels, Belgium

ABSTRACT

Ghrelin is the endogenous ligand for the growth hormone secretagogue receptor. Ghrelin is a peptide of 28 amino acids possessing an uncommon octanoyl moiety on the serine in position 3, which is crucial for its biological activity. Ghrelin is predominantly produced and secreted into the blood stream by the endocrine X/A like cells of the stomach mucosa. Besides, it is also expressed in other tissues like duodenum, jejunum, ileum, colon, lung, heart, pancreas, kidney, testis, pituitary and hypothalamus. Some of the major biological actions of ghrelin are the secretion of growth hormone, the stimulation of appetite and food intake, the regulation of gastric motility and acid secretion and the modulation of the endocrine and exocrine pancreatic functions. Ghrelin is an orexigenic peptide involved in the short-term regulation of appetite and food intake. The plasma ghrelin levels increase before meal and decrease strongly during the postprandial phase. Long-term body weight is also regulated by ghrelin, since it induces adiposity. The purpose of this chapter is to provide updated information on ghrelin, the role of ghrelin in the control of appetite, as well as the potential clinical applications of ghrelin agonists and antagonists in certain physiopathological conditions.

1. DISCOVERY OF GHRELIN

Growth hormone releasing hormone (GHRH) is known to activate the pituitary secretion of growth hormone, while somatostatin inhibits it. Endorphin-derived peptides were shown to stimulate GH secretion and this led to the development of peptidic and non-peptidic synthetic

---

* Corresponding author: Laboratory of Biological Chemistry and Nutrition, Faculty of Medicine, Université Libre de Bruxelles, Bat G/E, CP 611, 808 route de Lennik, B-1070 Brussels, Belgium. Tel: 32 2 555 62 10; Fax: 32 2 555 62 30; Email: cdelport@ulb.ac.be.

molecules named growth hormone secretagogues (GHS). Both GHRH and GHS stimulate GH secretion via the cAMP and the inositol triphosphates/calcium pathways, respectively, suggesting they are acting on distinct receptors. In 1996, GHS receptor (GHS-R 1a) was cloned from human pituitary and remained an orphan G-protein coupled receptor (GPCR) until the discovery, in 1999, of its natural ligand, ghrelin (Kojima et al., 1999; Kojima and Kangawa, 2008).

Ghrelin was purified from rat stomach and its structure is unprecedented as this 28 amino acid peptidic hormone contains a unique modification: a *n*-octanoylation of serine in position 3 (Kojima et al., 1999; Kojima et al., 2001) (figure 1). This modification turned out to be essential for its known biological activity encountered by its binding to the GHS-R 1a receptor.

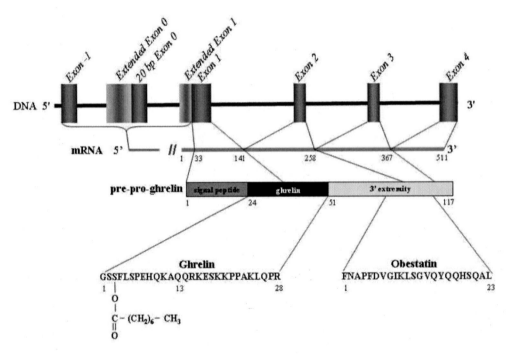

Figure 1. Human ghrelin gene structure contains 4 exons (boxes) and 3 introns (lines). After transcription, the mRNA is translated into prepro-ghrelin of 117 amino acids. Prepro-ghrelin is finally processed into ghrelin and/or obestatin.

2. HUMAN GHRELIN GENE STRUCTURE

The human ghrelin gene is located on chromosome 3 (3p25-26). Originally, human ghrelin gene was shown to contain a 20 bp non-coding exon, 4 coding exons and 3 introns and encoding a 511 bp mRNA (Kanamoto et al., 2004; Nakai et al., 2004). Very recently, the human ghrelin gene was shown to contain an additional novel exon (termed exon -1) and a 5' extension to exons 0 and 1 (Seim et al., 2007). Therefore, a revised exon-intron structure proposes that the human ghrelin gene spans 7.2 kb and consists of six rather than five exons (Seim et al., 2007) (figure 1). Mature ghrelin is encoded by exons 1 and 2. Prepro-ghrelin contains 117 amino acids (AA), the first 23 AA represent the signal peptide, followed by 94

AA coding pro-ghrelin (Korbonits et al., 2004). In 2005, another peptide, called obestatin, was shown to be derived from prepro-ghrelin (Zhang et al., 2005). The sequence of obestatin starts at the 25th AA downstream of ghrelin and consists of 23 AA (figure 1). Another ghrelin gene-derived mRNA transcript, not coding for ghrelin but that may encode for the C-terminal region of the full-length prepro-ghrelin, was also identified (Seim et al., 2007). Moreover, several spliced variants of human ghrelin gene were identified. A first group of transcripts include exons 1 to 4, coding for prepro-ghrelin, and varying only in the length of the sequence upstream of exon 1 (the prepro-ghrelin 5' untranslated region). Splice variant resulting from an alternative exon 2 splice site include des-Gln^{14}-ghrelin (Hosoda et al., 2000b). A second group of transcripts contain splice variants that include exon -1 in various combinations with exons downstream of exon 1 (exons 2 to 4) (Seim et al., 2007). Putative peptides encoded by these transcripts would include the sequence for C-ghrelin (exons -1, 2, 3, 4, including the coding sequence for obestatin as well) (Pemberton et al., 2003; Seim et al., 2007), the obestatin sequence (exons -1, 3, 4) (Seim et al., 2007; Zhang et al., 2005), and a novel C-terminal pro-ghrelin peptide lacking exon 3 (exons -1, 4) (Jeffery et al., 2005; Seim et al., 2007). Interestingly, this latter transcript has been shown to be upregulated in two cancers, i.e. breast cancer (Jeffery et al., 2005) and prostate cancer (Yeh et al., 2005). These various variants have been identified in different human tissues and cell lines, strongly suggesting a higher order of complexity of ghrelin gene expression. Indeed, an additional level of complexity may play an increasingly important role delivered by a third group of natural antisense transcripts (transcribed from the anti-sense strand), that were also recently identified (Seim et al., 2007), and subject as well to multiple transcription start sites and splice variants. However, these transcripts, to date do not seem to code for proteins, and may represent a source of non-coding RNAs implicated in gene regulation at the post-transcriptional and/or post-translational level.

Taken together, the data published to date on the human ghrelin gene structure strongly suggests that the ghrelin locus is far more complex than previously recognized. Further investigation will be necessary to understand the fine-tuning regulatory mechanisms that may be tissue specific, as well as dependent on physiological requirements. Likewise, it would be important to re-examine the ghrelin locus in order to identify and characterize novel peptides that may derive from it, and maybe other novel transcripts. This will raise challenging questions pertaining to their physiological functions in the light of ghrelin's pleiotropic actions. This in turn will open the way to their implication in various physiopathological conditions.

3. PREPRO-GHRELIN PROCESSING

Processing of the 117 AA prepro-ghrelin containing, containing pro-ghrelin (1-94), can lead to the formation of ghrelin 1-28 (in position 24-51 of prepro-ghrelin (Kojima et al., 1999), obestatin 1-23 (in position 76-98 of prepro-ghrelin) (Zhang et al., 2005), a C-terminal peptide of 66 AA (in position 52-117 of prepro-ghrelin) (Bang et al., 2007), and peptides derived from the 66 carboxy-terminal AA of pro-ghrelin (termed C-ghrelin) (Pemberton et al., 2003) (figure 2). Several enzymes responsible for processing the ghrelin precursor have been identified. Knockout mice for prohormone convertase 1/3 (PC 1/3), 2 (PC 2) and 5/6A (PC

5/6A) revealed that PC 1/3, but not PC 2 or PC 5/6A, is involved in the conversion of pro-ghrelin to ghrelin by cleaving at a single Arg residue in the stomach (Zhu et al., 2006) (figure 2). It is worth noting that the ghrelin sequence ends at Pro27 and Arg28, two amino acids corresponding to a processing signal. A cleavage most frequently occurs following Pro27-Arg28, and rarely after Pro27, generating respectively ghrelin 1-28 (Kojima et al., 1999) and ghrelin 1-27 (Hosoda et al., 2003). Cleavage following Pro27 is mostly the result of a carboxypeptidase-B like enzyme (Hosoda et al., 2003). Either ghrelin 1-28 or ghrelin 1-27 are then subjected to a particular post-translational modification: the acylation of the hydroxyl group of Ser3. The acylation most frequently occurs with an octanoyl group (C8:0), and more rarely with a decanoyl (C10:0) or a decenoyl (C10:1) group (Hosoda et al., 2003). Acylation of ghrelin can be increased by ingestion of either medium-chain fatty acids or medium chain triacylglycerols (Nishi et al., 2005).

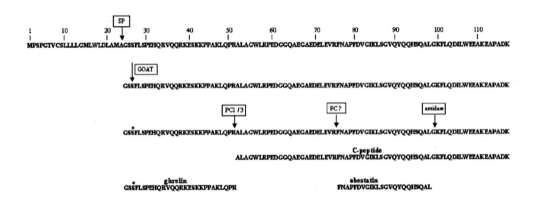

Figure 2. Processing of the prepro-ghrelin precursor. Prepro-ghrelin, composed of 117 amino acids, is processed into pro-ghrelin by the cleavage of the signal peptide by a signal peptidase (SP). In the endoplasmic reticulum, pro-ghrelin is octanoylated by the ghrelin O-acyl transferase (GOAT). Octanoylated pro-ghrelin is then processed into ghrelin and obestatin by prohormone convertase 1/3 (PC 1/3), followed by another prohormone convertase, and an amidase.

Very recently, the enzyme responsible for ghrelin octanoylation was simultaneously identified by two separate research groups as being an orphan membrane-bound O-acyl transferase (MBOAT) and renamed ghrelin O-acyl transferase (GOAT) (Gutierrez et al., 2008; Yang et al., 2008) (figure 2). Both teams based their reasoning on the same observations. Firstly, porcupine, an enzyme sharing structural similarities with MBOAT, is required for the acylation of serine in position 209 with palmitoleic acid and for transport of Wnt3a (member 3 of the wingless-type mouse mammary tumor virus integration site family) from the endoplasmic reticulum for secretion (Takada et al., 2006). Secondly, porcupine was localized in the same cellular compartment through which ghrelin is expected to pass during its processing. These observations led to the hypothesis that an acyl transferase of the MBOAT family could be involved in the acyl modification of ghrelin (Gutierrez et al., 2008; Yang et al., 2008). Like porcupine, all other MBOATs are believed to transfer only long-chain fatty acids of 16-18 carbons. Both teams discovered GOAT using slightly distinct approaches.

Gutierrez et al. (Gutierrez et al., 2008) beneficiated from the capacity of the human medullary thyroid carcinoma cells to produce ghrelin, allowing them to identify the ghrelin acyl transferase. Indeed, that cell line was used to perform gene-silencing of twelve candidate sequences. The selection was based on their similarity to known acyl transferases sequences, the presence of a human homologue, and the unknown function of the gene. Gene-silencing experiments revealed the knock-down of only one candidate gene encoding an uncharacterized protein containing structural motifs reminiscent of the MBOAT acyl transferase family. The authenticity of the human gene identified was verified using RT-PCR and 5' RACE reactions. The predicted protein encoded by the gene was named GOAT. Transient transfections of the GOAT cDNA were performed to assess the octanoylation of ghrelin. Mutation of the MBOAT-conserved histidine residue in position 338 of GOAT abolished the octanoylation of ghrelin. GOAT was also shown to acylate ghrelin with fatty acid ranging from C7 to C12.

Yang et al. (Yang et al., 2008) also sought for a cell line capable of octanoylating ghrelin in order to transfect cells with ghrelin cDNA and look at subsequent acylated ghrelin production by Western blot analysis. To confirm the presence of ghrelin in rat insulinoma Ins-1 cells, further transfections were performed using mutant forms of ghrelin cDNA encoding mutant forms of prepro-ghrelin with amino acid substitution at or near the arginine in position 28. To determine if any of the sixteen MBOATs, identified as containing 11 catalytic domains bearing conserved sequences, was capable of producing acylated ghrelin, Ins-1 cells were transfected with the corresponding sixteen MBOATs cDNA. Only one MBOAT cDNA led to ghrelin production. Furthermore, mutation of either serine in position 3 of ghrelin or of the MBOAT-conserved histidine residue in position 338 of GOAT abolished ghrelin acylation by GOAT. GOAT appears to be specific for medium chain fatty acids like octanoate. Moreover, (^{3}H)octanoate labeling experiments indicated that ghrelin is octanoylated before it translocates to the Golgi where it is cleaved by prohormone convertase 1/3 to form mature ghrelin. This suggested that GOAT is located in the endoplasmic reticulum.

GOAT, sharing structural similarities with members of the MBOAT family of acyl transferases (Chamoun et al., 2001; Hoffmann et al., 2000; Liang et al., 2004), is a highly hydrophobic protein with eight postulated membrane-spanning helices. Sequence conservation of GOAT across vertebrates and its tissue coexpression with ghrelin are consistent with the identification of ghrelin octanoylated forms in vertebrates. The presumed donor for octanoylation is octanoyl-CoA. However, how octanoyl Co-A gets into the endoplasmic reticulum lumen remains unclear. GOAT could possibly bind octanoyl CoA, and due to its hydrophobic nature, and allow transmembrane octanoylation of ghrelin

An in vitro biochemical assay for GOAT activity was recently developed using membranes from insect cells expressing mouse GOAT and purified recombinant pro-ghrelin as the acyl acceptor (Yang et al., 2008). Using that assay, it was shown that GOAT recognizes several amino acids in pro-ghrelin surrounding the octanoylation site on serine-3. Glycine-1, serine-3 and phenylalanine-4 represent the crucial residues for the GOAT activity, in consistency with their strict conservation among all vertebrate ghrelins (Kojima and Kangawa, 2008). A pentapeptide, corresponding to the first five N-terminal amino acids of ghrelin with its C-terminal end amidated, competitively inhibited GOAT activity and was used as a substrate by GOAT. A more efficient inhibition was obtained when the pentapeptide contained an octanoyl group linked to serine-3 by an amide linkage, instead of an ester linkage. A similar pentapeptide, but containing an alanine-3, instead of serine-3, also inhibited GOAT, was not used as a substrate by the enzyme. These data suggest that GOAT is subjected to end-product inhibition (Yang et al., 2008).

Very recently, it was shown that gastric GOAT mRNA levels were similar in fed and 48h-fasted rats, and that exogenous leptin administration to fasted rats markedly increased GOAT mRNA levels (Gonzalez et al., 2008). These data indicated that during fasting, low leptin levels prevent an increase in GOAT mRNA levels, and that GOAT is a leptin-regulated gene. Long-term chronic malnutrition (21 days) led to an increase in GOAT mRNA levels (Gonzalez et al., 2008) and this could represent the underlying mechanism responsible for increased acylated ghrelin levels in chronic undernutrition, such as anorexia nervosa (Soriano-Guillen et al., 2004).

GOAT knockout mice are therefore a valuable tool to determine the physiological consequences of a specific deficiency in acylated ghrelin. Moreover, GOAT represents a useful target for the development of anti-obesity and/or anti-diabetes drugs (Gualillo et al., 2008). Much work remains to be done to fully understand how GOAT fits into the control of energy homeostasis.

4. GHRELIN-RELATED PEPTIDES

Ghrelin peptides can be classified into two group based on the length, ghrelin 1-28 and ghrelin 1-27, or into four groups based on the nature of the acyl group on Ser3 (non-acylated, octanoylated, decanoylated, decenoylated). Although the major active form is octanoylated ghrelin 1-28, decanoyl ghrelin 1-28, decenoyl ghrelin 1-28, octanoyl ghrelin 1-27 and decanoyl ghrelin 1-27 were also found in the stomach and in plasma (Hosoda et al., 2003) (figure 3). In the stomach, decanoyl ghrelin 1-28, decanoyl ghrelin 1-27, octanoyl ghrelin 1-27 and decenoyl ghrelin 1-28 represent respectively only 17%, 8%, 17% and 8% of the biologically active ghrelin. In contrast to rat stomach, human stomach is devoid of des-Gln14 ghrelin (Hosoda et al., 2000b). It must be noted that the major circulating form of ghrelin is the des-acyl ghrelin, the so called biologically inactive form of ghrelin, at least on GHS-R 1a (Hosoda et al., 2000a). Besides, in human plasma, C-ghrelin also circulates at higher concentrations than octanoyl ghrelin (Pemberton et al., 2003).

A novel peptide derived from the carboxy-terminal of pro-ghrelin was identified in rat stomach and named obestatin, due to its appetite-suppressing potential (Zhang et al., 2005). Obestatin is a 23 AA peptide that is amidated, notably due to the presence of C-terminal Gly-Lys motif following the C-terminal AA of obestatin (Zhang et al., 2005). During the purification of obestatin from rat stomach, an obestatin truncated peptide was identified as containing the last 13 C-terminal AA of obestatin and named obestatin 11-23 (Zhang et al., 2005).

Ghrelin was identified in various mammalian species such as human (Kojima et al., 1999), rat (Kojima et al., 1999), mouse (Tanaka et al., 2001) (figure 4). In mammals, the first 10 N-terminal AA are identical and the acylation of Ser3 result principally in an octanoylation. Human ghrelin is identical to rat ghrelin, except for two AA in position 11 and

12. In ovines and bovines, ghrelin is composed of 27 AA, rather than 28, and is devoid of Gln14 similarly to rat des-Gln14-ghrelin.

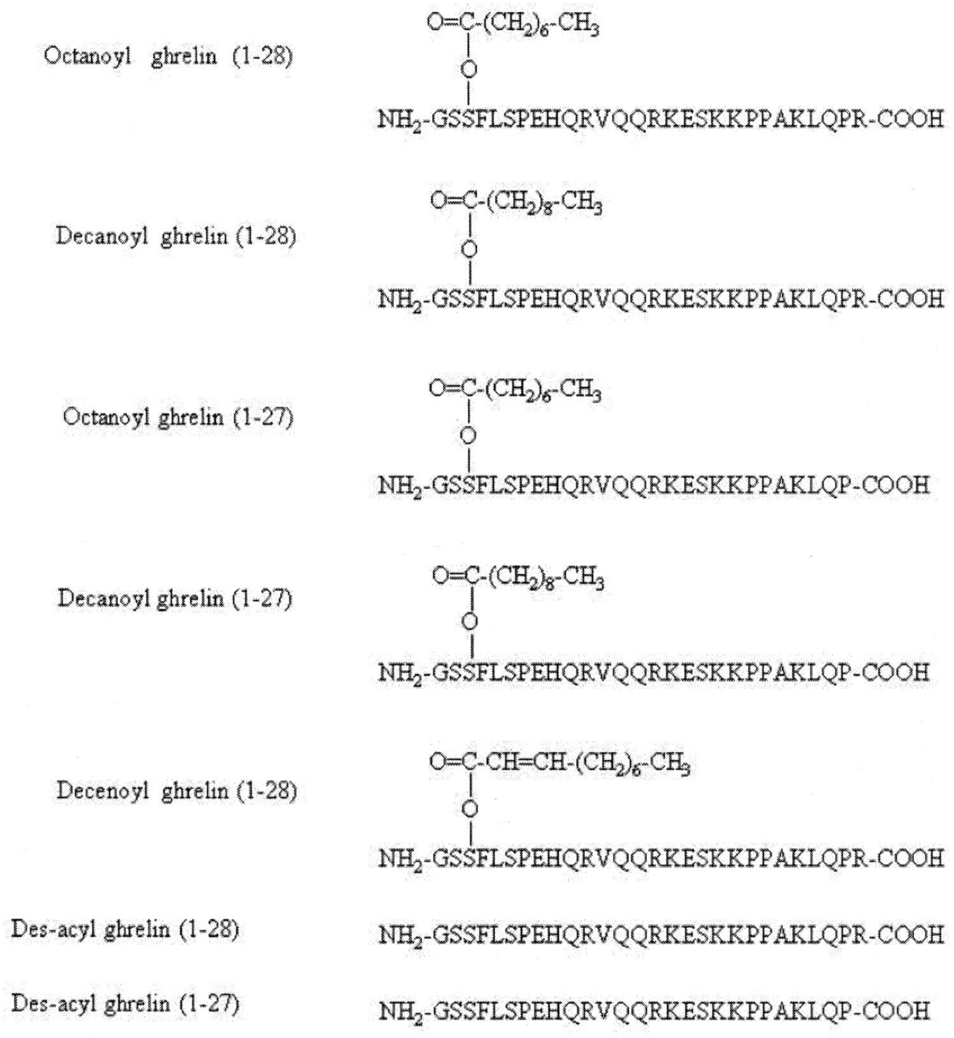

Octanoyl ghrelin (1-28)

$$O=C-(CH_2)_6-CH_3$$
$$|$$
$$O$$
$$|$$
NH$_2$-GSSFLSPEHQRVQQRKESKKPPAKLQPR-COOH

Decanoyl ghrelin (1-28)

$$O=C-(CH_2)_8-CH_3$$
$$|$$
$$O$$
$$|$$
NH$_2$-GSSFLSPEHQRVQQRKESKKPPAKLQPR-COOH

Octanoyl ghrelin (1-27)

$$O=C-(CH_2)_6-CH_3$$
$$|$$
$$O$$
$$|$$
NH$_2$-GSSFLSPEHQRVQQRKESKKPPAKLQP-COOH

Decanoyl ghrelin (1-27)

$$O=C-(CH_2)_8-CH_3$$
$$|$$
$$O$$
$$|$$
NH$_2$-GSSFLSPEHQRVQQRKESKKPPAKLQP-COOH

Decenoyl ghrelin (1-28)

$$O=C-CH=CH-(CH_2)_6-CH_3$$
$$|$$
$$O$$
$$|$$
NH$_2$-GSSFLSPEHQRVQQRKESKKPPAKLQPR-COOH

Des-acyl ghrelin (1-28)   NH$_2$-GSSFLSPEHQRVQQRKESKKPPAKLQPR-COOH

Des-acyl ghrelin (1-27)   NH$_2$-GSSFLSPEHQRVQQRKESKKPPAKLQP-COOH

Figure 3. Ghrelin forms identified from human stomach.

Very recently, ghrelin and des-acyl ghrelin were shown to be phosphorylated by protein kinase C on the Ser in position 18. While ghrelin and des-acyl ghrelin bind to phosphatidylcholine:phosphoserine sucrose-loaded vesicles in a phosphatidylserine-dependent manner, this binding capacity was greatly lowered when the peptides were phosphorylated. A possible explanation is the disruption of the amphipathic helix formed by about two third of the C-terminal part of the peptide (Dehlin et al., 2008). Further investigations will be required to determine if phosphorylation can occur in cells under specific conditions, and if so what would be the impact of such phosphorylation on the subcellular localization and function of the peptide.

Species	Sequence	Length
Equus-Caballus	GSSFLSPEHQKVQHRKSKGPAKLKR	28
Sus-Scrofa	GSSFLSPEHQKVQQRKSKGAAKLKP	28
Ailuropoda-Melanoleuca	GSSFLSPEHQKVQ-RKSKGPAKLQ	27
Felis-Catus	GSSFLSPEHQKVQQRKSKGPAKLQP	28
Homo-Sapiens	GSSFLSPEHQRVQQRKESKKPPAKLQP	28
Hylobates-Lar	GSSFLSPEHQRVQQRKESKKPPAKLQP	28
Pongo-Pygmaeus	GSSFLSPEHQRVQQRKESKKPPAKLQP	28
Pan-Troglodytes	GSSFLSPEHQRVQQRKESKKPPAKLQP	28
Erinaceus-Europaeus	GSSFLSPEHQRVQQRKSKGPAKLQP	28
Echinops-Telfairi	GSSFLSPEHQRVQQRKSKGPAKLQP	28
Dasypus-Novemcinctus	GSSFLSPEHQRVQHRKSKGPAKLQP	28
Macaca-Mulatta	GSSFLSPEHQRAQQRKSKGPAKLQP	28
Macaca-Fuscata	GSSFLSPEHQRAQQRKSKGPAKLQP	28
Papio-Hamadryas	GSSFLSPEHQRAQQRKSKGPAKLQP	28
Aotus-Trivirgatus	GSSFLSPEHQRIQQRKSKGPAKLQP	28
Saimiri-Sciureus	GSSFLSPEHQRIQQRKSKGPAKLQP	28
Cebus-Apella	GSSFLSPEHQRMQQRKSKGPAKLQS	28
Loxodonta-Africana	GSSFLSPEKNKLQQRKSKGPAKLQP	28
Canis-Familiaris	GSSFLSPEHQKLQQRKSKGPAKLQP	28
Otolemur-Garnettii	GSSFLSPDHQKIQQRKSKGPAKLQP	28
Microcebus-Murinus	GSSFLSPEHQKTQQRKSKGPAKLQP	28
Meriones-Unguiculatus	GSSFLSPEHQKTQQRKSKGPAKLQP	28
Mus-Musculus	GSSFLSPEHQKAQQRKSKGPAKLQP	28
Myotis-Lucifugus	GSSFLSPEHQKAQQRKDAKGPAKLQP	28
Rattus-Norvegicus	GSSFLSPEHQKAQQRKSKGPAKLQP	28
Tupaia-Belangeri	GSSFLSPEHQKAQQRKSKGPAKLQP	28
Ochotona-Princeps	GSSFLSPEHQKAQQRKAKGPAKLQP	28
Bubalus-Bubalis	GSSFLSPEHQKLQ-RKPKGSGRLKP	27
Capra-Hircus	GSSFLSPEHQKLQ-RKPKGSGRLKP	27
Cervus-Elaphus	GSSFLSPEHQKLQ-RKPKGSGRLKP	27
Odocoileu-Hemionu	GSSFLSPEHQKLQ-RKPKGSGRLKP	27
Odocoileus-Virginianus	GSSFLSPEHQKLQ-RKPKGSGRLKP	27
Ovis-Aries	GSSFLSPEHQKLQ-RKPKGSGRLKP	27
Rangifer-Tarandus	GSSFLSPEHQKLQ-RKPKGSGRLKP	27
Alces-Alces	GSSFLSPDHQKLQ-RKPKGSGRLKP	27
Bos-Taurus	GSSFLSPEHQKLQ-RKAKGSGRLKP	27
Kogia-Brevicep	GSSFLSPEHQKLQ-RKAKGSGRLKP	27
Monodelphis-Domestica	GSSFLSPEHPKTQ-RKTKGSVKLQP	27
Oryctolagus-Cuniculus	GSSFLSPEHQKAQQKDAKGPARLQP	28
Gallus-Gallus	GSSFLSPTYKNIQQKDTRKPTARLHR	28

Figure 4. Amino acid sequence homologies among mammalian ghrelin sequences. Multiple sequence alignment of 40 mammalian ghrelin peptide sequences, available to date in the two public sequence databases sets (*Ensembl* release 50 and *NCBI* Nucleotide). Dark gray shading are residues sharing 100% conserved identity (40/40 sequences), light gray shaded residues share at least 80% identity (i.e. identity in at least 32/40 sequences). Note that the amino terminal hepta-peptides is conserved with 100% identity. Every 10 amino acids are indicated by *. Peptide lengths are indicated in the rightmost column.

5. HUMAN GHRELIN RECEPTOR GENE STRUCTURE

The ghrelin receptor, termed GHS-R, belongs to the family of G-protein coupled receptor, characterized by seven transmembrane helix domains (Howard et al., 1996). GHS-R gene is located on chromosome 3 (3q26.2) and is composed of two exons separated by one intron. Exon 1 codes for the extracellular amino-terminal domain through to the fifth transmembrane helix of the GHSR. Exon 2 codes then for the sixth transmembrane helix through to the carboxy-terminal segment (McKee et al., 1997). GHS-R has two variants resulting from alternative splicing of its mRNA: GHS-R 1a and GHS-R 1b. GHS-R 1a mRNA, encoded by the two exons and from which the intron is excised by splicing, codes for a protein of 366 AA comprising the seven transmembrane helix domains. GHS-R 1b mRNA is coded only by exon 1 and and followed by the non-excised intron. Thereby, GHS-R 1b codes for a protein of 289 AA comprising only five transmembrane helix domains. The nucleotide sequences are identical for AA 1 to 265, thereafter GHS-R 1b mRNA nucleotide sequence is distinct from that of GHS-R 1a mRNA as of codon Leu265 and codes only for 24 additional AA using an alternative stop codon (McKee et al., 1997). Since the coupling of G-protein coupled receptor with the G-protein involves the third intracellular loop, GHS-R 1b is unable to couple to G-proteins. Though there is no obvious role for such a truncated receptor, it has recently been proposed to act as a dominant negative mutant of GHS-R 1a by heterodimerization (Leung et al., 2007), attenuating the latter's constitutive activity. GHS-R 1b was also detected in PBMCs, in the absence of the functional GHS-R 1a (Mager et al., 2008).

GHS-R 1a is not obviously related to known families of G-protein coupled receptors, although it is often included in a small family of the class A receptors for small polypeptides comprising the motilin receptor (52% homology), neurotensin receptor-1 and neurotensin receptor-2 (33-35% homology), neuromedin receptor-1 and neuromedin receptor-2 (± 30% homology), and the orphan GPR39 (27-32% homology) (McKee et al., 1997; Tan et al., 1998). Concerning GPR39, it must be cautioned that it was at first described as the receptor for obestatin (Zhang et al., 2005). Nevertheless, recent controversy over obestatin binding to GPR39 has lead to the conclusion that GPR39 is ultimately not the obestatin receptor (Lauwers et al., 2006; Tremblay et al., 2007).

Likewise, it must be noted that the scavenger receptor CD36, involved in the endocytosis of the pro-atherogenic oxidized low-density lipoproteins, is a pharmacologically and structurally distinct receptor for peptidyl GHSs, but not for ghrelin (Bodart et al., 1999; Bodart et al., 2002).

6. ACTIVATION MECHANISM OF GHRELIN RECEPTOR

Binding of GHSs and ghrelin to GHS-R 1a leads to phospholipase C activation. Phospholipase C activation induces the hydrolysis of phosphatidylinositol 4,5-biphosphate and the subsequent formation of diacylglycerol and inositol 1,4,5-trisphosphate. Diacylglycerol activates protein kinase C and inositol 1,4,5-trisphosphate induces a calcium release from the endoplasmic reticulum (Smith et al., 1996). Des-acyl ghrelin also seems to bind to GHS-R 1a but at very high concentration (micromolar range) (Gauna et al., 2007).

Neither ghrelin, nor GHSs, bind to GHS-R 1b, suggesting that GHS-R 1b is pharmacologically inactive (Howard et al., 1996). However, when GHS-R 1b is coexpressed with GHS-R 1a in HEK293 cells, the signal transduction of GHS-R 1a was decreased, suggesting that GHS-R 1b could form an heterodimer with GHS-R 1a (Chan and Cheng, 2004).

GHS-R 1a possesses constitutive activity (Holst et al., 2003) that might be mandatory for proper growth and development of the human body (Holst and Schwartz, 2006). In HEK293 cells, GHS-R 1a possesses constitutive activity that is about 50% of the maximal agonist-induced activity (Holst et al., 2003; Holst et al., 2006). The molecular basis for the constitutive activity appears to be related to three aromatic residues located in the sixth and seventh transmembrane helix domains that would promote the formation of a hydrophobic core between helices 6 and 7. This would ensure proper docking of the extracellular end of the seventh transmembrane helix domain into the sixth transmembrane domain, mimicking agonist activation and stabilizing the receptor in its active conformation (Holst et al., 2004). However, a naturally occurring non-conservative mutation, A204E, occurring surprisingly in the second extracellular loope, that eliminates the constitutive activity without impairing stimulation by ghrelin (Holliday et al., 2007; Pantel et al., 2006).

7. GENETIC POLYMORPHISM OF GHRELIN AND GHRELIN RECEPTOR

Interestingly, both ghrelin and its receptor (GHSR) genes are located on chromosome 3, and the regions have been linked to obesity (Kissebah et al., 2000; Yeh et al., 2005). A large number of polymorphisms have been identified in the ghrelin gene, not counting the transcript and splice variants described above. Several are found in the coding region of ghrelin, however a large number are in non-coding regions or in prepro-ghrelin but outside the ghrelin coding region.

Polymorphisms of both ghrelin and its receptor GHSR 1a have been studied in a wide series of disorders and pathologies, such as in obesity (Bing et al., 2005; Dardennes et al., 2007; Hinney et al., 2002; Korbonits et al., 2002; Larsen et al., 2005; Martin et al., 2008; Miraglia et al., 2004; Ukkola et al., 2001; Vivenza et al., 2004; Wang et al., 2004), in particular the Leu72Met polymorphism in prepro-ghrelin was associated with early onset of obesity (Korbonits et al., 2002; Miraglia et al., 2004; Ukkola et al., 2001; Ukkola et al., 2002). Another polymorphism, 3056T>C single nucleotide polymorphism (SNP), has been reported to be correlated, in Japanese women, to higher body mass index, fat mass and eating disorders (Ando et al., 2007). However, other studies yielded conflicting results (Bing et al., 2005; Hinney et al., 2002; Jo et al., 2005; Larsen et al., 2005). Another example of conflicting results, with respect to weight, is the Arg51Gln allele, for which a positive association was found (Ukkola et al., 2001), but no correlation was found in another study (Hinney et al., 2002). These authors also found that a frameshift mutation leading to ghrelin haplo-insufficiency was compatible with normal body weight. GH secretion was also studied in relation to short stature (height), as measured by IGF-1 and IGFBP-3 hepatic secretion in response to GH. A recent study showed lowered circulating levels of IGF-1 in ghrelin rs3755777 allele bearing subjects (Dossus et al., 2008), whereas decreased circulating levels of IGFBP-3 were correlated (though borderline) with the ghrelin rs2075356 SNP. Other studies, however, found no correlation (Ukkola et al., 2002; Vartiainen et al., 2004; Vivenza et al., 2004). On the other hand, 5 of the 15 alleles studied (Dossus et al., 2008) showed a correlation with height, whereas in a smaller study no significant association with genotype or haplotype were found with height, weight or body mass index (BMI) (Garcia et al., 2008). Likewise, a study of the Leu72Met, Gln90Leu and Arg51Gln proposed that ghrelin levels rather than ghrelin/obestatin polymorphism would play a role in GH deficiency and thus height (Zou et al., 2008). In contrast, the GHS-R 1a naturally occurring A204 mutation, leads to a loss of constitutive, activity, that decreases cell surface expression without impairing stimulation by ghrelin, and segregated with short stature in two unrelated families (Pantel et al., 2006). A correlation between Leu72Met and bing eating disorder was found (Monteleone et al., 2007), whereas no association of Leu72Met and Arg-51-Gln could be found with anorexia nervosa or bulimia nervosa (Monteleone et al., 2006). In contrast, the Leu72Met/Gln90Leu haplotype had an excess transmission in patients with anorexia nervosa (Dardennes et al., 2007). These authors invoke in the former study a lack of comparison between the clinical subtypes studied. However, they also argue, that ethnic and international variations in ghrelin gene polymorphism must be taken into account (Cellini et al., 2006; Miyasaka et al., 2006; Ukkola et al., 2002; Zou et al., 2008). Though, there is controversy as to the effects of ghrelin polymorphic variants on different disorders and pathologies, one must take into account the diversity of the subject panels used in the various studies, and the series of polymorphism investigated. The Leu72Met, as well other SNPs have been studied in relation to other disorders. The Leu72Met showed correlations with metabolic syndrome parameters, such as high-density-lipoproteins (HDL), triglycerides levels, blood pressure and increased risk for type 2 diabetes. However, in one report the levels of HDL/cholesterol were increased when compared to the Leu72Leu allele (Hubacek et al., 2007), whereas in another report it decreased in a study of older Amish (Steinle et al., 2005). Likewise, the risk factor was positively associated to ghrelin gene polymorphism in a Finnish study (Mager et al., 2006), and was not in a Korean study (Choi et al., 2006). Another study of 5 SNPs in exon 1, in introns and in the 3' untranslated region did not correlate with body fat percentage or serum lipid profiles (Martin et al., 2008). A GHS-R 1a polymorphism, rs2232165, has also been shown to be associated with alcohol-abuse (Landgren et al., 2008). Finally, ghrelin SNPs have been associated with various cancers, such as breast cancer (Dossus et al., 2008; Jeffery et al., 2005) and prostate cancer (Yeh et al., 2005).

In the light of an increasing body of data, displaying conflicting results, in the various areas investigated, a word of caution must be made regarding the polymorphisms in the prepro-ghrelin mRNA, outside of the ghrelin coding-region, e.g. Leu72Met. Indeed, these "mutated" sites may either affect proper processing of prepro-ghrelin, thereby potentially disrupting trafficking, posttranslational modification and secretion. However, most investigators did not see variations in circulating plasma levels. Though this may not be the best parameter, the acyl form is rapidly degraded in plasma and therefore plasma levels do not reflect local concentrations of the octanoylated form (De Vriese et al., 2004). Moreover, the recent discovery of novel peptides stemming from the prepro-ghrelin RNA (as discussed above), containing polymorphic differences studied previously, might have an impact on the cellular processing and physiological effects of these peptides, independently of ghrelin itself. Consequently, the study of prepro-ghrelin will link observed effects/correlations to ghrelin in a misleading manner; as the studies are conducted at the mRNA level and not at the protein(s) level. Clearly, in view of ghrelin's pleiotropic effects and the high level of complexity, in the ghrelin gene in terms of transcript variants, alternative splice variants, polymorphism, and multiple peptide products besides ghrelin, will require much more investigation and revisiting of previous studied areas. Furthermore, the polymorphic sites, thus far, described may affect the reverse strand transcript processing as well. Should the hypothesis that the anti-sense transcript harbor non-coding regulatory RNAs (Seim et al., 2007), such as microRNA, then such polymorphisms might alter considerably these regulatory molecules as well as potential target sequences on the sense strand. We speculate that these new findings will certainly open up future fascinating avenues of investigation in ghrelin gene expression and regulation.

8. Tissue Distribution of Ghrelin

In the digestive system, ghrelin is predominantly synthesized in the stomach (Ariyasu et al., 2001; Kojima et al., 1999). Five endocrine cell types have been identified in the gastric mucosa: enterochromaffin cells (EC), enterochromaffin-like cells (ECL), D cells, G cells and X/A like cells which respectively secrete serotonin, histamine, somatostatin, gastrin, GABA and ghrelin. Rat oxyntic cells display 60-70% of ECL cells, 20% of X/A-like cells, 2.5% of D-cells and 0-2% of EC and G cells. Human oxyntic endocrine cells display 30% of ECL cells, 20% of X/A-like cells, 22% of D-cells and 7% of EC and G cells (Simonsson et al., 1988; Solcia et al., 2000). X/A like cells are gastric endocrine cells located in the fundus (Date et al., 2000b; Rindi et al., 2002). They are round to ovoid cells, containing compact and dense secretory granules, located next to the capillary lumen, indicating ghrelin is secreted in an endocrine fashion into the plasma (Date et al., 2000b). Immunoreactive ghrelin cells have also been located in the duodenum, jejunum, ileum and colon (Date et al., 2000b; Hosoda et al., 2000a; Sakata et al., 2002). In the intestine, ghrelin concentration progressively decreases from the duodenum to the colon (Hosoda et al., 2000a). Circulating ghrelin arises in majority from the gastric mucosa and the intestine (Ariyasu et al., 2001; Krsek et al., 2002). In the endocrine pancreas, ghrelin-secreting cells have been colocalized with either glucagon in α-cells (Date et al., 2002b; Kageyama et al., 2005), or insulin in ß-cells (Volante et al., 2002), or in a new cell type called ϵ (Prado et al., 2004; Wierup et al., 2002; Wierup and Sundler, 2005). In the exocrine pancreas, ghrelin has been located to acinar cells (Lai et al., 2007).

In the central nervous system, ghrelin is found in low amounts (Hosoda et al., 2000a). However, neurons producing ghrelin have been identified in the arcuate nucleus of the hypothalamus, a region involved in the regulation of food intake (Kojima et al., 1999; Lu et al., 2002). Moreover, ghrelin has also been identified in a particular area in the hypothalamus. By sending their efferent fibers, ghrelin-containing neurons could stimulate the release of peptides from neurons containing neuropeptide Y (NPY) and the agouti-related protein (AGRP), orexins, pro-opiomelanocortin (POMC), and cocaïn- and amphetamine-regulated transcript (CART) (Cowley et al., 2003). Pituitary also contains ghrelin (Korbonits et al., 2001b; Korbonits et al., 2001a). In vivo studies indicated that ghrelin stimulates GH secretion, suggesting that somatotropic cells are target cells for ghrelin (Date et al., 2000a; Takaya et al., 2000). Furthermore, in the rat, ghrelin was found in cells secreting prolactin, GH, and thyroid stimulating hormone (Caminos et al., 2003).

Ghrelin is also expressed in other tissues such as in kidneys, adrenal glands, thyroid, breast, ovary, placenta, testis, prostate, liver, gallbladder, lung, skeletal muscle, myocardium, skin (Ghelardoni et al., 2006; Gnanapavan et al., 2002).

Studies related to tissue expression of obestatin remain limited. Obestatin expression was reported in the stomach, duodenum, jejunum, colon, myenteric plexus, pancreas, spleen, testis, cerebral cortex (Chanoine et al., 2006; Dun et al., 2006; Zhang et al., 2005; Zhao et al., 2008). In the stomach, most of obestatin-producing cells are distributed in the basal part of the oxyntic mucosa, and are with prepro-ghrelin-producing cells more numerous than ghrelin-producing cells (Zhao et al., 2008). In the pancreas, obestatin is present in the periphery of the islets, with a distribution distinct from that of α-cells, ß-cells, and δ-cells (Zhao et al., 2008).

9. GHRELIN IN CIRCULATION

Following surgical gastric mucosa removal, circulating ghrelin concentration is drastically reduced by about 80% in rat (Dornonville de la Cour et al., 2001) and human (Ariyasu et al., 2001; Jeon et al., 2004). Human plasma ghrelin-immunoreactivity consists of more than 90% of des-acyl ghrelin (Patterson et al., 2005). C-ghrelin also circulates at higher concentrations than octanoyl ghrelin in human plasma (Pemberton et al., 2003). It is presently not yet well understood if both ghrelin and des-acyl ghrelin, which are present in the stomach, are both secreted into the bloodstream via the same or differently regulated pathway(s). In rat stomach, ghrelin is degraded by deacylation, as well as by N-terminal proteolysis (De Vriese et al., 2004; Shanado et al., 2004), and lysophospholipase I was identified as a ghrelin deacylation enzyme (Shanado et al., 2004). Several mechanisms could account for the large presence of des-acyl ghrelin in the circulation: shorter half-life of ghrelin compared to des-acyl ghrelin (Akamizu et al., 2005) and plasma ghrelin deacylation (De Vriese et al., 2004; Hosoda et al., 2004). In serum, ghrelin desoctanoylation is achieved in human by butyrylcholinesterase and other esterase(s), such as platelet-activating factor acetylhydrolase, and in rat by carboxylesterase (De Vriese et al., 2004; De Vriese et al., 2007). Although paraoxonase was suggested to also participate to ghrelin deacylation (Beaumont et al., 2003), this hypothesis was not confirmed by us due to the lack of effect of EDTA on ghrelin deacylation in human serum and the negative correlation between des-acyl ghrelin and paraoxonase activity (De Vriese et al., 2004). Due to ghrelin degradation by serum, it is difficult to accurately determine the ghrelin level and consequently its physiological and pathophysiological roles. Therefore, we suggested that addition of inhibitors of esterases and proteases to blood collected samples would be critical to ensure ghrelin stability.

It is interesting to note that butyrylcholinesterase knockout mice fed with a normal standard 5% fat diet had normal body weight, while mice fed with high-fat diet (11% fat) became obese. Since the obesity could not be explained by increased ghrelin, caloric intake, or decreased exercise, it is hypothesized that butyrylcholinesterase plays a role in fat utilization (Li et al., 2008).

While des-acyl ghrelin mostly circulates as a free peptide, the majority of circulating acyl ghrelin is bound to larger molecules. In particular, ghrelin was found to bind to lipoproteins (Beaumont et al., 2003; De Vriese et al., 2007). The presence of the acyl group is necessary for ghrelin interaction with triglyceride-rich lipoproteins and low-density lipoprotein but not high-density lipoproteins and very high-density lipoproteins. Ghrelin interacts via its N- and C-terminal parts with high-density lipoproteins and very high-density lipoproteins. These data suggest that, whereas triglyceride-rich lipoproteins mostly transport acylated ghrelin, high-density lipoproteins and very high-density lipoproteins transport both ghrelin and des-acyl ghrelin (De Vriese et al., 2007).

10. GHRELIN- AND GHRELIN RECEPTOR-NULL MICE PHENOTYPES

The phenotype of ghrelin knockout mice is indistinguishable from that of wild-type mice. Indeed, no differences were noticed concerning the size, growth rate, body composition, food intake, reproduction, bone density, activity, development, organs weight, tissular pathology (De Smet et al., 2006; Sun et al., 2003; Wortley et al., 2004). Food intake of ghrelin knockout mice was similar to wild-type mice in response to starvation and to ghrelin injection. Though, in old ghrelin knockout mice interruption of the normal light/dark cycle triggers additional food intake (De Smet et al., 2006). Pre- and post- prandial concentrations of glucose, insulin, leptin and GH were similar.

Ghrelin knockout mice fed for six weeks with a high fat diet displayed a decrease in the respiratory quotient and in the fat mass, independently of any body weight change (Wortley et al., 2004). However, male ghrelin knockout mice submitted to a continuous high-fat diet three weeks after weaning (at approximately six weeks of age) are protected from the rapid weight gain occurring in wild-type mice (Wortley et al., 2005). Very recently, it was shown that congenic adult ghrelin knockout mice submitted to either a positive (high-fat diet) or negative (caloric restriction) energy balance displayed similar body weight as wild-type littermates (Sun et al., 2008). These contradictory data could be explained by differences in the mouse genetic backgrounds and/or the moment at which the high-fat diet was given to the animals. Further studies will be necessary to define the role of ghrelin in preventing or not preventing diet-induced obesity or weight gain after weight loss.

Ghrelin could modulate the type of metabolic substrate that is used preferentially to maintain energy balance, particularly under a high fat diet. These data are in agreement with the observed decreased use of fat in response to ghrelin administration in adult rats (Tschop et al., 2000). Furthermore, the lack of modification body weight in ghrelin-null mice as in NPY- or AGRP-null mice, and in NPY- and AGRP-null mice, strongly suggest the existence of compensatory mechanisms (Erickson et al., 1996; Herzog, 2003).

GHS-R knockout mice displayed a slightly smaller size, without any modification in appetite, food intake and body composition. Their ghrelin, insulin and leptin levels in response to starvation were similar to wild-type mice. In response to ghrelin injection, GHS-R-null mice do not release GH and do not increase their food intake, indicating that these effects are mediated by the GHS-R (Sun et al., 2004). A similar phenotype has been observed in transgenic rats expressing an antisense GHS-R mRNA, thereby attenuating GHS-R protein expression in the arcuate nucleus, also indicating that the GHS-R was involved in the regulation of GH secretion and food intake (Shuto et al., 2002). More recently, it was shown that GHS-R-null mice eat less food, metabolize more fat, become less adipose, and are more insulin-sensitive (Zigman et al., 2005). These latter data are consistent with the fact that ghrelin-null mice resist weight gain induced by early exposure to high fat diets (Wortley et al., 2005), but not with the fact that congenic adult knockout mice for GHS-R are not resisting diet-induced obesity or weight gain after weight loss (Sun et al., 2008). Interestingly, when fed with a standard chow diet, GHS-R and ghrelin double knockout mice display decreased body weight, increased energy expenditure, and increased motor activity (Pfluger et al., 2008).

Both ghrelin and GHS-R knockout mice submitted to caloric restriction displayed lower blood glucose levels, suggesting that the primary function of ghrelin in adult mice is to modulate glucose sensing and insulin sensitivity (Sun et al., 2008). This hypothesis was supported by the fact that GHS-R knockout mice fed with high-fat diet had several fold greater insulin sensitivity, no hepatic steatosis, and lower total cholesterol (Longo et al., 2008).

11. PHYSIOLOGICAL FUNCTIONS OF GHRELIN IN FEEDING

Appetite and Food Intake

The control of food intake is under the control of complex physiological mechanisms. Food intake is regulated by the hypothalamus but also directly influenced by gastrointestinal peptides, which respond to nutritional status and body composition. To defend against starvation, the organism replies in an integrative fashion using central brain centers, gastrointestinal peptides and adipose-derived signals (Baynes et al., 2006). In response to food intake, the concentrations of plasma glucose, free fatty acids and other nutrients increase, leading to hormones release. These hormones act on the tractus solitary nucleus, and on the arcuate nucleus of the hypothalamus to regulate the appetite and the energy metabolism at short and long terms. The arcuate nucleus of the hypothalamus contains two neuronal populations involved in the control of appetite: neurons synthesizing the neuropeptide Y (NPY) and agouti-related protein (AGRP) (their activation stimulates appetite) and neurons containing pro-opiomelanocortin (POMC), melanocortin (α-MSH) and cocaine- and amphetamine-regulated transcript (CART) (their activation inhibits appetite) (Ramos et al., 2005).

Intracerebroventricular, intravenous, or subcutaneous administration of ghrelin to rats leads to stimulation of food intake and decrease of energy expenditure, accounting for body weight increase (Kamegai et al., 2001; Nakazato et al., 2001; Shintani et al., 2001; Tschop et al., 2000; Wren et al., 2001). Intravenous ghrelin administration of ghrelin in humans also increases appetite and stimulates food intake (Wren et al., 2001). During fasting, before the onset of the meal, plasma ghrelin levels increase. After feeding, plasma ghrelin levels decrease strongly after 30 minutes (Cummings et al., 2001; Tschop et al., 2001). In fasting subjects, ghrelin levels display a circadian pattern similar to that described in people eating three meals per day (Natalucci et al., 2005). The preprandial increase and the postprandial decrease of plasma ghrelin levels strongly suggest that ghrelin might serve as a signal for meal initiation. Recently it has been demonstrated that the timing of ghrelin peaks is related to habitual meal patterns and may rise in anticipation of eating rather than eliciting feeding (Frecka and Mattes, 2008).

In contrast to ghrelin, most of the orexigenic peptides as NPY, AGRP, orexins, melanin-concentrating hormone (MCH) and galanin stimulate food intake when centrally administrated but not when peripherally administrated. Ghrelin is the only circulating hormone that stimulates appetite after systemic administration (table 1).

Among the anorexigenic peptides, several are synthesized in the hypothalamus, such as α-MSH, cocaine-and amphetamine-regulated transcript (CART), or corticotrophin-releasing hormone (CRH). Others are synthesized in endocrine cells of the gastrointestinal tractus, such as cholecystokinin (CCK), gastrin-related peptide (GRP), glucagon-like peptides (GLP-1 and GLP-2), pancreatic polypeptide (PP) and peptide YY (PYY). Leptin is synthesized in adipose tissue (table 1).

Table 1. Orexigenic and anorexigenic peptides

Orexigenic peptides	Anorexigenic peptides
Ghrelin	Melanocortin (α-MSH)
Neuropeptide Y (NPY)	Cocaïne- and amphetamine-regulated transcript (CART)
Agouti-related protein (AGRP)	Corticotropin-releasing hormone (CRH)
Melanin-concentrating hormone (MCH)	Cholecystokin (CCK)
Orexin A	Gastrin-related peptide (GRP)
Orexin B	Glucagon-like peptide 1 (GLP-1)
Galanin	Glucagon-like peptide 1 (GLP-2)
	Pancreatic polypeptide (PP)
	Peptide YY (PYY)
	Leptin

Mechanisms of Appetite Stimulation and Food Intake Control

Neurons expressing ghrelin have been identified in the arcuate nucleus of the hypothalamus, and in a previously uncharacterized group of neurons adjacent to the third ventricle between the dorsal, ventral, paraventricular, and arcuate hypothalamic nuclei. These neurons send efferents onto neurons producing NPY, AGRP, POMC, and CRH (Cowley et al., 2003). Ghrelin stimulates appetite and food intake through two different pathways:

1. Central Pathway

Ghrelin stimulates the activity of NPY/AGRP neurons (Cowley et al., 2003). In rats, intracerebroventricular injection of ghrelin induces overexpression of NPY and AGRP mRNAs (Kamegai et al., 2001). Inhibition of endogenous NPY and AGRP by anti-NPY and anti-AGRP antibodies, and by antagonists for Y1 and Y5 receptors abolished ghrelin-induced feeding (Nakazato et al., 2001). Similarly, in NPY or AGRP null-mice, ghrelin-induced feeding is weakly attenuated, but completely abolished in mice lacking both NPY and AGRP (Chen et al., 2004). Ablation of the NPY/AGRP neurons in mice completely suppress the feeding response to ghrelin (Luquet et al., 2007). In rats, peripheral injection of ghrelin also activates the dorsomedial hypothalamic nucleus, which is innervated by projections from other brain areas like NPY/AGRP fibers arising from the arcuate nucleus (Kobelt et al.,

2008). In NPY neurons, ghrelin interacts with the GHS-R and increases intracellular calcium via mechanisms depending on phospholipase C and adenylate cyclase-protein kinase A pathways (Kohno et al., 2007; Kohno et al., 2008). In humans, ghrelin increases circulating NPY levels (Coiro et al., 2006). All these data indicate that ghrelin activates hypothalamic NPY/AGRP neurons, stimulating the production of NPY and AGRP and therefore increasing food intake.

Intracerebroventricular administration of ghrelin activates not only the ARC but also the paraventricular nucleus and the lateral hypothalamus, including in orexin neurons (Scott et al., 2007). Ghrelin activates in vitro neurons expressing orexins (hypothalamic orexigenic neuropeptides) (Yamanaka et al., 2003). Appetite stimulation induced by ghrelin is inhibited in orexin-null mice and attenuated in mice pretreated with an anti-orexin antibody (Toshinai et al., 2003).

Peripheral ghrelin increases noradrenaline in the ARC and loss of neurons expressing dopamine β-hydroxylase abolishes ghrelin-induced feeding, suggesting that ghrelin stimulates food intake at least in part through the noradrenergic pathway (Date et al., 2006).

Ghrelin also inhibits POMC neurons, preventing the release of the anorexigenic peptide α-MSH (Riediger et al., 2003). CART inhibits food intake and is expressed by both vagal afferent and hypothalamic neurons. Ghrelin administration decreases CART expression in rat vagal afferents neurons (de Lartigue et al., 2007) while peripheral ghrelin blockade using a specific anti-ghrelin antibody increases the expression of CART in the hypothalamic paraventricular nucleus (Solomon et al., 2005).

Although GHS-R mRNA is expressed in the tuberomammilary nucleus, ghrelin does not affect histamine release, and increases food intake in histamine H(1)-receptor knock-out mice. Thus, ghrelin expresses its action in a histamine-independent manner (Ishizuka et al., 2006).

2. Vagal Pathway

Ghrelin may also stimulate appetite via the vagus nerve. Detection of the ghrelin receptor in afferent neurons of the rat and human nodose ganglion suggests that the vagus nerve may transmit ghrelin signal from the stomach to the brain (Burdyga et al., 2006; Sakata et al., 2003). In rats, blockade of the vagal afferent pathway, by vagotomy or perivagal application of an afferent neurotoxin, suppress ghrelin-induced feeding (Date et al., 2002a). In the same way, patients with vagotomy and oesophageal or gastric surgery are insensitive to the appetite stimulatory effect of ghrelin (le Roux et al., 2005; Takeno et al., 2004). Thus, through the activation of GHS-R on vagal afferent to the stomach, the signal induced by ghrelin may reach the nucleus of tractus solitarius, which communicates with the hypothalamus to increase food intake. However, intraperitoneal injection of ghrelin stimulates eating in rats with subdiaphragmatic vagal deafferentation, suggesting that the ghrelin signal does not involve vagal afferents (Arnold et al., 2006).

Regulation of Energy Homeostasis

In addition to its role in short-term regulation of food intake, ghrelin may also play a role in long-term body-weight regulation.

Plasma ghrelin levels are negatively correlated with BMI. Indeed, plasma ghrelin level is increased in anorexia nervosa and cachexia, and decreased in obesity. Moreover, ghrelin levels fluctuate in a compensatory manner to body weight variations (Soriano-Guillen et al., 2004). Ghrelin levels decrease with weight gain resulting from overfeeding (Williams et al., 2006), pregnancy (Palik et al., 2007), olanzapine treatment (Hosojima et al., 2006), or high fat diet (Otukonyong et al., 2005). Conversely, weight loss induces an increase of ghrelin levels. This effect is observed with weight loss resulting from food restriction (Purnell et al., 2007), long-term chronic exercise but not acute exercise (Kraemer and Castracane, 2007), cachectic states induced by anorexia nervosa (Soriano-Guillen et al., 2004), severe congestive heart failure (Nagaya et al., 2001), lung cancer (Shimizu et al., 2003), breast and colon cancers (Wolf et al., 2006). However, data on ghrelin levels after weight loss induced by gastric bypass surgery are controversial. Some studies found a decrease (Chan et al., 2006; Cummings et al., 2002b; Fruhbeck et al., 2004; Korner et al., 2006), no change (Couce et al., 2006; Mancini et al., 2006; Stenstrom et al., 2006) or an increase of ghrelin secretion (Haider et al., 2007; Mingrone et al., 2006; Stratis et al., 2006).

In vivo, chronic ghrelin administration induces adiposity (Tschop et al., 2000; Tsubone et al., 2005). Ghrelin increases body weight not only by stimulating food intake, but also by reducing energy expenditure, decreasing utilization of fat and increasing utilization of carbohydrates (Wortley et al., 2004). Ghrelin may thus influence adipocyte metabolism. In vitro, ghrelin stimulates differentiation of preadipocytes (Thompson et al., 2004), inhibits adipocyte apoptosis (Kim et al., 2004) and antagonizes lipolysis (Muccioli et al., 2004). Fat may be directed to either oxidation in skeletal muscle or brown adipose tissue, or to triglyceride storage in white adipose tissue. Chronic central infusion of ghrelin inhibits lipid oxidation and increases lipogenesis and triglyceride uptake in white adipocytes. An increase of the respiratory quotient indicates the decreased use of lipids for the generation of energy (Theander-Carrillo et al., 2006). Ghrelin has also been shown to shift food preference towards diets high in fat (Shimbara et al., 2004). Finally, ghrelin improves also lean body mass retention (Deboer et al., 2007). In elderly subjects and after diet-induced weight loss, ghrelin levels increase with reduction of fat-free mass, specially skeletal muscle mass, but not with changes in fat mass (Purnell et al., 2007). Recent data strongly support that ghrelin and des-acyl ghrelin modulate directly and positively adipogenesis and adipocyte function in rats, suggesting an important role for maintaining homeostasis (Giovambattista et al., 2008).

Ghrelin-null mice suggest a physiological role for ghrelin in energy homeostasis. The phenotype of ghrelin-null mice is similar to wild-type mice in terms of size, growth rate, food intake, body composition, reproduction, gross behavior, and tissue pathology (Sun et al., 2003). However, young ghrelin-null mice are protected from the weight gain induced by chronic exposure to a high-fat diet. These mice have lower adiposity, higher energy expenditure and locomotor activity. This suggests that ghrelin plays a role in excess dietary fat storage (Wortley et al., 2005; Wortley et al., 2004).

In patients with Prader-Willi syndrome (PWS), a genetic disorder characterized by mental retardation and hyperphagia leading to severe obesity, plasma ghrelin levels are higher than in healthy subjects and do not decrease after a meal (Cummings et al., 2002a; DelParigi et al., 2002). Other studies showed that ghrelin levels decreased postprandially in adult patients with PWS, but to a lesser extent than in obese and lean subjects (Gimenez-Palop et al., 2007; Paik et al., 2007). This lesser postprandial ghrelin suppression may be due to a blunted postprandial response of PYY, an anorexigenic peptide that decreases postprandial ghrelin levels. The low PYY levels could partially explain the high ghrelin levels observed in PWS (Gimenez-Palop et al., 2007). Interestingly, children (5 years of age and younger) with PWS have normal ghrelin levels. Since these children have not yet developed hyperphagia or excessive obesity, it suggests that ghrelin levels increase with the onset of hyperphagia (Erdie-Lalena et al., 2006; Haqq et al., 2008). In opposition with these data, Fiegerlova et al., showed that plasma ghrelin levels in children with PWS were elevated at any age, including the first years of life, thus preceding the development of obesity (Feigerlova et al., 2008). Thus, ghrelin may be responsible, at least partially, for the insatiable appetite and the obesity of these patients.

Relationships between Ghrelin and Obestatin

As opposed to ghrelin, which increases food intake and body weight gain, Zhan et al. reported that intraperitoneal or intracerebroventricular injection of obestatin to mice decreased food intake and body weight gain (Zhang et al., 2005). The initial observation that obestatin suppresses food intake in a time-dependent and dose-dependent manner ((Zhang et al., 2005) was reproduced in few studies ((Bresciani et al., 2006; Carlini et al., 2007; Green et al., 2007; Sibilia et al., 2006), but not by the majority of the studies carried out on rodents (Gourcerol et al., 2006; Gourcerol et al., 2007; Holst et al., 2007; Moechars et al., 2006; Nogueiras et al., 2007; Samson et al., 2007; Tremblay et al., 2007; Yamamoto et al., 2007; Zizzari et al., 2007). This issue in reproducing the effects of obestatin has been partially clarified by the existence of a U-shaped dose-response relationship between intraperitoneal administration of obestatin and suppression of food intake and body weight gain in rodent (Lagaud et al., 2007). The possible effect of obestatin on food intake might be secondary to an initial action in inhibiting thirst (Samson et al., 2007). However, if obestatin only minimally affects food intake, obestatin does not seem to modify energy metabolism in long-term administration to rats (Sibilia et al., 2006). In human, underweight anorectic and normal weight patients are characterized by higher plasma obestatin levels as well as an increased ghrelin to obestatin ratio, compared to obese patients. This suggests that obestatin might play a role in body weight regulation in these pathologies (Monteleone et al., 2008; Nakahara et al., 2008; Zamrazilova et al., 2008).

Relationships between Ghrelin and Leptin

Oppositely to ghrelin, leptin, a protein mainly produced by the adipose tissue, decreases food intake and increases energy expenditure to maintain the body fat stores. Fasting increases plasma ghrelin levels and decreases plasma leptin levels. Ghrelin expression in stomach cells, and plasma ghrelin levels are higher in leptin-null mice, the so called Ob/Ob mice which are hyperphagic and obese, than in healthy mice. However, ablation of ghrelin in Ob/Ob mice does not improve the obese phenotype, suggesting that the Ob/Ob phenotype is not a consequence of high ghrelin plasma levels (Sun et al., 2006).

After leptin administration, ghrelin concentration and food intake decrease, and energy expenditure increases (Nogueiras et al., 2008; Shintani et al., 2001). Ghrelin and leptin have thus opposite effects on food intake. Leptin activates POMC neurons, stimulating release of anorexigenic peptides α-MSH and CART, and inhibits NPY/AGRP neurons, preventing release of orexigenic peptides NPY and AGRP (Cowley et al., 2001). Moreover, inhibition of NPY/AGRP neurons induced by leptin prevents γ-aminobutyric acid (GABA) release, leading to activation of POMC neurons. Oppositely, ghrelin activates NPY neurons and increases GABA release, leading to POMC neurons inhibition (Cowley et al., 2003; Nogueiras et al., 2008). By activating NPY neurons, ghrelin increases intracellular calcium via mechanisms dependent on both the adenylate cyclase and phospholipase C (PLC) pathways. Leptin inhibits intracellular calcium increase induced by ghrelin via phosphatidylinositol 3-kinase- (PI3K) and phosphodiesterase 3- (PDE3) mediated pathways (Kohno et al., 2007). Therefore, leptin acts on hypothalamic neurons by inhibiting the effects of ghrelin. Finally, inverse variations of ghrelin and leptin levels are clearly critical for energy homeostasis regulation.

12. OTHER PHYSIOLOGICAL FUNCTIONS OF GHRELIN

The pleiotropic physiological functions of ghrelin are summarized in figure 5.

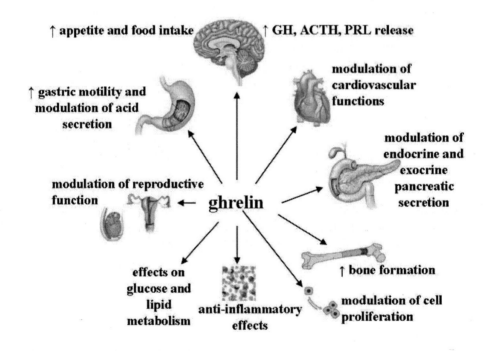

Figure 5. Pleiotropic biological functions of ghrelin. Major biological actions are summarized. GH: growth hormone; ACTH: adrenocorticotrophic hormone; PRL: prolactin.

Growth-Hormone Releasing Activity

Ghrelin strongly and dose-dependently stimulates growth hormone (GH) secretion, both in vivo and in vitro, in humans and animals by acting on GHS-R 1a present on pituitary somatotropic cells (Date et al., 2000a; Hataya et al., 2001; Malagon et al., 2003; Takaya et al.,

2000). To induce GH secretion from somatotropic cells, ghrelin activates the cGMP signal tranduction pathway but also requires activation of the nitric oxide synthase pathway (Rodriguez-Pacheco et al., 2008). Combined administration of ghrelin and GH-releasing hormone (GHRH) displays synergistic effects, rather than additive effects, on GH release. Ghrelin action on GH release also seems to be mediated by the hypothalamus as patients presenting organic lesions in the hypothalamus region are still able to release GH in response to ghrelin (Popovic et al., 2003). Apart from GH release, ghrelin stimulates adrenocorticotrophic hormone (ACTH), cortisol and prolactin (PRL) release ((Lengyel), 2006).

Des-acyl ghrelin is unable to stimulate GH secretion under physiological conditions, as it cannot bind to GHR-R. However, over-expression of des-acyl ghrelin in transgenic animals results in a small phenotype, maybe by modulation the GH-insulin growth factor 1 axis (Ariyasu et al., 2005).

Most studies have so far been unable to demonstrate that obestatin affects GH secretion in rats (Bresciani et al., 2006; Nogueiras et al., 2007; Samson et al., 2007; Yamamoto et al., 2007; Zhang et al., 2005). However, obestatin might inhibit ghrelin action on GH secretion under certain conditions, but this remains to be confirmed (Zizzari et al., 2007).

Gastrointestinal Functions

Ghrelin modulates gastric acid secretion. In anesthetized rats, intravenous administration of ghrelin dose-dependently increases gastric acid secretion (Asakawa et al., 2001; Masuda et al., 2000). This effect is abolished by vagotomy and by preliminary administration of atropine, suggesting that ghrelin might act through the vagus nerve (Masuda et al., 2000). The intracerebroventricular administration of ghrelin in anesthesized rats also stimulates gastric acid secretion (Date et al., 2001). However, other studies have shown that intracerebroventricular administration of ghrelin inhibited gastric acid secretion in conscious rats (Levin et al., 2005; Sibilia et al., 2002). Recently, it has been shown that simultaneous administration of ghrelin and gastrin induced a synergistic increase of gastric acid secretion (Fukumoto et al., 2008). Stimulatory or inhibitory effects of ghrelin on gastric acid secretion may depend on experimental conditions and models.

Ghrelin stimulates gastric motility by inducing the migrating motor complex and accelerating gastric emptying (Dass et al., 2003; Depoortere et al., 2005; Fujino et al., 2003; Peeters, 2003; Peeters, 2005). By its prokinetic effect, ghrelin is able to reverse gastric postoperative ileus in rat (Trudel et al., 2002).

Moreover, ghrelin exerts a gastroprotective effect against stress-, ethanol- and cysteamine-induced ulcers (Konturek et al., 2004; Sibilia et al., 2003). This effect depends on sensory nerve fiber integrity and is mediated by the nitric oxide system (Peeters, 2005).

Pancreatic Functions

Ghrelin seems to influence glucose metabolism. Acute ghrelin administration increases plasma glucose levels and amplifies the hyperglycemic effect of arginine. This effect could be due to glycogenolysis activation, indirectly by stimulation of catecholamine release, or directly by acting on hepatocytes where ghrelin might modulate neoglucogenesis. (Broglio et al., 2005; Gauna et al., 2005; Murata et al., 2002).

Ghrelin has been reported to influence the endocrine pancreatic function. Depending on the experimental conditions, ghrelin either stimulates (Adeghate and Ponery, 2002; Date et al., 2002b; Lee et al., 2002) or inhibits insulin secretion (Broglio et al., 2001; Colombo et al., 2003; Cui et al., 2008; Reimer et al., 2003). Salehi et al. suggest that the effect of ghrelin on insulin secretion depends on concentration: ghrelin might have an inhibitory effect at low concentratitis and a stimulating effect at high concentration (Salehi et al., 2004). Besides the direct effect of ghrelin on insulin secretion, a negative association between ghrelin secretion and insulin secretion has been observed (Ariyasu et al., 2001; Cummings et al., 2001; Saad et al., 2002; Toshinai et al., 2001). This could be explained by the increase of plasma ghrelin levels and the decrease of plasma insulin levels during fasting, but this does not involve a direct inhibitory effect on insulin secretion.

The effects of ghrelin on exocrine pancreatic function are also controversial. In rat pancreas, ghrelin was shown to inhibit pancreatic protein secretion or to increase protein output. These effects are indirect and may involve cholecystokinin and reflex vagal pathways (Jaworek, 2006).

Cardiovascular Functions

Ghrelin has diverse cardiovascular effects. In vitro, ghrelin inhibits apoptosis of cardiomyocytes and endothelial cells. Moreover, by inhibiting NF-κB activation in human endothelial cells and mononuclear cell adhesion, ghrelin might oppose inflammation of the cardiovascular system. Ghrelin exerts vasodilatory effects by an endothelium-independent mechanism. Administration of ghrelin decreases mean arterial pressure without changing the heart rate. Ghrelin improves cardiac contractility and left ventricular function in chronic heart failure and reduces infarct size (Isgaard and Johansson, 2005). In rats with myocardial infarction, ghrelin suppresses cardiac sympathetic activity and prevents early left ventricular remodeling, suggesting the potential usefulness of ghrelin as a new cardioprotective hormone early after myocardial infarction (Soeki et al., 2008).

Anti-Inflammatory Functions

Ghrelin has anti-inflammatory effects. Indeed, ghrelin inhibits production of proinflammatory cytokines in human endothelial cells, T cells, monocytes, and in a rat model of endotoxic shock (Chang et al., 2003; Dembinski et al., 2003; Dixit et al., 2004; Li et al., 2004; Nagaya et al., 2001; Xia et al., 2004). Also, ghrelin attenuates the development of acute pancreatitis in rats (Dembinski et al., 2003). Ghrelin dose-dependently inhibits proliferation of anti-CD3 activated splenic T lymphocytes in mice (Dixit and Taub, 2005). Ghrelin possesses a neutrophil-dependent anti-inflammatory effect that prevents burn-induced multiple organ injury and protects against oxidative organ damage (Sehirli et al., 2008). Ghrelin attenuates lipopolysaccharide-induced acute lung inflammation and suppresses lipopolysaccharide--induced proinflammatory cytokine production in lung macrophages, which is partially mediated by increased NO production (Chen et al., 2008).

Other Functions

Ghrelin participates in the regulation of the reproductive function. In the testis, ghrelin inhibits testosterone secretion. Besides having direct gonadal effects, ghrelin may participate in the regulation of gonadotropin secretion and may influence the timing of puberty. In the pituitary, ghrelin inhibits luteinizing hormone secretion (Garcia et al., 2007).

Ghrelin stimulates bone formation by stimulating in vitro osteoblastic cell proliferation and differentiation, inhibiting apoptosis, and increasing in vivo bone mineral density in both normal and GH-deficient rats (Fukushima et al., 2005).

In addition to these functions, ghrelin also modulates cell proliferation in various cell types (De Vriese et al., 2005; De Vriese and Delporte, 2007; Korbonits et al., 2004).

13. POTENTIAL CLINICAL APPLICATIONS OF GHRELIN

In search of GHS-R 1a agonists and antagonists, numerous structure-function studies have been performed using peptidic and non-peptidic ghrelin analogues. Given that ghrelin stimulates food intake, ghrelin agonists or antagonists are mainly developed for cachexia treatment and for obesity treatment, respectively. Although patients with cachexia have increased plasma ghrelin levels, reflecting a compensatory response to weight loss, ghrelin administration still improves food intake and weight gain in a rat model of cancer cachexia (Deboer et al., 2007), and in patients with congestive heart failure or chronic obstructive pulmonary disease (Nagaya et al., 2006). In patients with cachexia associated with anorexia nervosa, the effect of ghrelin administration is controversial (Miljic et al., 2006).

GHS-R 1a Agonists

As an alternative to growth hormone replacement therapy, an effort has been made to identify peptidomimetic and nonpeptidic small molecular growth hormone secretagogues (GHSs). Synthetic ghrelin agonists existed long before ghrelin was discovered. Indeed, in search for hypothalamic factor controlling the release of growth hormone, enkephalin analogues were synthesized as they induced weak GH release. This led to the discovery of GHSs, peptidic or non peptidic molecules inducing potent growth hormone release, such as growth hormone-releasing peptide-2 (GHRP-2), growth hormone-releasing peptide-6 (GHRP-6), hexarelin, MK-0677, CP-424,391 and NNC-26-073 (Smith et al., 1997; Smith et al., 2007; Wu et al., 1996). Several GHSs have advanced to clinical studies including MK-677 (Merck), CP-424391 (Pfizer), LY-444711 (Lilly).

In the full ghrelin sequence, the presence of the voluminous hydrophobic groups on Ser3 is critical for the biological activity of the peptide (Bednarek et al., 2000; Matsumoto et al., 2001). Maximal activity is reached with the acylation of Ser3 by an octanoyl group (C8:0). A substantial activity is maintained by the acylation of Ser3 by a decanoyl (C10:0), lauryl (C12:0) or palmitoyl (C16:0) group. However, the activity is largely decreased by the acylation of Ser3 by a butyryl (C4:0) or an acetyl (C2:0) group. Ser3 modification by a polyunsaturated fatty acid, such as 3-octenoyl (C8:1), or by a fatty acid containing a lateral chain, such as a 4-methylpentanoyl, maintain the activity (Matsumoto et al., 2001). Whereas the replacement of Ser3 by a Trp maintains the activity of ghrelin, its replacement by aliphatic AA such as Val, Leu or Ile totally inhibits the activity of ghrelin (Bednarek et al., 2000). Short peptides encompassing the first four or five residues of ghrelin remained functionally active, nearly as efficiently as the full-length ghrelin, on the on GHS-R 1a (Bednarek et al., 2000). Ala-scan of ghrelin 1-14 revealed the importance of the amino-terminal positive charge and Phe in position 4 for the receptor interaction. Furthermore, analogs of ghrelin 1-14 modified in position 8 (Glu) by Ala or Tyr were more potent that ghrelin 1-14 (Van Craenenbroeck et al., 2004).

BIM-28125, a peptidic analogue of ghrelin, was reported as a potent stimulator of growth hormone secretion (Rubinfeld et al., 2004). BIM-28131, a compound related to BIM-28125, induced body weight gain in rats (Strassburg et al., 2008). Certain oxindole derivatives such as SM-130686((+)-6-carbamoyl-3-(2-chlorophenyl)-2-diethylaminoethyl)-4-tri fluoro methyloxindo-le) had potent growth hormone releasing activity, and induced body weight as well as fat-free mass gain (Nagamine et al., 2001; Tokunaga et al., 2001). Structure-activity relationship of the C3-aromatic part of SM-130686 was examined and a series of 3-dichlorophenyl analogues were identified as potent ghrelin agonists (Tokunaga et al., 2005).

Among a series of GHS analogues synthesized based on the 1,2,4-triazole structure, some behaved as GHS-R 1a agonists such as JMV2873 (Demange et al., 2007). Some 3,4,5-trisubstituted 1,2,4-triazoles were synthesized and two possessed potent GHS-R 1a agonist activity (Moulin et al., 2008).

From a series of pseudopeptidic analogues derived from EP-51389, based on a gem-diamino structure, JMV1843 was identified as a potent GHS-R 1a agonist (Guerlavais et al., 2003). This molecule is currently under a phase III clinical trial in the US for the diagnosis of growth hormone deficiency in adults.

Diltiazem and some of its metabolites were reported to behave as GHS-R 1a agonists (Ma et al., 2007).

A series of small molecules GHS-R 1a agonists, SB-791016, were identified but suffered from poor oral absorption which may be attributed to the relatively high lipophilicity and poor solubility (Heightman et al., 2007). Subsequent structure-activity relationship optimization of these compounds and in vivo properties were recently reported, and a potent GHS-R 1a agonist was identified: GSK899490A (Witherington et al., 2008).

The potential use of GHS-R 1a agonists as therapeutic agents for the treatment of gastrointestinal motility disorders has also been investigated (Peeters, 2006). GHRP-6 is a GHS-R 1a agonist able to increase gastric emptying in normal rats (Depoortere et al., 2005), as well as in animal models of postoperative ileus (Trudel et al., 2002), septic ileus (De Winter et al., 2004), burn-induced slow gastrointestinal transit (Sallam et al., 2007), diabetes mellitus (Qiu et al., 2008a; Qiu et al., 2008b; Zheng et al., 2008). RC-1139, a GHS-R 1a agonist, was reported to behave as a potent gastrokinetic in rats, and it also reversed postoperative ileus, even in the presence of opiates (Poitras et al., 2005).

TZP-101, a small GHS-R 1a agonist displaying superior bioavailability than the ghrelin peptide, increases gastric emptying and intestinal transit in normal rats (Fraser et al., 2008), in a rat model of postoperative ileus (Venkova et al., 2007), and in patients with diabetic gastroparesis (Madsen et al., 2007). In a clinical phase I study, the safety, pharmacokinetics and pharmacodynamic of TZP-101 were recently evaluated in healthy volunteers and suggested that this compound could be used for gastrointestinal motility disorders (Lasseter et al., 2008).

GSK894281 (N-(5-(cis-3,5-dimethyl-1-piperazinyl)-2-(methyloxy)phenyl)-3-fluoro-4-(5-methyl-2-furanyl)benzenesulphonamide) is a GHS-R 1a agonist triggering defecation in rats (Shafton et al., 2008).

GHS-R 1a Antagonists

A GHS-R 1a antagonist, D-Lys^3-GHRP-6 delayed gastric emptying induced by GHS-R 1a agonist (Depoortere et al., 2006; Qiu et al., 2008a), but this could be due at least in part by interacting with the serotonergic 5-HT2B receptors (Depoortere et al., 2006).

The potential benefits of using GHS-R 1a antagonists for the treatment of type 2 diabetes and obesity, particularly in Prader-Willi syndrome, have been investigated. Ghrelin-receptor antagonists, as (D-Lys-3)GHRP-6, decrease food intake in lean mice and obese mice, and reduce weight gain (Asakawa et al., 2003; Beck et al., 2004).

Piperidine-substituted quinazolinone derivatives were identified as a novel class of small-molecules GHS-R 1a antagonists (Rudolph et al., 2007). Phenyl or phenoxy groups were identified as optimal substituents at position 6 of the quinazolinone core, and the replacement of phenyl groups in position 2 by small alkyl substituents were proven to be beneficial (Rudolph et al., 2007). YIL-781, a piperidine-substituted quinazolinone derivative acting as potent GHS-R 1a antagonist, was shown to improve glucose tolerance due to increased insulin secretion, to reduce food intake and to promote weight loss in diet-induced obese mice (Esler et al., 2007).

Among a series of GHS analogues synthesized based on the 1,2,4-triazole structure, some behaved as GHS-R 1a antagonists such as JMV2866 and JMV2844 (Demange et al., 2007). Some 3,4,5-trisubstituted 1,2,4-triazoles were synthesized and most of them possessed potent GHS-R 1a antagonist activity (Moulin et al., 2008).

Inverse Agonists

Consistent with the high constitutive activity of the ghrelin receptor, inverse agonists of the receptor, decreasing its constitutive activity, may be useful for the treatment of obesity (Holst et al., 2003). During long fasting, GHS-R 1a expression increases in the hypothalamus, leading to an increase of GHS-R 1a signaling, a higher appetite, and a decrease of energy expenditure. The decrease of the GHS-R 1a constitutive activity by an inverse agonist could increase the sensitivity to anorexigenic hormones like leptin or PYY, and prevent food intake between meals (Holst and Schwartz, 2004). (D-Arg^1, D-Phe^5, D-Trp7,9, Leu11)substance P was identified as an inverse agonist on GHS-R 1a (Holst et al., 2006). The use of inverse agonists of the GHS-R 1a in obesity treatment needs to be further investigated.

Others

Spiegelmers, antisense polyethylene glycol-modified L-oligonucleotides capable to specifically bind a target molecule, have been synthesized to neutralize ghrelin and inhibit its binding to the GHS-R 1a. The spiegelmer NOX-B11-2 decreased food intake and body weight in diet-induced obese mice (Asakawa et al., 2003; Kobelt et al., 2006; Shearman et al., 2006). Another Spiegelmer, NOX-B11-3 was also shown to inhibit ghrelin-induced GH release in rats (Helmling et al., 2004). NOX-B11-3 exerted long-lasting action after a single peripheral injection: it blocked ghrelin, but not fasting-induced neuronal activation in the hypothalamic arcuate nucleus (Becskei et al., 2008). The neutralization of circulating ghrelin by these Spiegelmers may be useful to treat diseases associated with high ghrelin levels such as the PWS.

Ghrelin hapten immunoconjugates lead to the production of antibodies specifically directed against acylated ghrelin. In rats with strong anti-ghrelin immune responses, body weight gain is reduced with preferential reduction of fat mass compared to lean mass, by decreasing feed efficiency (weight gain per kilocalorie of food) (Zorrilla et al., 2006).

Conclusion

The importance of ghrelin in appetite stimulation and body weight regulation is intensively investigated. The effect of ghrelin on appetite is mediated in hypothalamus through stimulation of NPY, AGRP and orexin release, and inhibition α-MSH and CART release, and through activation of GHS-R on vagal afferents in the stomach. The effect of ghrelin on body weight is mediated by stimulating food intake, but also by reducing energy expenditure and promoting adiposity. Ghrelin agonists seem useful for treatment of gastrointestinal motility disorders, cancer-induced cachexia, congestive heart failure or chronic obstructive pulmonary disease. Ghrelin-receptor antagonists, Spiegelmers and anti-ghrelin vaccine reduce body weight gain and might be useful for type 2 diabetes and obesity treatment, particularly in PWS. Recently, the enzyme responsible for the octanoylation of ghrelin, GOAT, was identified and could represent an additional interesting therapeutic target for the treatment of type 2 diabetes and obesity. All these clinical applications of ghrelin will require further intensive investigations.

Acknowledgments

This work was supported by grants 3.4510.03 and 3.4561.07 from the Fund for Medical Scientific Research (Belgium).

References

Adeghate, E. and Ponery, A. S. (2002). Ghrelin stimulates insulin secretion from the pancreas of normal and diabetic rats. *J. Neuroendocrinol. 14,* 555-560.

Akamizu, T., Shinomiya, T., Irako, T., Fukunaga, M., Nakai, Y., Nakai, Y., and Kangawa, K. (2005). Separate Measurement of Plasma Levels of Acylated and Desacyl Ghrelin in Healthy Subjects Using a New Direct ELISA Assay. *J. Clin. Endocrinol. Metab. 90,* 6-9.

Ando, T., Ichimaru, Y., Konjiki, F., Shoji, M., and Komaki, G. (2007). Variations in the preproghrelin gene correlate with higher body mass index, fat mass, and body dissatisfaction in young Japanese women. *Am. J. Clin. Nutr. 86,* 25-32.

Ariyasu, H., Takaya, K., Tagami, T., Ogawa, Y., Hosoda, K., Akamizu, T., Suda, M., Koh, T., Natsui, K., Toyooka, S., Shirakami, G., Usui, T., Shimatsu, A., Doi, K., Hosoda, H., Kojima, M., Kangawa, K., and Nakao, K. (2001). Stomach Is a Major Source of Circulating Ghrelin, and Feeding State Determines Plasma Ghrelin-Like Immunoreactivity Levels in Humans. *J. Clin. Endocrinol. Metab. 86,* 4753-4758.

Ariyasu, H., Takaya, K., Iwakura, H., Hosoda, H., Akamizu, T., Arai, Y., Kangawa, K., and Nakao, K. (2005). Transgenic mice overexpressing des-acyl ghrelin show small phenotype. *Endocrinology. 146,* 355-364.

Arnold, M., Mura, A., Langhans, W., and Geary, N. (2006). Gut vagal afferents are not necessary for the eating-stimulatory effect of intraperitoneally injected ghrelin in the rat. *J. Neurosci. 26,* 11052-11060.

Asakawa, A., Inui, A., Kaga, T., Yuzuriha, H., Nagata, T., Ueno, N., Makino, S., Fujimiya, M., Niijima, A., Fujino, M. A., and Kasuga, M. (2001). Ghrelin is an appetite-stimulatory signal from stomach with structural resemblance to motilin. *Gastroenterology. 120,* 337-345.

Asakawa, A., Inui, A., Kaga, T., Katsuura, G., Fujimiya, M., Fujino, M. A., and Kasuga, M. (2003). Antagonism of ghrelin receptor reduces food intake and body weight gain in mice. *Gut. 52,* 947-952.

Bang, A. S., Soule, S. G., Yandle, T. G., Richards, A. M., and Pemberton, C. J. (2007). Characterisation of proghrelin peptides in mammalian tissue and plasma. *J. Endocrinol. 192,* 313-323.

Baynes, K. C., Dhillo, W. S., and Bloom, S. R. (2006). Regulation of food intake by gastrointestinal hormones. *Curr. Opin. Gastroenterol. 22,* 626-631.

Beaumont, N. J., Skinner, V. O., Tan, T. M., Ramesh, B. S., Byrne, D. J., MacColl, G. S., Keen, J. N., Bouloux, P. M., Mikhailidis, D. P., Bruckdorfer, K. R., Vanderpump, M. P., and Srai, K. S. (2003). Ghrelin can bind to a species of high density lipoprotein associated with paraoxonase. *J. Biol. Chem. 278,* 8877-8880.

Beck, B., Richy, S., and Stricker-Krongrad, A. (2004). Feeding response to ghrelin agonist and antagonist in lean and obese Zucker rats. *Life Sci. 76,* 473-478.

Becskei, C., Bilik, K. U., Klussmann, S., Jarosch, F., Lutz, T. A., and Riediger, T. (2008). The anti-ghrelin Spiegelmer NOX-B11-3 blocks ghrelin- but not fasting-induced neuronal activation in the hypothalamic arcuate nucleus. *J. Neuroendocrinol. 20,* 85-92.

Bednarek, M. A., Feighner, S. D., Pong, S. S., McKee, K. K., Hreniuk, D. L., Silva, M. V., Warren, V. A., Howard, A. D., Van Der Ploeg, L. H., and Heck, J. V. (2000). Structure-function studies on the new growth hormone-releasing peptide, ghrelin: minimal sequence of ghrelin necessary for activation of growth hormone secretagogue receptor 1a. *J. Med. Chem. 43,* 4370-4376.

Bing, C., Ambye, L., Fenger, M., Jorgensen, T., Borch-Johnsen, K., Madsbad, S., and Urhammer, S. A. (2005). Large-scale studies of the Leu72Met polymorphism of the ghrelin gene in relation to the metabolic syndrome and associated quantitative traits. *Diabet Med. 22,* 1157-1160.

Bodart, V., Bouchard, J. F., McNicoll, N., Escher, E., Carriere, P., Ghigo, E., Sejlitz, T., Sirois, M. G., Lamontagne, D., and Ong, H. (1999). Identification and Characterization of a New Growth Hormone-Releasing Peptide Receptor in the Heart. *Circ. Res. 85,* 796-802.

Bodart, V., Febbraio, M., Demers, A., McNicoll, N., Pohankova, P., Perreault, A., Sejlitz, T., Escher, E., Silverstein, R. L., Lamontagne, D., and Ong, H. (2002). CD36 Mediates the Cardiovascular Action of Growth Hormone-Releasing Peptides in the Heart. *Circ. Res. 90,* 844-849.

Bresciani, E., Rapetti, D., Dona, F., Bulgarelli, I., Tamiazzo, L., Locatelli, V., and Torsello, A. (2006). Obestatin inhibits feeding but does not modulate GH and corticosterone secretion in the rat. *J. Endocrinol. Invest. 29,* RC16-RC18.

Broglio, F., Arvat, E., Benso, A., Gottero, C., Muccioli, G., Papotti, M., van der Lely, A. J., Deghenghi, R., and Ghigo, E. (2001). Ghrelin, a natural GH secretagogue produced by the stomach, induces hyperglycemia and reduces insulin secretion in humans. *J. Clin. Endocrinol. Metab. 86,* 5083-5086.

Broglio, F., Prodam, F., Me, E., Riganti, F., Lucatello, B., Granata, R., Benso, A., Muccioli, G., and Ghigo, E. (2005). Ghrelin: endocrine, metabolic and cardiovascular actions. *J. Endocrinol. Invest. 28,* 23-25.

Burdyga, G., Varro, A., Dimaline, R., Thompson, D. G., and Dockray, G. J. (2006). Ghrelin receptors in rat and human nodose ganglia: putative role in regulating CB-1 and MCH receptor abundance. *Am. J. Physiol. Gastrointest. Liver Physiol. 290,* G1289-G1297.

Caminos, J. E., Tena-Sempere, M., Gaytan, F., Sanchez-Criado, J. E., Barreiro, M. L., Nogueiras, R., Casanueva, F. F., Aguilar, E., and Dieguez, C. (2003). Expression of ghrelin in the cyclic and pregnant rat ovary. *Endocrinology. 144,* 1594-1602.

Carlini, V. P., Schioth, H. B., and Debarioglio, S. R. (2007). Obestatin improves memory performance and causes anxiolytic effects in rats. *Biochem. Biophys. Res. Commun. 352,* 907-912.

Cellini, E., Nacmias, B., Brecelj-Anderluh, M., Badia-Casanovas, A., Bellodi, L., Boni, C., Di Bella, D., Estivill, X., Fernandez-Aranda, F., Foulon, C., Friedel, S., Gabrovsek, M., Gorwood, P., Gratacos, M., Guelfi, J., Hebebrand, J., Hinney, A., Holliday, J., Hu, X., Karwautz, A., Kipman, A., Komel, R., Rotella, C. M., Ribases, M., Ricca, V., Romo, L., Tomori, M., Treasure, J., Wagner, G., Collier, D. A., and Sorbi, S. (2006). Case-control and combined family trios analysis of three polymorphisms in the ghrelin gene in European patients with anorexia and bulimia nervosa. *Psychiatr. Genet. 16,* 51-52.

Chamoun, Z., Mann, R. K., Nellen, D., von Kessler, D. P., Bellotto, M., Beachy, P. A., and Basler, K. (2001). Skinny Hedgehog, an Acyltransferase Required for Palmitoylation and Activity of the Hedgehog Signal. *Science. 293,* 2080-2084.

Chan, C. B. and Cheng, C. H. K. (2004). Identification and functional characterization of two alternatively spliced growth hormone secretagogue receptor transcripts from the pituitary of black seabream Acanthopagrus schlegeli. *Mol. Cell Endocrinol. 214,* 81-95.

Chan, J. L., Mun, E. C., Stoyneva, V., Mantzoros, C. S., and Goldfine, A. B. (2006). Peptide YY levels are elevated after gastric bypass surgery. *Obesity (Silver Spring), 14,* 194-198.

Chang, L., Zhao, J., Yang, J., Zhang, Z., Du, J., and Tang, C. (2003). Therapeutic effects of ghrelin on endotoxic shock in rats. *Eur. J. Pharmacol. 473,* 171-176.

Chanoine, J. P., Wong, A. C., and Barrios, V. (2006). Obestatin, acylated and total ghrelin concentrations in the perinatal rat pancreas. *Horm. Res. 66,* 81-88.

Chen, H. Y., Trumbauer, M. E., Chen, A. S., Weingarth, D. T., Adams, J. R., Frazier, E. G., Shen, Z., Marsh, D. J., Feighner, S. D., Guan, X. M., Ye, Z., Nargund, R. P., Smith, R. G., Van Der Ploeg, L. H., Howard, A. D., MacNeil, D. J., and Qian, S. (2004). Orexigenic action of peripheral ghrelin is mediated by neuropeptide Y and agouti-related protein. *Endocrinology. 145,* 2607-2612.

Chen, J., Liu, X., Shu, Q., Li, S., and Luo, F. (2008). Ghrelin attenuates lipopolysaccharide-induced acute lung injury through no pathway. *Med. Sci. Monit. 14,* BR141-BR146.

Choi, H. J., Cho, Y. M., Moon, M. K., Choi, H. H., Shin, H. D., Jang, H. C., Kim, S. Y., Lee, H. K., and Park, K. S. (2006). Polymorphisms in the ghrelin gene are associated with serum high-density lipoprotein cholesterol level and not with type 2 diabetes mellitus in Koreans. *J. Clin. Endocrinol. Metab. 91,* 4657-4663.

Coiro, V., Saccani-Jotti, G., Rubino, P., Manfredi, G., Melani, A., and Chiodera, P. (2006). Effects of ghrelin on circulating neuropeptide Y levels in humans. *Neuro Endocrinol. Lett. 27,* 755-757.

Colombo, M., Gregersen, S., Xiao, J., and Hermansen, K. (2003). Effects of ghrelin and other neuropeptides (CART, MCH, orexin A and B, and GLP-1) on the release of insulin from isolated rat islets. *Pancreas. 27,* 161-166.

Couce, M. E., Cottam, D., Esplen, J., Schauer, P., and Burguera, B. (2006). Is ghrelin the culprit for weight loss after gastric bypass surgery? A negative answer. *Obes. Surg. 16,* 870-878.

Cowley, M. A., Smart, J. L., Rubinstein, M., Cerdan, M. G., Diano, S., Horvath, T. L., Cone, R. D., and Low, M. J. (2001). Leptin activates anorexigenic POMC neurons through a neural network in the arcuate nucleus. *Nature. 411,* 480-484.

Cowley, M. A., Smith, R. G., Diano, S., Tschop, M., Pronchuk, N., Grove, K. L., Strasburger, C. J., Bidlingmaier, M., Esterman, M., Heiman, M. L., Garcia-Segura, L. M., Nillni, E. A., Mendez, P., Low, M. J., Sotonyi, P., Friedman, J. M., Liu, H., Pinto, S., Colmers, W. F., Cone, R. D., and Horvath, T. L. (2003). The distribution and mechanism of action of ghrelin in the CNS demonstrates a novel hypothalamic circuit regulating energy homeostasis. *Neuron. 37,* 649-661.

Cui, C., Ohnuma, H., Daimon, M., Susa, S., Yamaguchi, H., Kameda, W., Jimbu, Y., Oizumi, T., and Kato, T. (2008). Ghrelin infused into the portal vein inhibits glucose-stimulated insulin secretion in Wistar rats. *Peptides. 29,* 1241-1246.

Cummings, D. E., Purnell, J. Q., Frayo, R. S., Schmidova, K., Wisse, B. E., and Weigle, D. S. (2001). A preprandial rise in plasma ghrelin levels suggests a role in meal initiation in humans. *Diabetes. 50,* 1714-1719.

Cummings, D. E., Clement, K., Purnell, J. Q., Vaisse, C., Foster, K. E., Frayo, R. S., Schwartz, M. W., Basdevant, A., and Weigle, D. S. (2002a). Elevated plasma ghrelin levels in Prader-Willi syndrome. *Nat. Med. 8,* 643-644.

Cummings, D. E., Weigle, D. S., Frayo, R. S., Breen, P. A., Ma, M. K., Dellinger, E. P., and Purnell, J. Q. (2002b). Plasma ghrelin levels after diet-induced weight loss or gastric bypass surgery. *N. Engl. J. Med. 346,* 1623-1630.

Dardennes, R. M., Zizzari, P., Tolle, V., Foulon, C., Kipman, A., Romo, L., Iancu-Gontard, D., Boni, C., Sinet, P. M., Therese, B. M., Estour, B., Mouren, M. C., Guelfi, J. D., Rouillon, F., Gorwood, P., and Epelbaum, J. (2007). Family trios analysis of common polymorphisms in the obestatin/ghrelin, BDNF and AGRP genes in patients with Anorexia nervosa: association with subtype, body-mass index, severity and age of onset. *Psychoneuroendocrinology. 32,* 106-113.

Dass, N. B., Munonyara, M., Bassil, A. K., Hervieu, G. J., Osbourne, S., Corcoran, S., Morgan, M., and Sanger, G. J. (2003). Growth hormone secretagogue receptors in rat and human gastrointestinal tract and the effects of ghrelin. *Neuroscience. 120,* 443-453.

Date, Y., Murakami, N., Kojima, M., Kuroiwa, T., Matsukura, S., Kangawa, K., and Nakazato, M. (2000a). Central effects of a novel acylated peptide, ghrelin, on growth hormone release in rats. *Biochem. Biophys. Res. Commun. 275,* 477-480.

Date, Y., Kojima, M., Hosoda, H., Sawaguchi, A., Mondal, M. S., Suganuma, T., Matsukura, S., Kangawa, K., and Nakazato, M. (2000b). Ghrelin, a Novel Growth Hormone-Releasing Acylated Peptide, Is Synthesized in a Distinct Endocrine Cell Type in the Gastrointestinal Tracts of Rats and Humans. *Endocrinology. 141,* 4255-4261.

Date, Y., Nakazato, M., Murakami, N., Kojima, M., Kangawa, K., and Matsukura, S. (2001). Ghrelin acts in the central nervous system to stimulate gastric acid secretion. *Biochem. Biophys. Res. Commun. 280,* 904-907.

Date, Y., Murakami, N., Toshinai, K., Matsukura, S., Niijima, A., Matsuo, H., Kangawa, K., and Nakazato, M. (2002a). The role of the gastric afferent vagal nerve in ghrelin-induced feeding and growth hormone secretion in rats. *Gastroenterology. 123,* 1120-1128.

Date, Y., Nakazato, M., Hashiguchi, S., Dezaki, K., Mondal, M. S., Hosoda, H., Kojima, M., Kangawa, K., Arima, T., Matsuo, H., Yada, T., and Matsukura, S. (2002b). Ghrelin is present in pancreatic alpha-cells of humans and rats and stimulates insulin secretion. *Diabetes. 51,* 124-129.

Date, Y., Shimbara, T., Koda, S., Toshinai, K., Ida, T., Murakami, N., Miyazato, M., Kokame, K., Ishizuka, Y., Ishida, Y., Kageyama, H., Shioda, S., Kangawa, K., and Nakazato, M. (2006). Peripheral ghrelin transmits orexigenic signals through the noradrenergic pathway from the hindbrain to the hypothalamus. *Cell Metab. 4,* 323-331.

de Lartigue, G., Dimaline, R., Varro, A., and Dockray, G. J. (2007). Cocaine- and amphetamine-regulated transcript: stimulation of expression in rat vagal afferent neurons by cholecystokinin and suppression by ghrelin. *J. Neurosci. 27,* 2876-2882.

De Smet, B., Depoortere, I., Moechars, D., Swennen, Q., Moreaux, B., Cryns, K., Tack, J., Buyse, J., Coulie, B., and Peeters, T. L. (2006). Energy homeostasis and gastric emptying in ghrelin knockout mice. *J. Pharmacol. Exp. Ther. 316,* 431-439.

De Vriese, C., Gregoire, F., Lema-Kisoka, R., Waelbroeck, M., Robberecht, P., and Delporte, C. (2004). Ghrelin degradation by serum and tissue homogenates: identification of the cleavage sites. *Endocrinology. 145,* 4997-5005.

De Vriese, C., Gregoire, F., De Neef, P., Robberecht, P., and Delporte, C. (2005). Ghrelin is produced by the human erythroleukemic HEL cell line and involved in an autocrine pathway leading to cell proliferation. *Endocrinology. 146,* 1514-1522.

De Vriese, C. and Delporte, C. (2007). Autocrine proliferative effect of ghrelin on leukemic HL-60 and THP-1 cells. *J. Endocrinol. 192,* 199-205.

De Vriese, C., Hacquebard, M., Gregoire, F., Carpentier, Y., and Delporte, C. (2007). Ghrelin interacts with human plasma lipoproteins. *Endocrinology. 148,* 2355-2362.

De Winter, B. Y., De Man, J. G., Seerden, T. C., Depoortere, I., Herman, A. G., Peeters, T. L., and Pelckmans, P. A. (2004). Effect of ghrelin and growth hormone-releasing peptide 6 on septic ileus in mice. *Neurogastroenterol. Motil. 16,* 439-446.

Deboer, M. D., Zhu, X. X., Levasseur, P., Meguid, M. M., Suzuki, S., Inui, A., Taylor, J. E., Halem, H. A., Dong, J. Z., Datta, R., Culler, M. D., and Marks, D. L. (2007). Ghrelin treatment causes increased food intake and retention of lean body mass in a rat model of cancer cachexia. *Endocrinology. 148,* 3004-3012.

Dehlin, E., Liu, J., Yun, S. H., Fox, E., Snyder, S., Gineste, C., Willingham, L., Geysen, M., Gaylinn, B. D., and Sando, J. J. (2008). Regulation of ghrelin structure and membrane binding by phosphorylation. *Peptides. 29,* 904-911.

DelParigi, A., Tschop, M., Heiman, M. L., Salbe, A. D., Vozarova, B., Sell, S. M., Bunt, J. C., and Tataranni, P. A. (2002). High circulating ghrelin: a potential cause for hyperphagia and obesity in prader-willi syndrome. *J. Clin. Endocrinol. Metab. 87,* 5461-5464.

Demange, L., Boeglin, D., Moulin, A., Mousseaux, D., Ryan, J., Berge, G., Gagne, D., Heitz, A., Perrissoud, D., Locatelli, V., Torsello, A., Galleyrand, J. C., Fehrentz, J. A., and Martinez, J. (2007). Synthesis and pharmacological in vitro and in vivo evaluations of novel triazole derivatives as ligands of the ghrelin receptor. *J. Med. Chem. 50,* 1939-1957.

Dembinski, A., Warzecha, Z., Ceranowicz, P., Tomaszewska, R., Stachura, J., Konturek, S. J., and Konturek, P. C. (2003). Ghrelin attenuates the development of acute pancreatitis in rat. *J. Physiol. Pharmacol. 54,* 561-573.

Depoortere, I., De Winter, B., Thijs, T., De Man, J., Pelckmans, P., and Peeters, T. (2005). Comparison of the gastroprokinetic effects of ghrelin, GHRP-6 and motilin in rats in vivo and in vitro. *Eur. J. Pharmacol. 515,* 160-168.

Depoortere, I., Thijs, T., and Peeters, T. (2006). The contractile effect of the ghrelin receptor antagonist, D-Lys3-GHRP-6, in rat fundic strips is mediated through 5-HT receptors. *Eur. J. Pharmacol. 537,* 160-165.

Dixit, V. D., Schaffer, E. M., Pyle, R. S., Collins, G. D., Sakthivel, S. K., Palaniappan, R., Lillard, J. W., Jr., and Taub, D. D. (2004). Ghrelin inhibits leptin- and activation-induced proinflammatory cytokine expression by human monocytes and T cells. *J. Clin. Invest. 114,* 57-66.

Dixit, V. D. and Taub, D. D. (2005). Ghrelin and immunity: A young player in an old field. *Exp. Gerontol.*

Dornonville de la Cour, C., Bj÷rkqvist, M., Sandvik, A. K., Bakke, I., Zhao, C.-M., Chen, D., and Hskanson, R. (2001). A-like cells in the rat stomach contain ghrelin and do not operate under gastrin control. *Regulatory Peptides. 99,* 141-150.

Dossus, L., McKay, J. D., Canzian, F., Wilkening, S., Rinaldi, S., Biessy, C., Olsen, A., Tjonneland, A., Jakobsen, M. U., Overvad, K., Clavel-Chapelon, F., Boutron-Ruault, M. C., Fournier, A., Linseisen, J., Lukanova, A., Boeing, H., Fisher, E., Tricholpoulou, A., Georgila, C., Trichopoulos, D., Palli, D., Krogh, V., Tumino, R., Vineis, P., Quiros, J. R., Sala, N., Martinez-Garcia, C., Dorronsoro, M., Chirlaque, M. D., Barricarte, A., van Duijnhoven, F. J., Bueno-de-Mesquita, H. B., van Gils, C. H., Peeters, P. H., Hallmans, G., Lenner, P., Bingham, S., Khaw, K. T., Key, T. J., Travis, R. C., Ferrari, P., Jenab, M., Riboli, E., and Kaaks, R. (2008). Polymorphisms of genes coding for ghrelin and its receptor in relation to anthropometry, circulating levels of IGF-I and IGFBP-3, and breast cancer risk: a case-control study nested within the European Prospective Investigation into Cancer and Nutrition (EPIC). *Carcinogenesis. 29,* 1360-1366.

Dun, S. L., Brailoiu, G. C., Brailoiu, E., Yang, J., Chang, J. K., and Dun, N. J. (2006). Distribution and biological activity of obestatin in the rat. *J. Endocrinol. 191,* 481-489.

Erdie-Lalena, C. R., Holm, V. A., Kelly, P. C., Frayo, R. S., and Cummings, D. E. (2006). Ghrelin levels in young children with Prader-Willi syndrome. *J. Pediatr. 149,* 199-204.

Erickson, J. C., Clegg, K. E., and Palmiter, R. D. (1996). Sensitivity to leptin and susceptibility to seizures of mice lacking neuropeptide Y. *Nature. 381,* 415-421.

Esler, W. P., Rudolph, J., Claus, T. H., Tang, W., Barucci, N., Brown, S. E., Bullock, W., Daly, M., Decarr, L., Li, Y., Milardo, L., Molstad, D., Zhu, J., Gardell, S. J., Livingston, J. N., and Sweet, L. J. (2007). Small-molecule ghrelin receptor antagonists improve glucose tolerance, suppress appetite, and promote weight loss. *Endocrinology. 148,* 5175-5185.

Feigerlova, E., Diene, G., Conte-Auriol, F., Molinas, C., Gennero, I., Salles, J. P., Arnaud, C., and Tauber, M. (2008). Hyperghrelinemia precedes obesity in Prader-Willi syndrome. *J. Clin. Endocrinol. Metab. 93,* 2800-2805.

Fraser, G. L., Hoveyda, H. R., and Tannenbaum, G. S. (2008). Pharmacological Demarcation of the Growth Hormone, Gut Motility and Feeding Effects of Ghrelin Using a Novel Ghrelin Receptor Agonist. *Endocrinology.* en.

Frecka, J. M. and Mattes, R. D. (2008). Possible entrainment of ghrelin to habitual meal patterns in humans. *Am. J. Physiol. Gastrointest. Liver. Physiol. 294,* G699-G707.

Fruhbeck, G., Diez, C. A., and Gil, M. J. (2004). Fundus functionality and ghrelin concentrations after bariatric surgery. *N. Engl. J. Med. 350,* 308-309.

Fujino, K., Inui, A., Asakawa, A., Kihara, N., Fujimura, M., and Fujimiya, M. (2003). Ghrelin induces fasted motor activity of the gastrointestinal tract in conscious fed rats. *J. Physiol. 550,* 227-240.

Fukumoto, K., Nakahara, K., Katayama, T., Miyazatao, M., Kangawa, K., and Murakami, N. (2008). Synergistic action of gastrin and ghrelin on gastric acid secretion in rats. *Biochem. Biophys. Res. Commun. 374,* 60-63.

Fukushima, N., Hanada, R., Teranishi, H., Fukue, Y., Tachibana, T., Ishikawa, H., Takeda, S., Takeuchi, Y., Fukumoto, S., Kangawa, K., Nagata, K., and Kojima, M. (2005). Ghrelin directly regulates bone formation. *J. Bone Miner Res. 20,* 790-798.

Garcia, M. C., Lopez, M., Alvarez, C. V., Casanueva, F., Tena-Sempere, M., and Dieguez, C. (2007). Role of ghrelin in reproduction. *Reproduction. 133,* 531-540.

Garcia, E. A., Heude, B., Petry, C. J., Gueorguiev, M., Hassan-Smith, Z. K., Spanou, A., Ring, S. M., Dunger, D. B., Wareham, N., Sandhu, M., Ong, K. K., and Korbonits, M. (2008). Ghrelin receptor gene polymorphisms and body size in children and adults. *J. Clin. Endocrinol. Metab.*

Gauna, C., Delhanty, P. J., Hofland, L. J., Janssen, J. A., Broglio, F., Ross, R. J., Ghigo, E., and van der Lely, A. J. (2005). Ghrelin stimulates, whereas des-octanoyl ghrelin inhibits, glucose output by primary hepatocytes. *J. Clin. Endocrinol. Metab. 90,* 1055-1060.

Gauna, C., van de Zande, B., van Kerkwijk, A., Themmen, A. P. N., van der Lely, A. J., and Delhanty, P. J. D. (2007). Unacylated ghrelin is not a functional antagonist but a full agonist of the type 1a growth hormone secretagogue receptor (GHS-R). *Mol. Cell Endocrinol. 274,* 30-34.

Ghelardoni, S., Carnicelli, V., Frascarelli, S., Ronca-Testoni, S., and Zucchi, R. (2006). Ghrelin tissue distribution: comparison between gene and protein expression. *J. Endocrinol. Invest. 29,* 115-121.

Gimenez-Palop, O., Gimenez-Perez, G., Mauricio, D., Gonzalez-Clemente, J. M., Potau, N., Berlanga, E., Trallero, R., Laferrere, B., and Caixas, A. (2007). A lesser postprandial suppression of plasma ghrelin in Prader-Willi syndrome is associated with low fasting and a blunted postprandial PYY response. *Clin. Endocrinol. (Oxf), 66,* 198-204.

Giovambattista, A., Gaillard, R. C., and Spinedi, E. (2008). Ghrelin gene-related peptides modulate rat white adiposity. *Vitam. Horm. 77,* 171-205.

Gnanapavan, S., Kola, B., Bustin, S. A., Morris, D. G., McGee, P., Fairclough, P., Bhattacharya, S., Carpenter, R., Grossman, A. B., and Korbonits, M. (2002). The Tissue Distribution of the mRNA of Ghrelin and Subtypes of Its Receptor, GHS-R, in Humans. *J. Clin. Endocrinol. Metab. 87,* 2988.

Gonzalez, C., Vazquez, M., Lopez, M., and Dieguez, C. (2008). Influence of chronic undernutrition and leptin on GOAT mRNA levels in rat stomach mucosa. *J. Mol. Endocrinol.* JME-08-0102v2-JME-08-0102.

Gourcerol, G., Million, M., Adelson, D. W., Wang, Y., Wang, L., Rivier, J., St-Pierre, D. H., and Tache, Y. (2006). Lack of interaction between peripheral injection of CCK and obestatin in the regulation of gastric satiety signaling in rodents. *Peptides. 27,* 2811-2819.

Gourcerol, G., St Pierre, D. H., and Tache, Y. (2007). Lack of obestatin effects on food intake: Should obestatin be renamed ghrelin-associated peptide (GAP)? *Regulatory Peptides. 141,* 1-7.

Green, B. D., Irwin, N., and Flatt, P. R. (2007). Direct and indirect effects of obestatin peptides on food intake and the regulation of glucose homeostasis and insulin secretion in mice. *Peptides. 28,* 981-987.

Gualillo, O., Lago, F., and Dieguez, C. (2008). Introducing GOAT: a target for obesity and anti-diabetic drugs? *Trends Pharmacol. Sci. 29,* 398-401.

Guerlavais, V., Boeglin, D., Mousseaux, D., Oiry, C., Heitz, A., Deghenghi, R., Locatelli, V., Torsello, A., Ghe, C., Catapano, F., Muccioli, G., Galleyrand, J. C., Fehrentz, J. A., and Martinez, J. (2003). New active series of growth hormone secretagogues. *J. Med. Chem. 46,* 1191-1203.

Gutierrez, J. A., Solenberg, P. J., Perkins, D. R., Willency, J. A., Knierman, M. D., Jin, Z., Witcher, D. R., Luo, S., Onyia, J. E., and Hale, J. E. (2008). From the Cover: Ghrelin octanoylation mediated by an orphan lipid transferase. *Proc. Natl. Acad. Sci. U. S. A. 105,* 6320-6325.

Haider, D. G., Schindler, K., Prager, G., Bohdjalian, A., Luger, A., Wolzt, M., and Ludvik, B. (2007). Serum retinol-binding protein 4 is reduced after weight loss in morbidly obese subjects. *J. Clin. Endocrinol. Metab. 92,* 1168-1171.

Haqq, A. M., Grambow, S. C., Muehlbauer, M., Newgard, C. B., Svetkey, L. P., Carrel, A. L., Yanovski, J. A., Purnell, J. Q., and Freemark, M. (2008). Ghrelin concentrations in Prader-Willi Syndrome (PWS) infants and children: changes during development. *Clin. Endocrinol. (Oxf).*

Hataya, Y., Akamizu, T., Takaya, K., Kanamoto, N., Ariyasu, H., Saijo, M., Moriyama, K., Shimatsu, A., Kojima, M., Kangawa, K., and Nakao, K. (2001). A low dose of ghrelin stimulates growth hormone (GH) release synergistically with GH-releasing hormone in humans. *J. Clin. Endocrinol. Metab. 86,* 4552.

Heightman, T. D., Scott, J. S., Longley, M., Bordas, V., Dean, D. K., Elliott, R., Hutley, G., Witherington, J., Abberley, L., Passingham, B., Berlanga, M., de Los, F. M., Wise, A., Powney, B., Muir, A., McKay, F., Butler, S., Winborn, K., Gardner, C., Darton, J.,

Campbell, C., and Sanger, G. (2007). Potent achiral agonists of the ghrelin (growth hormone secretagogue) receptor. Part I: Lead identification. *Bioorg. Med. Chem. Lett. 17*, 6584-6587.

Helmling, S., Maasch, C., Eulberg, D., Buchner, K., Schroder, W., Lange, C., Vonhoff, S., Wlotzka, B., Tschop, M. H., Rosewicz, S., and Klussmann, S. (2004). Inhibition of ghrelin action in vitro and in vivo by an RNA-Spiegelmer. *Proc. Natl. Acad. Sci. U. S. A. 101*, 13174-13179.

Herzog, H. (2003). Neuropeptide Y and energy homeostasis: insights from Y receptor knockout models. *Eur. J. Pharmacol. 480*, 21-29.

Hinney, A., Hoch, A., Geller, F., Schafer, H., Siegfried, W., Goldschmidt, H., Remschmidt, H., and Hebebrand, J. (2002). Ghrelin gene: identification of missense variants and a frameshift mutation in extremely obese children and adolescents and healthy normal weight students. *J. Clin. Endocrinol. Metab. 87*, 2716-2719.

Hoffmann, N., Steinbuchel, A., and Rehm, B. H. (2000). The Pseudomonas aeruginosa phaG gene product is involved in the synthesis of polyhydroxyalkanoic acid consisting of medium-chain-length constituents from non-related carbon sources. *FEMS Microbiol. Lett. 184*, 253-259.

Holliday, N. D., Holst, B., Rodionova, E. A., Schwartz, T. W., and Cox, H. M. (2007). Importance of Constitutive Activity and Arrestin-Independent Mechanisms for Intracellular Trafficking of the Ghrelin Receptor. *Mol. Endocrinol. 21*, 3100-3112.

Holst, B. and Schwartz, T. W. (2004). Constitutive ghrelin receptor activity as a signaling set-point in appetite regulation. *Trends Pharmacol. Sci. 25*, 113-117.

Holst, B. and Schwartz, T. W. (2006). Ghrelin receptor mutations--too little height and too much hunger. *J. Clin. Invest. 116*, 637-641.

Holst, B., Cygankiewicz, A., Jensen, T. H., Ankersen, M., and Schwartz, T. W. (2003). High Constitutive Signaling of the Ghrelin Receptor--Identification of a Potent Inverse Agonist. *Mol. Endocrinol. 17*, 2201-2210.

Holst, B., Holliday, N. D., Bach, A., Elling, C. E., Cox, H. M., and Schwartz, T. W. (2004). Common Structural Basis for Constitutive Activity of the Ghrelin Receptor Family. *J. Biol. Chem. 279*, 53806-53817.

Holst, B., Lang, M., Brandt, E., Bach, A., Howard, A., Frimurer, T. M., Beck-Sickinger, A., and Schwartz, T. W. (2006). Ghrelin Receptor Inverse Agonists: Identification of an Active Peptide Core and Its Interaction Epitopes on the Receptor. *Mol. Pharmacol. 70*, 936-946.

Holst, B., Egerod, K. L., Schild, E., Vickers, S. P., Cheetham, S., Gerlach, L. O., Storjohann, L., Stidsen, C. E., Jones, R., Beck-Sickinger, A. G., and Schwartz, T. W. (2007). GPR39 signaling is stimulated by zinc ions but not by obestatin. *Endocrinology. 148*, 13-20.

Hosoda, H., Kojima, M., Matsuo, H., and Kangawa, K. (2000a). Ghrelin and des-acyl ghrelin: two major forms of rat ghrelin peptide in gastrointestinal tissue. *Biochem. Biophys. Res. Commun. 279*, 909-913.

Hosoda, H., Kojima, M., Matsuo, H., and Kangawa, K. (2000b). Purification and characterization of rat des-Gln14-Ghrelin, a second endogenous ligand for the growth hormone secretagogue receptor. *J. Biol. Chem. 275*, 21995-22000.

Hosoda, H., Kojima, M., Mizushima, T., Shimizu, S., and Kangawa, K. (2003). Structural divergence of human ghrelin. Identification of multiple ghrelin-derived molecules produced by post-translational processing. *J. Biol. Chem. 278*, 64-70.

Hosoda, H., Doi, K., Nagaya, N., Okumura, H., Nakagawa, E., Enomoto, M., Ono, F., and Kangawa, K. (2004). Optimum collection and storage conditions for ghrelin measurements: octanoyl modification of ghrelin is rapidly hydrolyzed to desacyl ghrelin in blood samples. *Clin. Chem. 50,* 1077-1080.

Hosojima, H., Togo, T., Odawara, T., Hasegawa, K., Miura, S., Kato, Y., Kanai, A., Kase, A., Uchikado, H., and Hirayasu, Y. (2006). Early effects of olanzapine on serum levels of ghrelin, adiponectin and leptin in patients with schizophrenia. *J. Psychopharmacol. 20,* 75-79.

Howard, A. D., Feighner, S. D., Cully, D. F., Arena, J. P., Liberator, P. A., Rosenblum, C. I., Hamelin, M., Hreniuk, D. L., Palyha, O. C., Anderson, J., Paress, P. S., Diaz, C., Chou, M., Liu, K. K., McKee, K. K., Pong, S. S., Chaung, L. Y., Elbrecht, A., Dashkevicz, M., Heavens, R., Rigby, M., Sirinathsinghji, D. J. S., Dean, D. C., Melillo, D. G., Patchett, A. A., Nargund, R., Griffin, P. R., DeMartino, J. A., Gupta, S. K., Schaeffer, J. M., Smith, R. G., and Van der Ploeg, L. H. T. (1996). A Receptor in Pituitary and Hypothalamus That Functions in Growth Hormone Release. *Science. 273,* 974-977.

Hubacek, J. A., Bohuslavova, R., Skodova, Z., and Adamkova, V. (2007). Variants within the ghrelin gene--association with HDL-cholesterol, but not with body mass index. *Folia Biol. (Praha), 53,* 202-206.

Isgaard, J. and Johansson, I. (2005). Ghrelin and GHS on cardiovascular applications/functions. *J. Endocrinol. Invest. 28,* 838-842.

Ishizuka, T., Nomura, S., Hosoda, H., Kangawa, K., Watanabe, T., and Yamatodani, A. (2006). A role of the histaminergic system for the control of feeding by orexigenic peptides. *Physiol. Behav. 89,* 295-300.

Jaworek, J. (2006). Ghrelin and melatonin in the regulation of pancreatic exocrine secretion and maintaining of integrity. *J. Physiol. Pharmacol. 57 Suppl 5,* 83-96.

Jeffery, P. L., Murray, R. E., Yeh, A. H., McNamara, J. F., Duncan, R. P., Francis, G. D., Herington, A. C., and Chopin, L. K. (2005). Expression and function of the ghrelin axis, including a novel preproghrelin isoform, in human breast cancer tissues and cell lines. *Endocr. Relat. Cancer. 12,* 839-850.

Jeon, T. Y., Lee, S., Kim, H. H., Kim, Y. J., Son, H. C., Kim, D. H., and Sim, M. S. (2004). Changes in plasma ghrelin concentration immediately after gastrectomy in patients with early gastric cancer. *J. Clin. Endocrinol. Metab. 89,* 5392-5396.

Jo, D. S., Kim, S. L., Kim, S. Y., Hwang, P. H., Lee, K. H., and Lee, D. Y. (2005). Preproghrelin Leu72Met polymorphism in obese Korean children. *J. Pediatr. Endocrinol. Metab. 18,* 1083-1086.

Kageyama, H., Funahashi, H., Hirayama, M., Takenoya, F., Kita, T., Kato, S., Sakurai, J., Lee, E. Y., Inoue, S., Date, Y., Nakazato, M., Kangawa, K., and Shioda, S. (2005). Morphological analysis of ghrelin and its receptor distribution in the rat pancreas. *Regul. Pept. 126,* 67-71.

Kamegai, J., Tamura, H., Shimizu, T., Ishii, S., Sugihara, H., and Wakabayashi, I. (2001). Chronic central infusion of ghrelin increases hypothalamic neuropeptide Y and Agouti-related protein mRNA levels and body weight in rats. *Diabetes. 50,* 2438-2443.

Kanamoto, N., Akamizu, T., Tagami, T., Hataya, Y., Moriyama, K., Takaya, K., Hosoda, H., Kojima, M., Kangawa, K., and Nakao, K. (2004). Genomic Structure and Characterization of the 5'-Flanking Region of the Human Ghrelin Gene. *Endocrinology. 145,* 4144-4153.

Kim, M. S., Yoon, C. Y., Jang, P. G., Park, Y. J., Shin, C. S., Park, H. S., Ryu, J. W., Pak, Y. K., Park, J. Y., Lee, K. U., Kim, S. Y., Lee, H. K., Kim, Y. B., and Park, K. S. (2004). The mitogenic and antiapoptotic actions of ghrelin in 3T3-L1 adipocytes. *Mol. Endocrinol. 18,* 2291-2301.

Kissebah, A. H., Sonnenberg, G. E., Myklebust, J., Goldstein, M., Broman, K., James, R. G., Marks, J. A., Krakower, G. R., Jacob, H. J., Weber, J., Martin, L., Blangero, J., and Comuzzie, A. G. (2000). Quantitative trait loci on chromosomes 3 and 17 influence phenotypes of the metabolic syndrome. *Proc. Natl. Acad. Sci. U. S. A. 97,* 14478-14483.

Kobelt, P., Helmling, S., Stengel, A., Wlotzka, B., Andresen, V., Klapp, B. F., Wiedenmann, B., Klussmann, S., and Monnikes, H. (2006). Anti-ghrelin Spiegelmer NOX-B11 inhibits neurostimulatory and orexigenic effects of peripheral ghrelin in rats. *Gut. 55,* 788-792.

Kobelt, P., Wisser, A. S., Stengel, A., Goebel, M., Inhoff, T., Noetzel, S., Veh, R. W., Bannert, N., van, d. V., I, Wiedenmann, B., Klapp, B. F., Tache, Y., and Monnikes, H. (2008). Peripheral injection of ghrelin induces Fos expression in the dorsomedial hypothalamic nucleus in rats. *Brain Res. 1204,* 77-86.

Kohno, D., Nakata, M., Maekawa, F., Fujiwara, K., Maejima, Y., Kuramochi, M., Shimazaki, T., Okano, H., Onaka, T., and Yada, T. (2007). Leptin suppresses ghrelin-induced activation of neuropeptide Y neurons in the arcuate nucleus via phosphatidylinositol 3-kinase- and phosphodiesterase 3-mediated pathway. *Endocrinology. 148,* 2251-2263.

Kohno, D., Sone, H., Minokoshi, Y., and Yada, T. (2008). Ghrelin raises [Ca2+]i via AMPK in hypothalamic arcuate nucleus NPY neurons. *Biochem. Biophys. Res. Commun. 366,* 388-392.

Kojima, M. and Kangawa, K. (2008). Structure and function of ghrelin. *Results Probl. Cell Differ. 46,* 89-115.

Kojima, M., Hosoda, H., Date, Y., Nakazato, M., Matsuo, H., and Kangawa, K. (1999). Ghrelin is a growth-hormone-releasing acylated peptide from stomach. *Nature. 402,* 656-660.

Kojima, M., Hosoda, H., Matsuo, H., and Kangawa, K. (2001). Ghrelin: discovery of the natural endogenous ligand for the growth hormone secretagogue receptor. *Trends Endocrinol. Metab. 12,* 118-122.

Konturek, P. C., Brzozowski, T., Pajdo, R., Nikiforuk, A., Kwiecien, S., Harsch, I., Drozdowicz, D., Hahn, E. G., and Konturek, S. J. (2004). Ghrelin-a new gastroprotective factor in gastric mucosa. *J. Physiol. Pharmacol. 55,* 325-336.

Korbonits, M., Bustin, S. A., Kojima, M., Jordan, S., Adams, E. F., Lowe, D. G., Kangawa, K., and Grossman, A. B. (2001a). The expression of the growth hormone secretagogue receptor ligand ghrelin in normal and abnormal human pituitary and other neuroendocrine tumors. *J. Clin. Endocrinol. Metab. 86,* 881-887.

Korbonits, M., Kojima, M., Kangawa, K., and Grossman, A. B. (2001b). Presence of ghrelin in normal and adenomatous human pituitary. *Endocrine. 14,* 101-104.

Korbonits, M., Gueorguiev, M., O'Grady, E., Lecoeur, C., Swan, D. C., Mein, C. A., Weill, J., Grossman, A. B., and Froguel, P. (2002). A variation in the ghrelin gene increases weight and decreases insulin secretion in tall, obese children. *J. Clin. Endocrinol. Metab. 87,* 4005-4008.

Korbonits, M., Goldstone, A. P., Gueorguiev, M., and Grossman, A. B. (2004). Ghrelin--a hormone with multiple functions. *Frontiers in Neuroendocrinology. 25,* 27-68.

Korner, J., Inabnet, W., Conwell, I. M., Taveras, C., Daud, A., Olivero-Rivera, L., Restuccia, N. L., and Bessler, M. (2006). Differential effects of gastric bypass and banding on circulating gut hormone and leptin levels. *Obesity (Silver Spring), 14,* 1553-1561.

Kraemer, R. R. and Castracane, V. D. (2007). Exercise and humoral mediators of peripheral energy balance: ghrelin and adiponectin. *Exp. Biol. Med. (Maywood), 232,* 184-194.

Krsek, M., Rosicka, M., Haluzik, M., Svobodova, J., Kotrlikova, E., Justova, V., Lacinova, Z., and Jarkovska, Z. (2002). Plasma ghrelin levels in patients with short bowel syndrome. *Endocr. Res. 28,* 27-33.

Lagaud, G. J., Young, A., Acena, A., Morton, M. F., Barrett, T. D., and Shankley, N. P. (2007). Obestatin reduces food intake and suppresses body weight gain in rodents. *Biochem. Biophys. Res. Commun. 357,* 264-269.

Lai, K. C., Cheng, C. H., and Leung, P. S. (2007). The ghrelin system in acinar cells: localization, expression, and regulation in the exocrine pancreas. *Pancreas. 35,* e1-e8.

Landgren, S., Jerlhag, E., Zetterberg, H., Gonzalez-Quintela, A., Campos, J., Olofsson, U., Nilsson, S., Blennow, K., and Engel, J. A. (2008). Association of Pro-Ghrelin and GHS-R1A Gene Polymorphisms and Haplotypes With Heavy Alcohol Use and Body Mass. *Alcohol. Clin. Exp. Res. 32,* 1-8.

Larsen, L. H., Gjesing, A. P., Sorensen, T. I., Hamid, Y. H., Echwald, S. M., Toubro, S., Black, E., Astrup, A., Hansen, T., and Pedersen, O. (2005). Mutation analysis of the preproghrelin gene: no association with obesity and type 2 diabetes. *Clin. Biochem. 38,* 420-424.

Lasseter, K. C., Shaughnessy, L., Cummings, D., Pezzullo, J. C., Wargin, W., Gagnon, R., Oliva, J., and Kosutic, G. (2008). Ghrelin agonist (TZP-101): safety, pharmacokinetics and pharmacodynamic evaluation in healthy volunteers: a phase I, first-in-human study. *J. Clin. Pharmacol. 48,* 193-202.

Lauwers, E., Landuyt, B., Arckens, L., Schoofs, L., and Luyten, W. (2006). Obestatin does not activate orphan G protein-coupled receptor GPR39. *Biochem. Biophys. Res. Commun, 351,* 21-25.

le Roux, C. W., Neary, N. M., Halsey, T. J., Small, C. J., Martinez-Isla, A. M., Ghatei, M. A., Theodorou, N. A., and Bloom, S. R. (2005). Ghrelin does not stimulate food intake in patients with surgical procedures involving vagotomy. *J. Clin. Endocrinol. Metab. 90,* 4521-4524.

Lee, H. M., Wang, G., Englander, E. W., Kojima, M., and Greeley, G. H., Jr. (2002). Ghrelin, A New Gastrointestinal Endocrine Peptide that Stimulates Insulin Secretion: Enteric Distribution, Ontogeny, Influence of Endocrine, and Dietary Manipulations. *Endocrinology. 143,* 185-190.

Lengyel, A. M. (2006). From growth hormone-releasing peptides to ghrelin: discovery of new modulators of GH secretion. *Arq. Bras. Endocrinol. Metabol. 50,* 17-24.

Leung, P. K., Chow, K. B., Lau, P. N., Chu, K. M., Chan, C. B., Cheng, C. H., and Wise, H. (2007). The truncated ghrelin receptor polypeptide (GHS-R1b) acts as a dominant-negative mutant of the ghrelin receptor. *Cell Signal. 19,* 1011-1022.

Levin, F., Edholm, T., Ehrstrom, M., Wallin, B., Schmidt, P. T., Kirchgessner, A. M., Hilsted, L. M., Hellstrom, P. M., and Naslund, E. (2005). Effect of peripherally administered ghrelin on gastric emptying and acid secretion in the rat. *Regul. Pept. 131,* 59-65.

Li, B., Duysen, E. G., and Lockridge, O. (2008). The butyrylcholinesterase knockout mouse is obese on a high-fat diet. *Chem. Biol. Interact. 175,* 88-91.

Li, W. G., Gavrila, D., Liu, X., Wang, L., Gunnlaugsson, S., Stoll, L. L., McCormick, M. L., Sigmund, C. D., Tang, C., and Weintraub, N. L. (2004). Ghrelin inhibits proinflammatory responses and nuclear factor-kappaB activation in human endothelial cells. *Circulation. 109,* 2221-2226.

Liang, J. J., Oelkers, P., Guo, C., Chu, P. C., Dixon, J. L., Ginsberg, H. N., and Sturley, S. L. (2004). Overexpression of Human Diacylglycerol Acyltransferase 1, Acyl-CoA:Cholesterol Acyltransferase 1, or Acyl-CoA:Cholesterol Acyltransferase 2 Stimulates Secretion of Apolipoprotein B-containing Lipoproteins in McA-RH7777 Cells. *J. Biol. Chem. 279,* 44938-44944.

Longo, K. A., Charoenthongtrakul, S., Giuliana, D. J., Govek, E. K., McDonagh, T., Qi, Y., Distefano, P. S., and Geddes, B. J. (2008). Improved insulin sensitivity and metabolic flexibility in ghrelin receptor knockout mice. *Regul. Pept. 150,* 55-61.

Lu, S., Guan, J. L., Wang, Q. P., Uehara, K., Yamada, S., Goto, N., Date, Y., Nakazato, M., Kojima, M., Kangawa, K., and Shioda, S. (2002). Immunocytochemical observation of ghrelin-containing neurons in the rat arcuate nucleus. *Neurosci. Lett. 321,* 157-160.

Luquet, S., Phillips, C. T., and Palmiter, R. D. (2007). NPY/AgRP neurons are not essential for feeding responses to glucoprivation. *Peptides. 28,* 214-225.

Ma, J. N., Schiffer, H. H., Knapp, A. E., Wang, J., Wong, K. K., Currier, E. A., Owens, M., Nash, N. R., Gardell, L. R., Brann, M. R., Olsson, R., and Burstein, E. S. (2007). Identification of the atypical L-type Ca2+ channel blocker diltiazem and its metabolites as ghrelin receptor agonists. *Mol. Pharmacol. 72,* 380-386.

Madsen, J. L., Madsbad, S., Shaughnessy, L., Jensen, T. H., Pezzullo, J. C., and Kosutic, G. (2007). Ghrelin Agonist (TZP-101) Gastroprokinetic Action in Diabetic Patients with Gastroparesis: A Pilot Study. *Am. Diabetes Ass.* Abst 0599-P.

Mager, U., Lindi, V., Lindstrom, J., Eriksson, J. G., Valle, T. T., Hamalainen, H., Ilanne-Parikka, P., Keinanen-Kiukaanniemi, S., Tuomilehto, J., Laakso, M., Pulkkinen, L., and Uusitupa, M. (2006). Association of the Leu72Met polymorphism of the ghrelin gene with the risk of Type 2 diabetes in subjects with impaired glucose tolerance in the Finnish Diabetes Prevention Study. *Diabet. Med. 23,* 685-689.

Mager, U., Kolehmainen, M., de Mello, V. D., Schwab, U., Laaksonen, D. E., Rauramaa, R., Gylling, H., Atalay, M., Pulkkinen, L., and Uusitupa, M. (2008). Expression of ghrelin gene in peripheral blood mononuclear cells and plasma ghrelin concentrations in patients with metabolic syndrome. *Eur. J. Endocrinol. 158,* 499-510.

Malagon, M. M., Luque, R. M., Ruiz-Guerrero, E., Rodriguez-Pacheco, F., Garcia-Navarro, S., Casanueva, F. F., Gracia-Navarro, F., and Castano, J. P. (2003). Intracellular signaling mechanisms mediating ghrelin-stimulated growth hormone release in somatotropes. *Endocrinology. 144,* 5372-5380.

Mancini, M. C., Costa, A. P., de Melo, M. E., Cercato, C., Giannella-Neto, D., Garrido, A. B., Jr., Rosberg, S., Albertsson-Wikland, K., Villares, S. M., and Halpern, A. (2006). Effect of gastric bypass on spontaneous growth hormone and ghrelin release profiles. *Obesity. (Silver Spring), 14,* 383-387.

Martin, G. R., Loredo, J. C., and Sun, G. (2008). Lack of Association of Ghrelin Precursor Gene Variants and Percentage Body Fat or Serum Lipid Profiles. *Obesity. 16,* 908-912.

Masuda, Y., Tanaka, T., Inomata, N., Ohnuma, N., Tanaka, S., Itoh, Z., Hosoda, H., Kojima, M., and Kangawa, K. (2000). Ghrelin Stimulates Gastric Acid Secretion and Motility in Rats. *Biochem. Biophys. Res. Commun. 276,* 905-908.

Matsumoto, M., Hosoda, H., Kitajima, Y., Morozumi, N., Minamitake, Y., Tanaka, S., Matsuo, H., Kojima, M., Hayashi, Y., and Kangawa, K. (2001). Structure-activity relationship of ghrelin: pharmacological study of ghrelin peptides. *Biochem. Biophys. Res. Commun. 287,* 142-146.

McKee, K. K., Palyha, O. C., Feighner, S. D., Hreniuk, D. L., Tan, C. P., Phillips, M. S., Smith, R. G., Van der Ploeg, L. H. T., and Howard, A. D. (1997). Molecular Analysis of Rat Pituitary and Hypothalamic Growth Hormone Secretagogue Receptors. *Mol. Endocrinol. 11,* 415-423.

Miljic, D., Pekic, S., Djurovic, M., Doknic, M., Milic, N., Casanueva, F. F., Ghatei, M., and Popovic, V. (2006). Ghrelin has partial or no effect on appetite, growth hormone, prolactin, and cortisol release in patients with anorexia nervosa. *J. Clin. Endocrinol. Metab. 91,* 1491-1495.

Mingrone, G., Granato, L., Valera-Mora, E., Iaconelli, A., Calvani, M. F., Bracaglia, R., Manco, M., Nanni, G., and Castagneto, M. (2006). Ultradian ghrelin pulsatility is disrupted in morbidly obese subjects after weight loss induced by malabsorptive bariatric surgery. *Am. J. Clin. Nutr. 83,* 1017-1024.

Miraglia, d. G., Santoro, N., Cirillo, G., Raimondo, P., Grandone, A., D'Aniello, A., Di Nardo, M., and Perrone, L. (2004). Molecular screening of the ghrelin gene in Italian obese children: the Leu72Met variant is associated with an earlier onset of obesity. *Int. J. Obes. Relat. Metab. Disord. 28,* 447-450.

Miyasaka, K., Hosoya, H., Sekime, A., Ohta, M., Amono, H., Matsushita, S., Suzuki, K., Higuchi, S., and Funakoshi, A. (2006). Association of ghrelin receptor gene polymorphism with bulimia nervosa in a Japanese population. *J. Neural. Transm. 113,* 1279-1285.

Moechars, D., Depoortere, I., Moreaux, B., De, S. B., Goris, I., Hoskens, L., Daneels, G., Kass, S., Ver, D. L., Peeters, T., and Coulie, B. (2006). Altered gastrointestinal and metabolic function in the GPR39-obestatin receptor-knockout mouse. *Gastroenterology. 131,* 1131-1141.

Monteleone, P., Tortorella, A., Castaldo, E., Di Filippo, C., and Maj, M. (2006). No association of the Arg51Gln and Leu72Met polymorphisms of the ghrelin gene with anorexia nervosa or bulimia nervosa. *Neurosci. Lett. 398,* 325-327.

Monteleone, P., Tortorella, A., Castaldo, E., Di Filippo, C., and Maj, M. (2007). The Leu72Met polymorphism of the ghrelin gene is significantly associated with binge eating disorder. *Psychiatr. Genet. 17,* 13-16.

Monteleone, P., Serritella, C., Martiadis, V., Scognamiglio, P., and Maj, M. (2008). Plasma obestatin, ghrelin, and ghrelin/obestatin ratio increase in underweight patients with anorexia nervosa but not in symptomatic patients with bulimia nervosa. *J. Clin. Endocrinol. Metab.* in press doi:10.1210/jc.2008-1138.

Moulin, A., Demange, L., Ryan, J., M'Kadmi, C., Galleyrand, J. C., Martinez, J., and Fehrentz, J. A. (2008). Trisubstituted 1,2,4-triazoles as ligands for the ghrelin receptor: on the significance of the orientation and substitution at position 3. *Bioorg. Med. Chem. Lett. 18,* 164-168.

Muccioli, G., Pons, N., Ghe, C., Catapano, F., Granata, R., and Ghigo, E. (2004). Ghrelin and des-acyl ghrelin both inhibit isoproterenol-induced lipolysis in rat adipocytes via a non-type 1a growth hormone secretagogue receptor. *Eur. J. Pharmacol. 498,* 27-35.

Murata, M., Okimura, Y., Iida, K., Matsumoto, M., Sowa, H., Kaji, H., Kojima, M., Kangawa, K., and Chihara, K. (2002). Ghrelin modulates the downstream molecules of insulin signaling in hepatoma cells. *J. Biol. Chem. 277*, 5667-5674.

Nagamine, J., Nagata, R., Seki, H., Nomura-Akimaru, N., Ueki, Y., Kumagai, K., Taiji, M., and Noguchi, H. (2001). Pharmacological profile of a new orally active growth hormone secretagogue, SM-130686. *J. Endocrinol. 171*, 481-489.

Nagaya, N., Uematsu, M., Kojima, M., Date, Y., Nakazato, M., Okumura, H., Hosoda, H., Shimizu, W., Yamagishi, M., Oya, H., Koh, H., Yutani, C., and Kangawa, K. (2001). Elevated circulating level of ghrelin in cachexia associated with chronic heart failure: relationships between ghrelin and anabolic/catabolic factors. *Circulation. 104*, 2034-2038.

Nagaya, N., Kojima, M., and Kangawa, K. (2006). Ghrelin, a novel growth hormone-releasing peptide, in the treatment of cardiopulmonary-associated cachexia. *Intern. Med. 45*, 127-134.

Nakahara, T., Harada, T., Yasuhara, D., Shimada, N., Amitani, H., Sakoguchi, T., Kamiji, M. M., Asakawa, A., and Inui, A. (2008). Plasma obestatin concentrations are negatively correlated with body mass index, insulin resistance index, and plasma leptin concentrations in obesity and anorexia nervosa. *Biol. Psychiatry. 64*, 252-255.

Nakai, N., Kaneko, M., Nakao, N., Fujikawa, T., Nakashima, K., Ogata, M., and Tanaka, M. (2004). Identification of promoter region of ghrelin gene in human medullary thyroid carcinoma cell line. *Life Sci. 75*, 2193-2201.

Nakazato, M., Murakami, N., Date, Y., Kojima, M., Matsuo, H., Kangawa, K., and Matsukura, S. (2001). A role for ghrelin in the central regulation of feeding. *Nature. 409*, 194-198.

Natalucci, G., Riedl, S., Gleiss, A., Zidek, T., and Frisch, H. (2005). Spontaneous 24-h ghrelin secretion pattern in fasting subjects: maintenance of a meal-related pattern. *Eur. J. Endocrinol. 152*, 845-850.

Nishi, Y., Hiejima, H., Hosoda, H., Kaiya, H., Mori, K., Fukue, Y., Yanase, T., Nawata, H., Kangawa, K., and Kojima, M. (2005). Ingested Medium-Chain Fatty Acids Are Directly Utilized for the Acyl Modification of Ghrelin. *Endocrinology. 146*, 2255-2264.

Nogueiras, R., Pfluger, P., Tovar, S., Arnold, M., Mitchell, S., Morris, A., Perez-Tilve, D., Vazquez, M. J., Wiedmer, P., Castaneda, T. R., DiMarchi, R., Tschop, M., Schurmann, A., Joost, H. G., Williams, L. M., Langhans, W., and Dieguez, C. (2007). Effects of obestatin on energy balance and growth hormone secretion in rodents. *Endocrinology. 148*, 21-26.

Nogueiras, R., Tschop, M. H., and Zigman, J. M. (2008). Central nervous system regulation of energy metabolism: ghrelin versus leptin. *Ann. N. Y. Acad. Sci. 1126*, 14-19.

Otukonyong, E. E., Dube, M. G., Torto, R., Kalra, P. S., and Kalra, S. P. (2005). High-fat diet-induced ultradian leptin and insulin hypersecretion are absent in obesity-resistant rats. *Obes. Res. 13*, 991-999.

Paik, K. H., Lee, M. K., Jin, D. K., Kang, H. W., Lee, K. H., Kim, A. H., Kim, C., Lee, J. E., Oh, Y. J., Kim, S., Han, S. J., Kwon, E. K., and Choe, Y. H. (2007). Marked suppression of ghrelin concentration by insulin in Prader-willi syndrome. *J. Korean Med. Sci. 22*, 177-182.

Palik, E., Baranyi, E., Melczer, Z., Audikovszky, M., Szocs, A., Winkler, G., and Cseh, K. (2007). Elevated serum acylated (biologically active) ghrelin and resistin levels associate with pregnancy-induced weight gain and insulin resistance. *Diabetes Res. Clin. Pract. 76,* 351-357.

Pantel, J., Legendre, M., Cabrol, S., Hilal, L., Hajaji, Y., Morisset, S., Nivot, S., Vie-Luton, M. P., Grouselle, D., de Kerdanet, M., Kadiri, A., Epelbaum, J., Le Bouc, Y., and Amselem, S. (2006). Loss of constitutive activity of the growth hormone secretagogue receptor in familial short stature. *J. Clin. Invest. 116,* 760-768.

Patterson, M., Murphy, K. G., le Roux, C. W., Ghatei, M. A., and Bloom, S. R. (2005). Characterization of Ghrelin-Like Immunoreactivity in Human Plasma. *J. Clin. Endocrinol. Metab. 90,* 2205-2211.

Peeters, T. L. (2003). Central and peripheral mechanisms by which ghrelin regulates gut motility. *J. Physiol. Pharmacol. 54 Suppl. 4,* 95-103.

Peeters, T. L. (2005). Ghrelin: a new player in the control of gastrointestinal functions. *Gut. 54,* 1638-1649.

Peeters, T. L. (2006). Potential of ghrelin as a therapeutic approach for gastrointestinal motility disorders. *Curr. Opin. Pharmacol. 6,* 553-558.

Pemberton, C., Wimalasena, P., Yandle, T., Soule, S., and Richards, M. (2003). C-terminal pro-ghrelin peptides are present in the human circulation. *Biochem. Biophys. Res. Commun. 310,* 567-573.

Pfluger, P. T., Kirchner, H., Gunnel, S., Schrott, B., Perez-Tilve, D., Fu, S., Benoit, S. C., Horvath, T., Joost, H. G., Wortley, K. E., Sleeman, M. W., and Tschop, M. H. (2008). Simultaneous deletion of ghrelin and its receptor increases motor activity and energy expenditure. *Am. J. Physiol. Gastrointest. Liver Physiol. 294,* G610-G618.

Poitras, P., Polvino, W. J., and Rocheleau, B. (2005). Gastrokinetic effect of ghrelin analog RC-1139 in the rat. Effect on post-operative and on morphine induced ileus. *Peptides. 26,* 1598-1601.

Popovic, V., Miljic, D., Micic, D., Damjanovic, S., Arvat, E., Ghigo, E., Dieguez, C., and Casanueva, F. F. (2003). Ghrelin main action on the regulation of growth hormone release is exerted at hypothalamic level. *J. Clin. Endocrinol. Metab. 88,* 3450-3453.

Prado, C. L., Pugh-Bernard, A. E., Elghazi, L., Sosa-Pineda, B., and Sussel, L. (2004). Ghrelin cells replace insulin-producing beta cells in two mouse models of pancreas development. *Proc. Natl. Acad. Sci. U. S. A. 101,* 2924-2929.

Purnell, J. Q., Cummings, D., and Weigle, D. S. (2007). Changes in 24-h area-under-the-curve ghrelin values following diet-induced weight loss are associated with loss of fat-free mass, but not with changes in fat mass, insulin levels or insulin sensitivity. *Int. J. Obes. (Lond), 31,* 385-389.

Qiu, W. C., Wang, Z. G., Wang, W. G., Yan, J., and Zheng, Q. (2008a). Gastric motor effects of ghrelin and growth hormone releasing peptide 6 in diabetic mice with gastroparesis. *World J. Gastroenterol. 14,* 1419-1424.

Qiu, W. C., Wang, Z. G., Wang, W. G., Yan, J., and Zheng, Q. (2008b). Therapeutic effects of ghrelin and growth hormone releasing peptide 6 on gastroparesis in streptozotocin-induced diabetic guinea pigs in vivo and in vitro. *Chin. Med. J. (Engl.), 121,* 1183-1188.

Ramos, E. J., Meguid, M. M., Campos, A. C., and Coelho, J. C. (2005). Neuropeptide Y, alpha-melanocyte-stimulating hormone, and monoamines in food intake regulation. *Nutrition. 21,* 269-279.

Reimer, M. K., Pacini, G., and Ahren, B. (2003). Dose-dependent inhibition by ghrelin of insulin secretion in the mouse. *Endocrinology. 144,* 916-921.

Riediger, T., Traebert, M., Schmid, H. A., Scheel, C., Lutz, T. A., and Scharrer, E. (2003). Site-specific effects of ghrelin on the neuronal activity in the hypothalamic arcuate nucleus. *Neurosci. Lett. 341,* 151-155.

Rindi, G., Necchi, V., Savio, A., Torsello, A., Zoli, M., Locatelli, V., Raimondo, F., Cocchi, D., and Solcia, E. (2002). Characterisation of gastric ghrelin cells in man and other mammals: studies in adult and fetal tissues. *Histochem. Cell Biol. 117,* 511-519.

Rodriguez-Pacheco, F., Luque, R. M., Tena-Sempere, M., Malagon, M. M., and Castano, J. P. (2008). Ghrelin induces growth hormone secretion via a nitric oxide/cGMP signalling pathway. *J. Neuroendocrinol. 20,* 406-412.

Rubinfeld, H., Hadani, M., Taylor, J. E., Dong, J. Z., Comstock, J., Shen, Y., DeOliveira, D., Datta, R., Culler, M. D., and Shimon, I. (2004). Novel ghrelin analogs with improved affinity for the GH secretagogue receptor stimulate GH and prolactin release from human pituitary cells. *Eur. J. Endocrinol. 151,* 787-795.

Rudolph, J., Esler, W. P., O'connor, S., Coish, P. D., Wickens, P. L., Brands, M., Bierer, D. E., Bloomquist, B. T., Bondar, G., Chen, L., Chuang, C. Y., Claus, T. H., Fathi, Z., Fu, W., Khire, U. R., Kristie, J. A., Liu, X. G., Lowe, D. B., McClure, A. C., Michels, M., Ortiz, A. A., Ramsden, P. D., Schoenleber, R. W., Shelekhin, T. E., Vakalopoulos, A., Tang, W., Wang, L., Yi, L., Gardell, S. J., Livingston, J. N., Sweet, L. J., and Bullock, W. H. (2007). Quinazolinone derivatives as orally available ghrelin receptor antagonists for the treatment of diabetes and obesity. *J. Med. Chem. 50,* 5202-5216.

Saad, M. F., Bernaba, B., Hwu, C. M., Jinagouda, S., Fahmi, S., Kogosov, E., and Boyadjian, R. (2002). Insulin regulates plasma ghrelin concentration. *J. Clin. Endocrinol. Metab. 87,* 3997-4000.

Sakata, I., Nakamura, K., Yamazaki, M., Matsubara, M., Hayashi, Y., Kangawa, K., and Sakai, T. (2002). Ghrelin-producing cells exist as two types of cells, closed- and opened-type cells, in the rat gastrointestinal tract. *Peptides. 23,* 531-536.

Sakata, I., Yamazaki, M., Inoue, K., Hayashi, Y., Kangawa, K., and Sakai, T. (2003). Growth hormone secretagogue receptor expression in the cells of the stomach-projected afferent nerve in the rat nodose ganglion. *Neurosci. Lett. 342,* 183-186.

Salehi, A., Dornonville, d. l. C., Hakanson, R., and Lundquist, I. (2004). Effects of ghrelin on insulin and glucagon secretion: a study of isolated pancreatic islets and intact mice. *Regul. Pept. 118,* 143-150.

Sallam, H. S., Oliveira, H. M., Gan, H. T., Herndon, D. N., and Chen, J. D. (2007). Ghrelin improves burn-induced delayed gastrointestinal transit in rats. *Am. J. Physiol. Regul. Integr. Comp. Physiol. 292,* R253-R257.

Samson, W. K., White, M. M., Price, C., and Ferguson, A. V. (2007). Obestatin acts in brain to inhibit thirst. *Am. J. Physiol. Regul. Integr. Comp. Physiol. 292,* R637-R643.

Scott, V., McDade, D. M., and Luckman, S. M. (2007). Rapid changes in the sensitivity of arcuate nucleus neurons to central ghrelin in relation to feeding status. *Physiol. Behav. 90,* 180-185.

Sehirli, O., Sener, E., Sener, G., Cetinel, S., Erzik, C., and Yegen, B. C. (2008). Ghrelin improves burn-induced multiple organ injury by depressing neutrophil infiltration and the release of pro-inflammatory cytokines. *Peptides. 29,* 1231-1240.

Seim, I., Collet, C., Herington, A., and Chopin, L. (2007). Revised genomic structure of the human ghrelin gene and identification of novel exons, alternative splice variants and natural antisense transcripts. *BMC Genomics. 8,* 298.

Shafton, A. D., Sanger, G. J., Witherington, J., Brown, J. D., Muir, A., Butler, S., Abberley, L., Shimizu, Y., and Furness, J. B. (2008). Oral administration of a centrally acting ghrelin receptor agonist to conscious rats triggers defecation. *Neurogastroenterol. Motil.* in press doi:10.1111/j.1365-2982.2008.01176.x.

Shanado, Y., Kometani, M., Uchiyama, H., Koizumi, S., and Teno, N. (2004). Lysophospholipase I identified as a ghrelin deacylation enzyme in rat stomach. *Biochem. Biophys. Res. Commun. 325,* 1487-1494.

Shearman, L. P., Wang, S. P., Helmling, S., Stribling, D. S., Mazur, P., Ge, L., Wang, L., Klussmann, S., Macintyre, D. E., Howard, A. D., and Strack, A. M. (2006). Ghrelin neutralization by a ribonucleic acid-SPM ameliorates obesity in diet-induced obese mice. *Endocrinology. 147,* 1517-1526.

Shimbara, T., Mondal, M. S., Kawagoe, T., Toshinai, K., Koda, S., Yamaguchi, H., Date, Y., and Nakazato, M. (2004). Central administration of ghrelin preferentially enhances fat ingestion. *Neurosci. Lett. 369,* 75-79.

Shimizu, Y., Nagaya, N., Isobe, T., Imazu, M., Okumura, H., Hosoda, H., Kojima, M., Kangawa, K., and Kohno, N. (2003). Increased plasma ghrelin level in lung cancer cachexia. *Clin. Cancer Res. 9,* 774-778.

Shintani, M., Ogawa, Y., Ebihara, K., izawa-Abe, M., Miyanaga, F., Takaya, K., Hayashi, T., Inoue, G., Hosoda, K., Kojima, M., Kangawa, K., and Nakao, K. (2001). Ghrelin, an endogenous growth hormone secretagogue, is a novel orexigenic peptide that antagonizes leptin action through the activation of hypothalamic neuropeptide Y/Y1 receptor pathway. *Diabetes. 50,* 227-232.

Shuto, Y., Shibasaki, T., Otagiri, A., Kuriyama, H., Ohata, H., Tamura, H., Kamegai, J., Sugihara, H., Oikawa, S., and Wakabayashi, I. (2002). Hypothalamic growth hormone secretagogue receptor regulates growth hormone secretion, feeding, and adiposity. *J. Clin. Invest. 109,* 1429-1436.

Sibilia, V., Pagani, F., Guidobono, F., Locatelli, V., Torsello, A., Deghenghi, R., and Netti, C. (2002). Evidence for a central inhibitory role of growth hormone secretagogues and ghrelin on gastric acid secretion in conscious rats. *Neuroendocrinology. 75,* 92-97.

Sibilia, V., Rindi, G., Pagani, F., Rapetti, D., Locatelli, V., Torsello, A., Campanini, N., Deghenghi, R., and Netti, C. (2003). Ghrelin protects against ethanol-induced gastric ulcers in rats: studies on the mechanisms of action. *Endocrinology. 144,* 353-359.

Sibilia, V., Bresciani, E., Lattuada, N., Rapetti, D., Locatelli, V., De, L., V, Dona, F., Netti, C., Torsello, A., and Guidobono, F. (2006). Intracerebroventricular acute and chronic administration of obestatin minimally affect food intake but not weight gain in the rat. *J. Endocrinol. Invest. 29,* RC31-RC34.

Simonsson, M., Eriksson, S., Hakanson, R., Lind, T., Lonroth, H., Lundell, L., O'Connor, D. T., and Sundler, F. (1988). Endocrine cells in the human oxyntic mucosa. A histochemical study. *Scand. J. Gastroenterol. 23,* 1089-1099.

Smith, R. G., Pong, S. S., Hickey, G., Jacks, T., Cheng, K., Leonard, R., Cohen, C. J., Arena, J. P., Chang, C. H., Drisko, J., Wyvratt, M., Fisher, M., Nargund, R., and Patchett, A. (1996). Modulation of pulsatile GH release through a novel receptor in hypothalamus and pituitary gland. *Recent Prog. Horm. Res. 51,* 261-285.

Smith, R. G., Van Der Ploeg, L. H., Howard, A. D., Feighner, S. D., Cheng, K., Hickey, G. J., Wyvratt, M. J., Jr., Fisher, M. H., Nargund, R. P., and Patchett, A. A. (1997). Peptidomimetic regulation of growth hormone secretion. *Endocr. Rev. 18,* 621-645.

Smith, R. G., Sun, Y., Jiang, H., barran-Zeckler, R., and Timchenko, N. (2007). Ghrelin receptor (GHS-R1A) agonists show potential as interventive agents during aging. *Ann. N. Y. Acad. Sci. 1119,* 147-164.

Soeki, T., Kishimoto, I., Schwenke, D. O., Tokudome, T., Horio, T., Yoshida, M., Hosoda, H., and Kangawa, K. (2008). Ghrelin suppresses cardiac sympathetic activity and prevents early left ventricular remodeling in rats with myocardial infarction. *Am. J. Physiol. Heart Circ. Physiol. 294,* H426-H432.

Solcia, E., Rindi, G., Buffa, R., Fiocca, R., and Capella, C. (2000). Gastric endocrine cells: types, function and growth. *Regul. Pept. 93,* 31-35.

Solomon, A., De Fanti, B. A., and Martinez, J. A. (2005). Peripheral ghrelin participates in glucostatic feeding mechanisms and in the anorexigenic signalling mediated by CART and CRF neurons. *Nutr. Neurosci. 8,* 287-295.

Soriano-Guillen, L., Barrios, V., Campos-Barros, A., and Argente, J. (2004). Ghrelin levels in obesity and anorexia nervosa: effect of weight reduction or recuperation. *J. Pediatr. 144,* 36-42.

Steinle, N. I., Pollin, T. I., O'Connell, J. R., Mitchell, B. D., and Shuldiner, A. R. (2005). Variants in the ghrelin gene are associated with metabolic syndrome in the Old Order Amish. *J. Clin. Endocrinol. Metab. 90,* 6672-6677.

Stenstrom, B., Zhao, C. M., Tommeras, K., Arum, C. J., and Chen, D. (2006). Is gastrin partially responsible for body weight reduction after gastric bypass? *Eur. Surg. Res. 38,* 94-101.

Strassburg, S., Anker, S. D., Castaneda, T. R., Burget, L., Perez-Tilve, D., Pfluger, P. T., Nogueiras, R., Halem, H., Dong, J. Z., Culler, M. D., Datta, R., and Tschop, M. H. (2008). Long-term effects of ghrelin and ghrelin receptor agonists on energy balance in rats. *Am. J. Physiol. Endocrinol. Metab. 295,* E78-E84.

Stratis, C., Alexandrides, T., Vagenas, K., and Kalfarentzos, F. (2006). Ghrelin and peptide YY levels after a variant of biliopancreatic diversion with Roux-en-Y gastric bypass versus after colectomy: a prospective comparative study. *Obes. Surg. 16,* 752-758.

Sun, Y., Asnicar, M., Saha, P. K., Chan, L., and Smith, R. G. (2006). Ablation of ghrelin improves the diabetic but not obese phenotype of ob/ob mice. *Cell Metab. 3,* 379-386.

Sun, Y., Wang, P., Zheng, H., and Smith, R. G. (2004). Ghrelin stimulation of growth hormone release and appetite is mediated through the growth hormone secretagogue receptor. *Proc. Natl. Acad. Sci. U. S. A. 101,* 4679-4684.

Sun, Y., Butte, N. F., Garcia, J. M., and Smith, R. G. (2008). Characterization of adult ghrelin and ghrelin receptor knockout mice under positive and negative energy balance. *Endocrinology. 149,* 843-850.

Sun, Y., Ahmed, S., and Smith, R. G. (2003). Deletion of Ghrelin Impairs neither Growth nor Appetite. *Mol. Cell Biol. 23,* 7973-7981.

Takada, R., Satomi, Y., Kurata, T., Ueno, N., Norioka, S., Kondoh, H., Takao, T., and Takada, S. (2006). Monounsaturated fatty acid modification of Wnt protein: its role in Wnt secretion. *Dev. Cell. 11,* 791-801.

Takaya, K., Ariyasu, H., Kanamoto, N., Iwakura, H., Yoshimoto, A., Harada, M., Mori, K., Komatsu, Y., Usui, T., Shimatsu, A., Ogawa, Y., Hosoda, K., Akamizu, T., Kojima, M., Kangawa, K., and Nakao, K. (2000). Ghrelin strongly stimulates growth hormone release in humans. *J. Clin. Endocrinol. Metab. 85,* 4908-4911.

Takeno, R., Okimura, Y., Iguchi, G., Kishimoto, M., Kudo, T., Takahashi, K., Takahashi, Y., Kaji, H., Ohno, M., Ikuta, H., Kuroda, Y., Obara, T., Hosoda, H., Kangawa, K., and Chihara, K. (2004). Intravenous administration of ghrelin stimulates growth hormone secretion in vagotomized patients as well as normal subjects. *Eur. J. Endocrinol. 151,* 447-450.

Tan, C. P., McKee, K. K., Liu, Q., Palyha, O. C., Feighner, S. D., Hreniuk, D. L., Smith, R. G., and Howard, A. D. (1998). Cloning and Characterization of a Human and Murine T-Cell Orphan G-Protein-Coupled Receptor Similar to the Growth Hormone Secretagogue and Neurotensin Receptors. *Genomics. 52,* 223-229.

Tanaka, M., Hayashida, Y., Iguchi, T., Nakao, N., Nakai, N., and Nakashima, K. (2001). Organization of the mouse ghrelin gene and promoter: occurrence of a short noncoding first exon. *Endocrinology. 142,* 3697-3700.

Theander-Carrillo, C., Wiedmer, P., Cettour-Rose, P., Nogueiras, R., Perez-Tilve, D., Pfluger, P., Castaneda, T. R., Muzzin, P., Schurmann, A., Szanto, I., Tschop, M. H., and Rohner-Jeanrenaud, F. (2006). Ghrelin action in the brain controls adipocyte metabolism. *J. Clin. Invest. 116,* 1983-1993.

Thompson, N. M., Gill, D. A., Davies, R., Loveridge, N., Houston, P. A., Robinson, I. C., and Wells, T. (2004). Ghrelin and des-octanoyl ghrelin promote adipogenesis directly in vivo by a mechanism independent of the type 1a growth hormone secretagogue receptor. *Endocrinology. 145,* 234-242.

Tokunaga, T., Hume, W. E., Umezome, T., Okazaki, K., Ueki, Y., Kumagai, K., Hourai, S., Nagamine, J., Seki, H., Taiji, M., Noguchi, H., and Nagata, R. (2001). Oxindole derivatives as orally active potent growth hormone secretagogues. *J. Med. Chem. 44,* 4641-4649.

Tokunaga, T., Hume, W. E., Nagamine, J., Kawamura, T., Taiji, M., and Nagata, R. (2005). Structure-activity relationships of the oxindole growth hormone secretagogues. *Bioorg. Med. Chem. Lett. 15,* 1789-1792.

Toshinai, K., Mondal, M. S., Nakazato, M., Date, Y., Murakami, N., Kojima, M., Kangawa, K., and Matsukura, S. (2001). Upregulation of Ghrelin expression in the stomach upon fasting, insulin-induced hypoglycemia, and leptin administration. *Biochem. Biophys. Res. Commun. 281,* 1220-1225.

Toshinai, K., Date, Y., Murakami, N., Shimada, M., Mondal, M. S., Shimbara, T., Guan, J. L., Wang, Q. P., Funahashi, H., Sakurai, T., Shioda, S., Matsukura, S., Kangawa, K., and Nakazato, M. (2003). Ghrelin-induced food intake is mediated via the orexin pathway. *Endocrinology. 144,* 1506-1512.

Tremblay, F., Perreault, M., Klaman, L. D., Tobin, J. F., Smith, E., and Gimeno, R. E. (2007). Normal Food Intake and Body Weight in Mice Lacking the G Protein-Coupled Receptor GPR39. *Endocrinology. 148,* 501-506.

Trudel, L., Tomasetto, C., Rio, M. C., Bouin, M., Plourde, V., Eberling, P., and Poitras, P. (2002). Ghrelin/motilin-related peptide is a potent prokinetic to reverse gastric postoperative ileus in rat. *Am. J. Physiol. Gastrointest. Liver Physiol. 282,* G948-G952.

Tschop, M., Smiley, D. L., and Heiman, M. L. (2000). Ghrelin induces adiposity in rodents. *Nature. 407,* 908-913.

Tschop, M., Wawarta, R., Riepl, R. L., Friedrich, S., Bidlingmaier, M., Landgraf, R., and Folwaczny, C. (2001). Post-prandial decrease of circulating human ghrelin levels. *J. Endocrinol. Invest. 24,* RC19-RC21.

Tsubone, T., Masaki, T., Katsuragi, I., Tanaka, K., Kakuma, T., and Yoshimatsu, H. (2005). Ghrelin regulates adiposity in white adipose tissue and UCP1 mRNA expression in brown adipose tissue in mice. *Regul. Pept. 130,* 97-103.

Ukkola, O., Ravussin, E., Jacobson, P., Snyder, E. E., Chagnon, M., Sjostrom, L., and Bouchard, C. (2001). Mutations in the preproghrelin/ghrelin gene associated with obesity in humans. *J. Clin. Endocrinol. Metab. 86,* 3996-3999.

Ukkola, O., Ravussin, E., Jacobson, P., Perusse, L., Rankinen, T., Tschop, M., Heiman, M. L., Leon, A. S., Rao, D. C., Skinner, J. S., Wilmore, J. H., Sjostrom, L., and Bouchard, C. (2002). Role of ghrelin polymorphisms in obesity based on three different studies. *Obes. Res. 10,* 782-791.

Van Craenenbroeck, M., Gregoire, F., De Neef, P., Robberecht, P., and Perret, J. (2004). Ala-scan of ghrelin (1-14): interaction with the recombinant human ghrelin receptor. *Peptides. 25,* 959-965.

Vartiainen, J., Poykko, S. M., Raisanen, T., Kesaniemi, Y. A., and Ukkola, O. (2004). Sequencing analysis of the ghrelin receptor (growth hormone secretagogue receptor type 1a) gene. *Eur. J. Endocrinol. 150,* 457-463.

Venkova, K., Fraser, G., Hoveyda, H. R., and Greenwood-Van, M. B. (2007). Prokinetic effects of a new ghrelin receptor agonist TZP-101 in a rat model of postoperative ileus. *Dig. Dis. Sci. 52,* 2241-2248.

Vivenza, D., Rapa, A., Castellino, N., Bellone, S., Petri, A., Vacca, G., Aimaretti, G., Broglio, F., and Bona, G. (2004). Ghrelin gene polymorphisms and ghrelin, insulin, IGF-I, leptin and anthropometric data in children and adolescents. *Eur. J. Endocrinol. 151,* 127-133.

Volante, M., Allia, E., Gugliotta, P., Funaro, A., Broglio, F., Deghenghi, R., Muccioli, G., Ghigo, E., and Papotti, M. (2002). Expression of ghrelin and of the GH secretagogue receptor by pancreatic islet cells and related endocrine tumors. *J. Clin. Endocrinol. Metab. 87,* 1300-1308.

Wang, H. J., Geller, F., Dempfle, A., Schauble, N., Friedel, S., Lichtner, P., Fontenla-Horro, F., Wudy, S., Hagemann, S., Gortner, L., Huse, K., Remschmidt, H., Bettecken, T., Meitinger, T., Schafer, H., Hebebrand, J., and Hinney, A. (2004). Ghrelin receptor gene: identification of several sequence variants in extremely obese children and adolescents, healthy normal-weight and underweight students, and children with short normal stature. *J. Clin. Endocrinol. Metab. 89,* 157-162.

Wierup, N., Svensson, H., Mulder, H., and Sundler, F. (2002). The ghrelin cell: a novel developmentally regulated islet cell in the human pancreas. *Regul. Pept. 107,* 63-69.

Wierup, N. and Sundler, F. (2005). Ultrastructure of islet ghrelin cells in the human fetus. *Cell Tissue Res. 319,* 423-428.

Williams, D. L., Grill, H. J., Cummings, D. E., and Kaplan, J. M. (2006). Overfeeding-induced weight gain suppresses plasma ghrelin levels in rats. *J. Endocrinol. Invest. 29,* 863-868.

Witherington, J., Abberley, L., Briggs, M. A., Collis, K., Dean, D. K., Gaiba, A., King, N. P., Kraus, H., Shuker, N., Steadman, J. G., Takle, A. K., Sanger, G., Wadsworth, G., Butler, S., McKay, F., Muir, A., Winborn, K., and Heightman, T. D. (2008). Potent achiral agonists of the growth hormone secretagogue (ghrelin) receptor. Part 2: Lead optimisation. *Bioorg. Med. Chem. Lett. 18,* 2203-2205.

Wolf, I., Sadetzki, S., Kanety, H., Kundel, Y., Pariente, C., Epstein, N., Oberman, B., Catane, R., Kaufman, B., and Shimon, I. (2006). Adiponectin, ghrelin, and leptin in cancer cachexia in breast and colon cancer patients. *Cancer. 106,* 966-973.

Wortley, K. E., Anderson, K. D., Garcia, K., Murray, J. D., Malinova, L., Liu, R., Moncrieffe, M., Thabet, K., Cox, H. J., Yancopoulos, G. D., Wiegand, S. J., and Sleeman, M. W. (2004). Genetic deletion of ghrelin does not decrease food intake but influences metabolic fuel preference. *Proc. Natl. Acad. Sci. U. S. A. 101,* 8227-8232.

Wortley, K. E., del Rincon, J. P., Murray, J. D., Garcia, K., Iida, K., Thorner, M. O., and Sleeman, M. W. (2005). Absence of ghrelin protects against early-onset obesity. *J. Clin. Invest. 115,* 3573-3578.

Wren, A. M., Seal, L. J., Cohen, M. A., Brynes, A. E., Frost, G. S., Murphy, K. G., Dhillo, W. S., Ghatei, M. A., and Bloom, S. R. (2001). Ghrelin Enhances Appetite and Increases Food Intake in Humans. *J. Clin. Endocrinol. Metab. 86,* 5992.

Wu, D., Chen, C., Zhang, J., Bowers, C. Y., and Clarke, I. J. (1996). The effects of GH-releasing peptide-6 (GHRP-6) and GHRP-2 on intracellular adenosine 3',5'-monophosphate (cAMP) levels and GH secretion in ovine and rat somatotrophs. *J. Endocrinol. 148,* 197-205.

Xia, Q., Pang, W., Pan, H., Zheng, Y., Kang, J. S., and Zhu, S. G. (2004). Effects of ghrelin on the proliferation and secretion of splenic T lymphocytes in mice. *Regul. Pept. 122,* 173-178.

Yamamoto, D., Ikeshita, N., Daito, R., Herningtyas, E. H., Toda, K., Takahashi, K., Iida, K., Takahashi, Y., Kaji, H., Chihara, K., and Okimura, Y. (2007). Neither intravenous nor intracerebroventricular administration of obestatin affects the secretion of GH, PRL, TSH and ACTH in rats. *Regul. Pept. 138,* 141-144.

Yamanaka, A., Beuckmann, C. T., Willie, J. T., Hara, J., Tsujino, N., Mieda, M., Tominaga, M., Yagami, K., Sugiyama, F., Goto, K., Yanagisawa, M., and Sakurai, T. (2003). Hypothalamic orexin neurons regulate arousal according to energy balance in mice. *Neuron. 38,* 701-713.

Yang, J., Brown, M. S., Liang, G., Grishin, N. V., and Goldstein, J. L. (2008). Identification of the Acyltransferase that Octanoylates Ghrelin, an Appetite-Stimulating Peptide Hormone. *Cell. 132,* 387-396.

Yeh, A. H., Jeffery, P. L., Duncan, R. P., Herington, A. C., and Chopin, L. K. (2005). Ghrelin and a novel preproghrelin isoform are highly expressed in prostate cancer and ghrelin activates mitogen-activated protein kinase in prostate cancer. *Clin. Cancer Res. 11,* 8295-8303.

Zamrazilova, H., Hainer, V., Sedlackova, D., Papezova, H., Kunesova, M., Bellisle, F., Hill, M., and Nedvidkova, J. (2008). Plasma obestatin levels in normal weight, obese and anorectic women. *Physiol. Res. 57 Suppl 1,* S49-S55.

Zhang, J. V., Ren, P. G., Avsian-Kretchmer, O., Luo, C. W., Rauch, R., Klein, C., and Hsueh, A. J. W. (2005). Obestatin, a Peptide Encoded by the Ghrelin Gene, Opposes Ghrelin's Effects on Food Intake. *Science. 310,* 996-999.

Zhao, C. M., Furnes, M. W., Stenstrom, B., Kulseng, B., and Chen, D. (2008). Characterization of obestatin- and ghrelin-producing cells in the gastrointestinal tract and pancreas of rats: an immunohistochemical and electron-microscopic study. *Cell Tissue Res. 331,* 575-587.

Zheng, Q., Qiu, W. C., Yan, J., Wang, W. G., Yu, S., Wang, Z. G., and Ai, K. X. (2008). Prokinetic effects of a ghrelin receptor agonist GHRP-6 in diabetic mice. *World J. Gastroenterol. 14,* 4795-4799.

Zhu, X., Cao, Y., Voodg, K., and Steiner, D. F. (2006). On the Processing of Proghrelin to Ghrelin. *J. Biol. Chem. 281,* 38867-38870.

Zigman, J. M., Nakano, Y., Coppari, R., Balthasar, N., Marcus, J. N., Lee, C. E., Jones, J. E., Deysher, A. E., Waxman, A. R., White, R. D., Williams, T. D., Lachey, J. L., Seeley, R. J., Lowell, B. B., and Elmquist, J. K. (2005). Mice lacking ghrelin receptors resist the development of diet-induced obesity. *J. Clin. Invest. 115,* 3564-3572.

Zizzari, P., Longchamps, R., Epelbaum, J., and Bluet-Pajot, M. T. (2007). Obestatin Partially Affects Ghrelin Stimulation of Food Intake and GH Secretion in Rodents. *Endocrinology. 148,* 1648-1653.

Zorrilla, E. P., Iwasaki, S., Moss, J. A., Chang, J., Otsuji, J., Inoue, K., Meijler, M. M., and Janda, K. D. (2006). Vaccination against weight gain. *Proc. Natl. Acad. Sci. U. S. A. 103,* 13226-13231.

Zou, C. C., Huang, K., Liang, L., and Zhao, Z. Y. (2008). Polymorphisms of the ghrelin/obestatin gene and ghrelin levels in Chinese children with short stature. *Clinical Endocrinology. 69,* 99-104.

INDEX

A

AA, 218, 219, 222, 225, 240
absorption, 240
acceptor, 221
accounting, 231
acid, xi, 217, 218, 220, 221, 224, 236, 237, 239, 246, 248, 250, 253, 259, 260
ACTH, 236, 237, 263
activation, 225, 226, 231, 233, 236, 237, 238, 242, 243, 247, 252, 254, 259
active ingredients, viii, 55, 67, 182, 187
acute, 234, 238, 245, 247, 259
acute lung injury, 245
acyl transferase, 220, 221
acylation, 220, 221, 222, 239
Adams, 245, 252
adenosine, 263
adhesion, 238
adipocyte, 234, 261
adipocytes, 234, 252, 255
adiponectin, 251, 253
adipose, 230, 231, 232, 234, 235, 262
adipose tissue, 232, 234, 235, 262
adipose tissue reserves, viii, 56
adiposity, xii, 217, 234, 242, 249, 259, 261, 262
administration, 222, 230, 231, 232, 233, 234, 235, 237, 239, 259, 261, 263
adolescents, 250, 262
adrenal gland, 228
adrenal glands, 228
adult, 230, 231, 234, 258, 260
adults, 240, 248
afferent nerve, 258
age, 230, 235, 246
agents, 240, 260
aging, 260

agonist, 226, 240, 241, 243, 248, 253, 259, 262, 264
alanine, 222
alcohol, 227
allele, 226
alleles, 226
alpha, 246, 257
alternative, 219, 225, 227, 239, 258
amide, 222
amino, xi, 217, 218, 220, 221, 224, 225, 240
amino acid, xi, 217, 218, 220, 221, 224
amino acids, xi, 217, 218, 220, 221, 224
amphetamine, 228, 231, 232, 246
anabolic, 256
analog, 257
animal models, 240
animals, 230, 236, 237
anorexia, 222, 227, 234, 239, 244, 255, 256, 260
anorexia nervosa, 222, 227, 234, 239, 255, 256, 260
anorexia nervosa (AN), ix, 97
antagonist, 241, 243, 247, 248
antagonists, xii, 217, 232, 239, 241, 242, 248, 258
anthropometry, 247
antiapoptotic, 252
antibody, 233
antisense, 219, 230, 242, 258
anti-sense, 219
anti-sense, 228
anxiolytic, 244
apoptosis, 234, 238, 239
appetite, xi, 217, 222, 230, 231, 232, 233, 235, 241, 242, 243, 248, 250, 255, 260
appetite control, vii, viii, 30, 43, 44, 49, 55, 56, 57, 58, 69
appetite regulation, vii, viii, 1, 2, 3, 4, 5, 6, 7, 8, 9, 10, 13, 14, 16, 17, 19, 41, 43, 44, 55, 56, 57, 58, 62, 64, 67, 187, 210, 250

appetite suppressant, viii, 42, 56, 180, 187, 188, 189, 212
appetite suppression, viii, 55, 56, 65, 177, 187, 208
application, 233
ARC, 233
arginine, 221, 237
arousal, 263
ART, 245
atropine, 237
authenticity, 221
autocrine, 246

B

Badia, 244
bariatric surgery, 248, 255
BDNF, 246
behavior, 234
Belgium, 217, 242
benefits, 241
beta cell, 257
biliopancreatic, 260
biliopancreatic diversion, 260
binding, 218, 223, 225, 242, 247, 249
binge eating disorder, 255
bioavailability, 240
biological activity, xi, 217, 218, 239, 248
blocks, 243
blood, xi, 217, 227, 229, 231, 251, 254
blood glucose, 231
blood pressure, 227
blood stream, xi, 217
bloodstream, 229
blot, 221
body composition, 230, 231, 234
body dissatisfaction, 243
body fat, 227, 235
body mass index (BMI), ix, 75, 182, 227
body size, 248
body weight, xii, 217, 226, 229, 230, 231, 234, 235, 240, 242, 243, 251, 253, 260
Boeing, 247
bone density, 230
borderline, 226
bowel, 253
brain, 231, 232, 233, 258, 261
breast cancer, 219, 227, 247, 251
Brussels, 217
bulimia, 227, 244, 255
bulimia nervosa, 227, 244, 255
burn, 238, 240, 258
bypass, 234, 244, 245, 253, 254, 260

C

Ca^{2+}, 252, 254
cachexia, 234, 239, 242, 247, 256, 259, 263
calcium, 218, 225, 233, 236
caloric intake, 229
caloric restriction, 230, 231
cAMP, 218, 263
cancer, x, 2, 29, 30, 31, 44, 48, 52, 64, 84, 95, 121, 135, 136, 137, 138, 139, 140, 142, 144, 145, 146, 147, 149, 150, 151, 173, 191, 195, 214, 219, 227, 234, 239, 242, 247, 251, 259, 263
capillary, 228
carbohydrates, 234
carbon, 250
carcinoma, 221, 256
cardiomyocytes, 238
cardiopulmonary, 256
cardiovascular system, 238
catabolic, 256
catecholamine, 237
cDNA, 221
cell, 219, 221, 227, 228, 238, 239, 246, 251, 256, 262
cell line, 219, 221, 246, 251, 256
cell lines, 219, 251
cell surface, 227
central melanocortin system, x, 135, 136, 137, 141, 142, 143, 144, 145, 149
central nervous system, 228, 246
cerebral cortex, 229
cerebrospinal fluid (CSF), ix, 97, 102
channel blocker, 254
children, 235, 248, 249, 250, 251, 252, 255, 262, 264
cholecystokinin, 232, 238, 246
cholesterol, 227, 231, 245, 251
chromosome, 218, 225, 226
chromosomes, 252
chronic heart failure, x, 135, 136, 144, 145, 148, 149, 151, 238, 256
chronic kidney disease, x, 135, 136, 138, 139, 140, 143, 144, 145, 147, 151
chronic obstructive pulmonary disease, 239, 242
circadian, 231
circulation, 229, 257
cis, 241
cleavage, 220, 246
clinical trial, 240
CNS, 245
Co, 221, 261
cocaine, 231, 232
codes, 225
coding, 218, 226, 227, 247

codon, 225
colectomy, 260
colon, xi, 217, 228, 229, 234, 263
colon cancer, 234, 263
complexity, 219, 227
compounds, 240
concentration, 225, 228, 229, 235, 238, 251, 256, 258
congestive heart failure, 234, 239, 242
conservation, 221
control, xii, 217, 222, 231, 244, 247, 251, 257
conversion, 220
correlation, 226, 229
correlations, 227
corticosterone, 244
cortisol, 237, 255
coupling, 225
CP, 217, 239
CRH, 232
C-terminal, 219, 221, 222, 223, 229, 257
cytokine, 238, 247
cytokines, 238, 258

D

dairy products,, viii, 40, 56
defecation, 241, 259
deficiency, 222, 227, 240
degradation, 229, 246
delayed gastric emptying, 241
density, 227, 229, 230, 239, 245
derivatives, 240, 241, 247, 258, 261
diabetes, 222, 227, 240, 241, 242, 253, 254, 258
diabetes mellitus, 240
diacylglycerol, 225
diet, 229, 230, 231, 234, 241, 242, 245, 253, 256, 257, 259, 264
diet restriction (DR), ix, 97, 102
dietary, 234
dietary fat, 234
diets, 230, 234
differentiation, 234, 239
Discovery, 217
diseases, 242
disorder, 227, 234, 255
distribution, 229, 245, 248, 251
divergence, 250
diversity, 227
donor, 221
dopamine, 233
dose-response relationship, 235
downstream molecules, 256
drugs, 222, 249

duodenum, xi, 217, 228, 229

E

eating, 226, 231, 233, 243, 255
eating behaviour traits, vii, 1, 4, 17, 18, 19
eating disorders, 226
elderly, 234
electron, 263
ELISA, 243
encoding, 218, 221
endocrine, xi, 217, 228, 232, 238, 244, 260, 262
endocytosis, 225
endogenous ligand, xi, 217, 250, 252
endoplasmic reticulum, 220, 221, 225
endothelial cell, 238, 254
endothelial cells, 238, 254
endothelium, 238
energy, 222, 230, 231, 234, 235, 241, 242, 245, 250, 253, 256, 257, 260, 263
energy expenditure, vii, viii, xi, 2, 29, 30, 32, 37, 43, 44, 51, 52, 55, 56, 58, 61, 72, 80, 81, 82, 83, 84, 85, 87, 94, 136, 137, 139, 146, 147, 148, 153, 165, 173, 176, 184, 199, 205, 206, 209, 216, 231, 234, 235, 241, 242, 257
enterochromaffin cells, 228
enzymes, 219
ester, 222
esterase, 229
esterases, 229
ethanol, 237, 259
Evaluation and Nurturing Relationship Issues, Communication and Happiness (ENRICH), x, 125, 129
exercise, 229, 234
exocrine, xi, 217, 228, 238, 251, 253
Exon 2, 225
exons, 218, 225, 258
experimental condition, 237, 238
exposure, 230, 234

F

familial, 257
family, 220, 221, 224, 225, 244
fasting, 222, 231, 238, 241, 242, 243, 249, 256, 261
Fasting, 235
fat, 226, 229, 230, 231, 234, 240, 242, 243, 253, 256, 257, 259
fatty acids, 220, 221, 231
feeding, 231, 232, 233, 244, 246, 251, 254, 256, 258, 259, 260

feeding environment, vii, 1, 2, 8, 9, 10, 17
feeding practices, vii, 1, 2, 8, 11, 12, 13, 14, 16, 18, 19, 20, 21, 22, 27, 170
feeling of satiety, viii, 55, 177
fetal, 258
fetal tissue, 258
fetus, 262
fiber, 237
fibers, 228, 232
flexibility, 254
food, xi, 217, 228, 230, 231, 232, 233, 234, 235, 239, 241, 242, 243, 247, 249, 253, 257, 259, 261, 263
food pattern, viii, 55
food utilization, viii, 56
Fox, 247
frameshift mutation, 226, 250
fuel, 263
fundus, 228

G

G protein, 253
GABA, 228, 236
gallbladder, 228
ganglia, 244
ganglion, 233, 258
gastrectomy, 251
gastric, xi, 217, 222, 228, 229, 233, 234, 237, 240, 241, 244, 245, 246, 248, 249, 251, 252, 253, 254, 258, 259, 260, 261
gastric mucosa, 228, 229, 252
gastric ulcer, 259
gastrin, 228, 232, 237, 247, 248, 260
gastrointestinal, 231, 232, 240, 241, 242, 243, 246, 248, 250, 255, 257, 258, 263
gastrointestinal tract, 232, 246, 248, 258, 263
gastro-intestinal tract, viii, 56
gastroparesis, 240, 257
gene, 218, 219, 221, 222, 225, 226, 227, 243, 244, 245, 248, 249, 250, 251, 252, 253, 254, 255, 256, 258, 260, 261, 262, 264
gene expression, 219, 228
generation, 234
genes, 226, 246, 247
genomic, 258
genotype, 227
GH, 217, 226, 228, 230, 236, 237, 239, 240, 241, 242, 244, 247, 249, 253, 258, 259, 262, 263, 264
GLP-1, 232, 245
glucagon, 228, 232, 258
glucose, 230, 231, 237, 241, 245, 248, 249, 254
glucose metabolism, 237
glucose tolerance, 241, 248, 254
glycol, 242
gonadotropin, 239
gonadotropin secretion, 239
GPCR, 218
G-protein, 218, 224, 225
grants, 242
granules, 228
groups, 220, 222, 239, 241
growth, xi, 217, 226, 230, 234, 236, 237, 239, 240, 243, 244, 246, 248, 249, 250, 252, 253, 254, 255, 256, 257, 258, 259, 260, 261, 262
growth factor, 237
growth hormone, xi, 217, 236, 239, 240, 243, 244, 246, 248, 249, 250, 252, 253, 254, 255, 256, 257, 258, 259, 260, 261, 262
growth rate, 230, 234
gut, 253, 257

H

half-life, 229
haplotype, 227
harmonal levels, viii, 55
HDL, 227, 251
heart, xi, 217, 234, 238, 239, 242, 256
Heart, 244, 260
heart failure, 238, 256
heart rate, 238
height, 226, 250
helix, 223, 224, 226
hepatocytes, 238, 248
hepatoma, 256
heterodimer, 226
high density lipoprotein, 243
high fat, 230, 234
high-density lipoprotein, 229, 245
high-fat, 229, 230, 231, 234, 253
histamine, 228, 233
histidine, 221
histochemical, 259
homeostasis, 222, 234, 236, 245, 246, 249, 250
homology, 225
hormone, xi, 217, 218, 228, 231, 232, 236, 237, 238, 239, 240, 243, 244, 246, 248, 249, 250, 252, 253, 254, 255, 256, 257, 258, 259, 260, 261, 262
hormones, 231, 241, 243
human, 218, 219, 221, 222, 223, 226, 229, 233, 235, 238, 244, 246, 247, 250, 251, 252, 253, 254, 256, 257, 258, 259, 261, 262
humans, 231, 233, 236, 244, 245, 246, 248, 249, 260, 262
hydrolysis, 225
hydrolyzed, 251

hydrophobic, 221, 226, 239
hydrophobic groups, 239
hydroxyl, 220
hyperglycemia, 244
hypoglycemia, 261
hypothalamic, 232, 233, 236, 239, 242, 243, 245, 251, 252, 257, 258, 259
hypothalamus, ix, xi, 1, 26, 58, 61, 84, 97, 100, 101, 102, 103, 106, 109, 111, 136, 137, 141, 142, 143, 144, 172, 174, 175, 185, 186, 188, 189, 192, 198, 199, 208, 212, 217, 228, 231, 232, 233, 237, 241, 242, 246, 259
hypothesis, 220, 228, 229, 231

I

identification, 221, 246, 250, 258, 262
identity, 224
IGF, 226, 247, 262
IGF-1, 226
IGF-I, 247, 262
ileum, xi, 217, 228
immune response, 242
immunity, 247
immunohistochemical, 263
immunoreactivity, 229
impaired glucose tolerance, 254
in vitro, 221, 233, 236, 239, 247, 250, 257
in vivo, 236, 239, 240, 247, 250, 257, 261
inactive, 222, 225
indirect effect, 249
infants, 249
infarction, 238
inflammation, 238
inflammatory, 238, 258
ingestion, 220, 259
inhibition, 221, 236, 242, 257
inhibitors, 229
inhibitory, 237, 238, 259
inhibitory effect, 237, 238
initiation, 231, 245
injection, 230, 232, 233, 235, 242, 249, 252
injury, 238, 245, 258
inositol, 218, 225
insulin, 228, 230, 231, 237, 238, 241, 242, 244, 245, 246, 249, 252, 254, 256, 257, 258, 261, 262
insulin resistance, 256, 257
insulin sensitivity, 231, 254, 257
insulin signaling, 256
insulinoma, 221
integration, 220
integrity, 237, 251
interaction, 229, 240, 249, 262

intestine, 228
intraperitoneal, 233, 235
intravenous, 231, 237, 263
intron, 218, 225
introns, 218, 227
ions, 250

J

Japanese, 226, 243, 255
Japanese women, 226, 243
jejunum, xi, 217, 228, 229
Jordan, 252

K

kidney, xi, 217
kidneys, 228
kinase, 223, 225, 233, 236, 252
King, 262
knockout, 222, 229, 230, 231, 246, 250, 253, 254, 255, 260
Korean, 227, 251, 256

L

L1, 252
labeling, 221
lean body mass, 234, 247
left ventricular, 238, 260
leptin, viii, ix, 42, 55, 61, 62, 63, 67, 70, 71, 73, 74, 75, 84, 85, 86, 87, 88, 91, 92, 93, 94, 95, 139, 147, 150, 174, 175, 179, 185, 193, 194, 197, 198, 210, 222, 230, 235, 241, 247, 248, 249, 251, 253, 256, 259, 261, 262, 263
lesions, 237
leukemic, 246
Liberator, 251
ligand, xi, 217, 218, 250, 252
ligands, 247, 255
linkage, 222
lipid, 227, 234, 249
Lipid, 254
lipid oxidation, 234
lipid profile, 227
lipids, 234
lipolysis, 234, 255
lipopolysaccharide, 238, 245
lipoprotein, 229, 243
lipoproteins, 227, 229, 246
lipostatic signal, viii, 56
liver, 228

localization, 223, 253
locomotor activity, 234
locus, 219
low-density, 225, 229
low-density lipoprotein, 225, 229
lumen, 221, 228
lung, xi, 217, 228, 234, 238, 245, 259
lung cancer, 234, 259
luteinizing hormone, 239

mucosa, xi, 217, 228, 229, 249, 252, 259
multiple linear regression, ix, 75
muscle, 228, 234
muscle mass, 234
mutant, 221, 225, 253
mutation, 221, 226, 227, 250
mutations, 250
myocardial infarction, 238, 260
myocardium, 228

M

macrophages, 238
maintenance, 256
malabsorptive, 255
malnutrition, 222
mammals, 222, 258
Martial Satisfaction Scale (EMS), x, 125, 129
meals, 231, 241
mean arterial pressure, 238
mediators, 253
melanin, 231
melatonin, 251
membranes, 221
memory, 244
memory performance, 244
mental retardation, 234
Merck, 239
metabolic, 227, 230, 244, 252, 254, 255, 260, 263
metabolic information, viii, 56
metabolic syndrome, 227, 244, 252, 254, 260
metabolism, 231, 234, 235, 237, 256, 261
metabolites, 240, 254
mice, 219, 222, 229, 230, 231, 232, 233, 234, 235, 238, 241, 242, 243, 246, 248, 249, 254, 257, 258, 259, 260, 262, 263, 264
mimicking, 226
misleading, 227
mitogen, 263
mitogen-activated protein kinase, 263
mitogenic, 252
models, 237, 240, 250, 257
modulation, xi, 217, 237
molecules, 218, 228, 229, 239, 240, 241, 250, 256
monocytes, 238, 247
mononuclear cell, 238, 254
mononuclear cells, 254
Moon, 245
morphine, 257
motor activity, 231, 248, 257
mouse, 220, 221, 222, 230, 253, 255, 257, 261
mouse model, 257
mRNA, 218, 222, 225, 227, 230, 233, 249, 251, 262

N

Nash, 254
natural, 218, 219, 244, 252, 258
nerve, 233, 237, 246
nervous system, 256
network, 245
neural events, viii, 55
neural network, 245
neuroendocrine, 252
neurons, 228, 231, 232, 233, 235, 245, 246, 252, 254, 258, 260, 263
neuropeptide, 228, 231, 245, 248, 251, 252, 259
Neuropeptide Y, 232, 250, 257
neuropeptides, 233, 245
neurotensin, 225
neutralization, 242, 259
neutrophil, 238, 258
NF-κB, 238
Ni, 220, 256
nitric oxide, 237, 258
nitric oxide synthase, 237
NO, 238
noradrenaline, 233
normal, 226, 229, 230, 235, 239, 240, 242, 250, 252, 261, 262, 263
N-terminal, 221, 222, 229
nuclear, 254
nuclei, 232
nucleotide sequence, 225
nucleus, 228, 230, 231, 232, 233, 242, 243, 245, 252, 254, 258
nutrients, 231

O

obese, 229, 234, 235, 241, 242, 243, 249, 250, 251, 252, 253, 255, 259, 260, 262, 263
obese patients, 235
obesity, 222, 226, 229, 230, 234, 239, 241, 242, 247, 248, 249, 253, 255, 256, 258, 259, 260, 262, 263, 264

Index

obesity in later childhood, vii, 1
observations, 220
olanzapine, 234, 251
olibra, viii, 56
oligonucleotides, 242
opiates, 240
opposition, 235
optimization, 240
oral, 240
orexigenic neuropeptides, 233
orexin A, 245
organ, 238, 258
organic, 237
organism, 231
orientation, 255
ovary, 228, 244
oxidation, 234
oxidative, 238
oxide, 237, 258

P

pancreas, xi, 217, 228, 229, 238, 242, 245, 251, 253, 257, 262, 263
pancreatic, xi, 217, 232, 238, 246, 251, 258, 262
pancreatic islet, 258, 262
pancreatitis, 238, 247
parameter, 227
paraoxonase, 229, 243
paraventricular, 232, 233
paraventricular nucleus, 233
parenting behavior, vii
passive components, viii, 55
pathology, 230, 234
pathophysiological, 229
pathways, 218, 232, 233, 236, 238
patients, 227, 233, 234, 235, 237, 239, 240, 244, 246, 251, 253, 254, 255, 261, 263
PCR, 221
peptidase, 220
peptide, xi, 217, 218, 219, 220, 222, 223, 224, 227, 229, 232, 233, 234, 239, 240, 243, 246, 249, 250, 252, 256, 257, 259, 260, 261, 263
Peptide, 217, 224, 232, 244, 246, 250, 253, 263
peptides, 217, 219, 222, 223, 224, 227, 228, 231, 232, 236, 240, 243, 249, 251, 253, 255, 257
perinatal, 245
Peripheral, 233, 246, 252, 260
peripheral blood, 254
peripheral blood mononuclear cell, 254
pharmacokinetics, 240, 253
pharmacological, 247, 255
phenotype, 230, 234, 235, 237, 243, 260

phenotypes, 252
phenylalanine, 221
phosphatidylcholine, 223
phosphatidylserine, 223
phosphodiesterase, 236, 252
phospholipase C, 225, 233, 236
phosphorylation, 223, 247
physiological, 219, 222, 227, 229, 231, 234, 236, 237
physiological body constitution, viii, 55
PI3K, 236
pigs, 257
pituitary, xi, 217, 236, 239, 244, 252, 258, 259
pituitary gland, 259
placenta, 228
plant extracts (phytochemicals), xi, 171
plasma, xii, 217, 222, 227, 228, 229, 231, 234, 235, 237, 238, 239, 243, 245, 246, 249, 251, 254, 256, 258, 259, 262
plasma levels, 227, 235
platelet, 229
platelet-activating factor, 229
play, 219, 227, 233, 235
PLC, 236
plexus, 229
polycarbohydrates, viii, 55
polyethylene, 242
polymorphism, 226, 227, 243, 251, 254, 255
polymorphisms, 226, 227, 244, 246, 248, 255, 262
polypeptide, 232, 253
polypeptides, 225
polyunsaturated fat, 239
polyunsaturated fatty acid, 239
poor, 240
population, 255
portal vein, 245
postoperative, 237, 240, 261, 262
post-translational, 219, 220, 250
Prader-Willi syndrome, 234, 241, 248, 249
preference, 234, 263
pregnancy, 234, 257
pregnant, 244
pressure, 227, 238
pro-atherogenic, 225
production, 221, 233, 238, 242
proinflammatory, 238, 247, 254
pro-inflammatory, 258
prolactin, 228, 236, 237, 255, 258
proliferation, 238, 239, 246, 263
promoter, 256, 261
promoter region, 256
prostate, 219, 227, 228, 263
prostate cancer, 219, 227, 263
proteases, 229

protein, 221, 223, 225, 227, 228, 230, 231, 232, 233, 235, 238, 245, 248, 249, 251, 260
protein kinase C, 223, 225
proteins, 219, 225
proteolysis, 229
Pseudomonas, 250
Pseudomonas aeruginosa, 250
puberty, 239
public, 224
purification, 222

Q

Quantitative trait loci, 252
quantum of food, viii, 55

R

range, 225
rat, 218, 221, 222, 228, 229, 233, 237, 238, 239, 240, 243, 244, 245, 246, 247, 248, 249, 250, 251, 253, 254, 255, 257, 258, 259, 261, 262, 263
rats, 222, 230, 231, 232, 233, 234, 235, 237, 238, 239, 240, 241, 242, 243, 244, 246, 247, 248, 251, 252, 256, 258, 259, 260, 262, 263
RC, 240, 257
reasoning, 220
receptor agonist, 254, 259, 260, 262, 264
receptors, 218, 225, 232, 241, 244, 246, 247, 264
regulation, xi, 217, 219, 228, 230, 233, 235, 236, 239, 242, 249, 250, 251, 253, 256, 257, 259
relationship, 235, 240, 255
relationships, 256, 261
remodeling, 238, 260
reproduction, 230, 234, 248
residues, 221, 224, 226, 240
resistance, 256, 257
resistin, 256
respiratory, 230, 234
retention, 234, 247
reticulum, 220, 221, 225
retinol, 249
retinol-binding protein, 249
ribonucleic acid, 259
risk, 227, 247, 254
RNA, 227, 250
rodent, 235
rodents, 235, 249, 253, 256, 261
RP, 264

S

safety, 240, 253
scavenger, 225
schizophrenia, 251
Schmid, 258
search, 239
secrete, 228
secretion, xi, 217, 220, 226, 227, 228, 230, 234, 236, 237, 238, 239, 240, 241, 242, 244, 245, 246, 248, 249, 251, 252, 253, 256, 257, 258, 259, 260, 261, 263
seizures, 248
sensing, 231
sensitivity, 231, 241, 254, 257, 258
series, 226, 240, 241, 249
serine, xi, 217, 218, 220, 221
serotonergic, 241
serotonin, 228
Hydroxytryptamine (5-HT, ix, 97
serum, 227, 229, 245, 246, 251, 256
serum cholesterol, ix, 75, 76, 79, 83, 84, 91
serum triacylglycerol, ix, 75, 76, 91
severity, 246
sharing, 220, 221, 224
shock, 238, 244
short-term, xii, 217, 233
signal peptide, 218, 220
signal transduction, 225
signaling, 241, 249, 250, 254, 256
signalling, 258, 260
signals, 231, 246
similarity, 221
single nucleotide polymorphism, 226
sites, 219, 227, 246
skeletal muscle, 228, 234
skin, 228
SNP, 226
SNPs, 227
solubility, 240
somatostatin, 217, 228
SP, 220, 259
species, 222, 243
spleen, 229
stability, 229
starvation, 230, 231
stomach, xi, 217, 218, 220, 222, 223, 228, 229, 233, 235, 242, 243, 244, 247, 249, 252, 258, 259, 261
storage, 234, 251
stress, 237
students, 250, 262
substitution, 221, 255
sucrose, 223

Sun, 230, 231, 234, 235, 254, 260
suppression, 234, 235, 246, 249, 256
surgery, 233, 234, 244, 245
surgical, 229, 253
susceptibility, 248
sympathetic, 238, 260
syndrome, 245, 247, 253, 256
synergistic, 237
synergistic effect, 237
synthesis, 250

T

T cell, 238, 247
T cells, 238, 247
T lymphocyte, 238, 263
T lymphocytes, 238, 263
testis, xi, 217, 228, 229, 239
testosterone, 239
therapeutic agents, 240
therapy, 239
thyroid, 221, 228, 256
thyroid carcinoma, 221, 256
thyroid stimulating hormone, 228
time, 235
timing, 231, 239
tissue, 219, 221, 229, 232, 234, 235, 243, 246, 248, 250, 262
Togo, 251
tolerance, 241, 248
total cholesterol, 231
traits, 244
transcript, 219, 226, 227, 228, 231, 232, 246
transcription, 218, 219
transcriptional, 219
transcripts, 219, 244, 258
transfer, 220
transgenic, 230, 237
Transgenic, 243
transmembrane, 221, 224, 226
transmission, 227
transmits, 246
transport, 220, 229
triacylglycerols, 220
trial, 240
triggers, 230, 259
triglyceride, 229, 234

triglycerides, 227
Trp, 240
TSH, 263
tumor, 220
tumors, 252, 262
type 2 diabetes, 227, 241, 242, 245, 253
type 2 diabetes mellitus, 245

U

undernutrition, 222, 249

V

Vaccination, 264
vaccine, 242
vagal nerve, 246
vagus, 233, 237
vagus nerve, 233, 237
values, 257
variation, 252
ventricle, 232
vertebrates, 221
virus, 220

W

waist circumference, ix, 28, 75, 79, 82, 84, 90, 91, 93, 94, 182, 189, 194, 195
waist-to-hip ratio, ix, 75, 79, 82, 84, 91, 93
weather conditions, viii, 55
weight gain, 230, 234, 235, 239, 241, 242, 257, 259, 262, 264
weight loss, 230, 234, 239, 241, 245, 248, 249, 255, 257
weight management, xi, 37, 44, 46, 133, 171, 185, 197, 199, 201, 203
weight reduction, 260
Wistar rats, 245
women, 263

Z

zinc, 250